Dedication

To our Fathers

Sherman Sachs
who understood that natures heals and
loving care is for all creatures great and small.
1918–1995
&
Percy Brown
a gentleman with the hands of a healer and
a courageous heart intent on caring
1921–2004

Ayurvedic Spa

*Treatments for large and small spas
as well as home care to help everyone
become healthy, happy,
and feel inspired.*

By Melanie and Robert Sachs

LOTUS
PRESS
TWIN LAKES, WI

DISCLAIMER
This is a reference work that is not intended to treat, diagnose or prescribe. The information contained herein is in no way to be considered a substitute for consultation or treatment by a duly licensed health care professional.

Composition/Layout: Trice Atkinson
Illustrations:
    Still life—Alyson LeBlanc of LeBlanc Studios (neodiva@gmail.com)
    Background peony pattern—Robert Beer

Printed in the United States of America

ISBN: 978-0-9409-8596-4

Library of Congress Control Number: 2007930322

Published by:
Lotus Press, P.O. Box 325, Twin Lakes, Wisconsin 53181
web: www.lotuspress.com
e-mail: lotuspress@lotuspress.com
800-824-6396

Acknowledgements

*T*his book has been almost two years in the making, with a good deal of thought that went into even thinking about doing it at all. But here it is. We celebrate the fact that we did it! And there are some others who also deserve acknowledgement for their efforts here as well.

First and foremost, we want to thank Lotus Press for encouraging and supporting this project. Deadlines were set and reset as life has a way of letting you know that all things come in their own time and much happens along the way. We thank Santosh Krinsky and Cathy Hoselton for their understanding and kind and generous hearts.

Then there are the models. You are going to find a good number of useful pictures throughout this book. We wish to thank our son, Jabeth, for enduring two very driven parents and being willing to get in a steam box and offer his feet when needed. We also wish to thank Carmela Vignocchi for her patience, grace, and humor in our first photo shoot. Then there is our beautiful surfer couple, Charlie Clingman and Betsy Ball. Besides being devoted to surfing, Charlie is a great artist (go to www.ForeverStoked.com) and Betsy does the marketing. When our project was at its most intense, they reminded us that you can be "forever stoked" and relax and have fun.

In the portion of the book devoted to marketing, there is a very special contribution from Uta Birkmayer of X-sense. She is one of the top innovative marketing professionals in the nation and has done brilliant work with the spa industry. Her approach is so in keeping with the spirit of Ayurveda and we feel that her contribution will help all of you bring greater success into your businesses.

We would like to acknowledge Marianne Lang whose broken heart bought her America and whose skill, patience and enthusiasm helped us first formulate a number of these treatments and in the process was renewed herself. She is very recently happily married so the treatments do work! And again to Germany many thanks to all at Primavera-Life whose generosity helped us first get a lot of these ideas on paper and whose support allowed us to learn from many great German students.

Very special thanks to those who have connected so strongly with Ayurveda and these treatments and who now teach for us. Jon Alan Vice, fondly now known as "bowl boy," has mastered working the kansa vataki bowl and has supported us and made us look good in so many ways. To Dawn Tardif whose beauty and business ethics inspire us and whose knowledge and skill contributes so much. And Becky Eivens whose soul was touched by shirodhara in the heart of Texas and has showed us that Ayurveda can thrive in even in the more conservative parts of the USA.

We want to acknowledge the spa industry for being so enthusiastic about our work and really beginning the process of bringing Ayurveda to the general public. Some thought it was all going to be a fad. In this regard, special thanks must go to the editor, Monica Schuloff-Smith and staff of Les Nouvelle Esthestique who have supported our writing and made us so welcome at their shows. They were some of the first to say that Ayurveda is the holistic spa paradigm for the twenty-first century. Others who contributed to bringing out our work in Ayurveda to the spa and beauty industry also include Jane Wurwand of International Dermal Institute, Marianne Uban of The Sterling Silver Institute, Guy Jonkman of Spa Management and Melinda Taschetta-Millane of Skin, Inc. And there are so many more treatments and lifestyle gifts from Ayurveda still to come!

A special mention, warm hug and thanks go to Tara Grodjesk who pioneered Ayurveda in the spa industry. Her welcome, respect, and interest in our work means a lot to us.

In the tradition of Ayurveda we formally thank all our teachers great and small. We stand on your shoulders and feel surrounded by your love. We have you to thank for all we have and all we are able to do.

Lastly, we want to thank you, the readers. Many have asked for this book. And whether this is the first book you have seen about Ayurveda or just part of your collection, we feel confident that whether you are at home, in a day spa, or a destination spa, Ayurvedic Spa will offer you a new way of experiencing your body and mind, and will transform your life and work.

Table of Contents

Foreword

*A*yurvedic Spa is a remarkably comprehensive resource for any-one in the home, day, or destination spa business. Melanie and Robert Sachs draw their knowledge from a deep well of diverse training in Indian and Tibetan Ayurveda. Their training has given them the ability to see Ayurveda for what it truly is. While Ayurveda is rich in therapies, lifestyles and constitutional recommendations, what Ayurve-da "is" as the Sachs have so eloquently written, is a universal body of knowledge designed as a system of medicine to purify the physical and subtle bodies and prepare the body/mind to experience its full physical and spiritual potential. It is not only for Hindus nor is it Hindu. It is not a vegetarian system or connected to any other such dogma. It is, by definition, the study of life and therefore all life, be it plant, animal, or human must live in harmony with each other. Nature, the climate, geo-graphical location, seasons, and ethnicity all determine the natural laws that humans have been forced to follow in order to survive. Ayurvedic Spa has taken this precious knowledge of Ayurveda and formatted it for us to successfully introduce into the spa industry and thus the main stream of our culture.

Ayurveda may be thousands of years old, ancient and even consid-ered out-dated by some, but the reason Ayurveda is becoming more and more popular is because it offers our modern culture the missing pieces to our health care puzzle. Each of the therapies offered in *Ayurvedic Spa* establishes both a physical detoxification of the body and a silencing of the mind. It is from this silence that the body gleans the awareness to heal. Ayurveda is designed to lower the metabolism, enhance self aware-ness, and establish an inner calm that allows the client to handle day-to-day stressors like water off a duck's back. When the body and mind are both quieted in the way these Ayurvedic therapies do, a deep and permanent hub of silence is established as the source of our thoughts, actions, and desires. Much like a hurricane—the bigger the eye, the bigger the silence--the more powerful the winds, the more productive we become. This is a law of nature and it appears that it will be through the spa industry and books like *Ayurvedic Spa* that this precious knowledge of Ayurveda will be revealed.

—DR. JOHN DOUILLARD

John Douillard, D.C., Ph.D. has written four books on Ayurveda including his best selling *Body, Mind and Sport* and his most recent, *The Encyclopedia of Ayurvedic Massage*. He practices Ayurveda in Boulder Colorado where he lives with his wife and six children. He can be reached at lifespa.com.

Over the last 30 years, spas in the U.S. have evolved from "Fat Farms" to Wellness Centers. In the 70's and early 80's spas were places where wealthy women went to lose weight. By the mid 80's spas were advertising themselves as "pampering palaces", the "ultimate in luxury". Going to the spa was considered a luxury only available to the elite. In the United States, most spas of that time aspired to be called a "European Spa" which was the defining factor to be credible. U.S. Spas wanted to mirror European spas but did not have the support from our medical system to be supervised and run by medical doctors, nor were spa vacations covered by health insurance, as had been true in Europe. As the fitness movement grew, the U.S. strength was not found in medical integration for spas, but in fitness and beauty. Most resort and hotel spas had well-developed fitness club facilities and offered basic beauty services and Swedish massage. Thus, American spas became amenities to big hotels and resorts, with only a small number of destination spas offering substantial wellness programs that truly encouraged healthy lifestyle change.

Originally, there were only a handful of destination spas that created an experience for guests that represented an integrated approach to wellness: healthy food, exercise, massage and beauty treatments, and relaxation time all in a beautiful environment, and inspiring change. The original Golden Door, Rancho La Puerta and Canyon Ranch were the icons for the spa industry. Today, there are numerous reputable destination spas where individuals go during times of life transition to seek change physically, emotionally and spiritually.

Dr. Vasant Lad was one of the first Ayurvedic Physicians to come to the U.S. to teach Ayurveda. I feel so very blessed and honored to have been one of his first students in 1981. Also a student of Dr. Lad's, Melanie too was inspired by his profound gift for teaching. It is perhaps the seeds he sowed in both of us that allowed us to take Ayurveda to spas, massage therapists, and aestheticians throughout the world. Pratima Raichur, Deepak Chopra, Bri Maya Twirari, David Frawley, and Melanie's life partner, Bob, along with others, have helped to educate the masses about Ayurveda. I remain in awe of the movement that we created in the spa industry, to bring the wisdom of Ayurveda where it had never been before. By introducing basic Ayurvedic concepts and spa treatments inspired by or derived from Ayurvedic therapies, we as individual practitioners could touch not just 20 or 30 clients a week, but could now reach thousands and thousands of individuals seeking profound relaxation, healing, or perhaps the most dynamic life change.

Ayurveda had its first introduction to hotel, resort, and destination spas in the late 80's. Ayurvedic-derived spa treatments were introduced to top spas such as the famed Sonoma Mission Inn, Marriott's Desert Springs Resort, and Claremont Hotel and Spa. The Day Spa boom had not yet taken off. Most Massage Therapists being trained had never heard of the word "Ayurveda". We introduced treatments that were adapted from Ayurvedic therapies. The spa guests responded to the balancing effects of the treatments. These treatments became best-selling services, even though the spa-goer had not been familiar with Ayurveda at all, a tribute to the powerful healing affects of the herbs, oils and techniques.

So many of the alternative healing modalities that have resurfaced today and gained popularity in spas are rooted in Ayurveda. Gem and Crystal therapy, Aromatherapy, Herbal Therapy, Reflexology, Homeopathy, Polarity Therapy, Colonic therapy, Color Therapy . . . . and on and on. Ayurveda has so much to offer spas as they mature from "beauty and pampering" to "wellness and longevity". Ayurveda's integrative approach to health and healing provides the threads needed to be woven into the fabric of wellness programs in spas throughout the world. Ayurvedic spa treatments are now becoming the core to spa programming in the majority of top spas today. I celebrate this growth. We have truly made a difference in the world! Through education provided by dedicated teachers such as Melanie and Bob Sachs, we have expanded spa programming to include Ayurvedic therapies and incorporated Ayurvedic principles to treat each client as the unique individual they are. With gratitude and respect I honor The Mother of all Healing. With sincerest appreciation, I honor Melanie and Bob Sachs for their untiring commitment to continue to weave Ayurveda into the fabric of the spa community.

—TARA GRODJESK

TARA SPA THERAPY

Section One

What You Need to Know and Just in Case You Wanted to Know

*Modern man associates himself
with the ancient world not in order to reflect it
like a mirror, but to capture its spirit
and apply it in a modern way.*

PALLADIO

CHAPTER 1

Our Story

One of the very first conversations I remember having with Bob happened when we were sitting together in the grounds of a very large psychiatric hospital on the south side of London. I was training as an occupational therapist and Bob had arrived for a placement from a counseling college. I wanted to feel him out on a matter that was eating at me. I cannot remember my exact words, but what I was basically asking him was, "Am I crazy or is it this place, this health care system, this view of the body/mind system? And, if it is IT, not me that's crazy, what is the alternative and what can we do about it?" That was nearly thirty years ago and our marriage and journey through our work lives together has been all about answering this question.

Along the way we have been lucky enough to have had some of the most wonderful teachers. Thinking through our journey together and remembering these amazing people made us realize that as wonderful as we thought they all were at the time of our meeting, the world at large, especially those endorsing the contemporary health care model, seemed to considered our mentors as fringe, weird, wild, and even totally mad. We felt they were all teaching the truth.

Our first teacher was Rex Lassalle. We met at a Tibetan Buddhist retreat center in Scotland in 1975. He was there with a friend meditating, taking long runs in the pouring rain, cooking and eating only buckwheat and hijiki (Japanese seaweed). We met in the kitchen and he invited me to come to his first class in macrobiotics. A month later we met in a small room above "The Gentle Ghost," one of London's first natural food restaurants and we continued to meet every Monday for the next nine weeks. I became vegetarian and ate very little besides brown rice and vegetables. For the first time in my life I was free of eczema and had no trouble with asthma, but my occupational therapy college tutors were very worried that I had gone mad or joined a cult. So they sent a school representative on a 200-mile train journey to check on me. That's a very long way from a British perspective.

Bob at this time was working just outside London near Hampton Court in a halfway house for those who had been in long term psychiatric hospital or would need that kind of hospital care if they were not at the house. He had completed his degree at the University of Lancaster and was now training in group therapy. The Richmond Fellowship for which he worked offered a unique approach to caring for people after leaving mental hospitals. But as progressive as they were, this organization was still working with conventional psychiatrists. For his own peace of mind, but also because of his broader interests in eastern thought, Bob started his study of yoga with a retired executive of the English milk marketing board. Jonathan O'Dell was a prince of a man and at 70 demonstrated a vigor and clarity that few people half his age possessed. Later on, Bob studied with Johanna Auld of Staines and eventually completed his certification with the All India Board under her tutelage. Bob tried to introduce yogic stretching and breathing into the halfway house where he worked. It worked beautifully for the patients in helping them to deal with stress and anxiety, but it caused stress and anxiety for their psychiatrists. During this same time, Rex and Bob became close friends and our information about oriental medicine and diet grew together in a life we were beginning to create as a couple.

1976 almost saw a door fling open for us both with respect to an interest that was beginning to consume both of us. Soon after we decided to get married in the spring, we heard of an Ayurvedic program being offered in London with Dr. Shyam Singh and Dr. Jack Lowzdan of the White Cross Society. Dr. Singh was one of the physicians to Bhagwan Sri Rajneesh, later known as Osho. He was wild even by our standards, and his remedies were pretty cathartic but amazingly effective. He gave me my first acupuncture treatment. While the needles were in I could neither move nor speak. It was pretty frightening but gave me a real experience of body energetics that I will never forget. It is he we have to thank for the antidoted Ayurvedic coffee recipe we now use in our classes.

That same summer Rex introduced us to Michio Kushi, the principle master of macrobiotics at the time. We took a week long professional training program with him. Interestingly enough, the class and meals were held at Mandeer, an excellent vegetarian Indian restaurant. Macrobiotics really seemed to work for me but I was the thinnest I had ever been, weighing only 96 lbs. It was hard to find a wedding dress that didn't make me look like Orphan Annie!

Soon after the end of the program with Michio, we were married. After our civil ceremony we had a Tibetan Buddhist marriage blessing followed by an all-macrobiotic reception, catered by Rex. We imagine that most of our guests felt like they had been invited to a picnic on the moon; rice salads with seaweed, miso tahini spreads, breads made just with flour and water. At the time, we didn't think that we were being weird or fringe, just introducing friends and loved ones to a new way of eating. I don't think we got many converts, though.

Bob and I stayed involved with macrobiotics because it was, at the time, the most recognized and popular form of oriental medicine available in Western Europe. We were attracted to Ayurveda, but other than Dr. Singh, there were few teachers that we were aware of. There was even a Tibetan medicine study group that we joined for a while, headed by osteopath Dr. Tom Dummer. But then again, there were also at that time few Tibetan doctors in the west to learn from.

That fall we left England and traveled to Boulder, Colorado. We traveled from London to New York on a Russian cruise ship that has since sunk off the coast of Australia. It was the classic immigrant experience for me, sailing up the Hudson. We carried some of our own macrobiotically prepared food, a habit we still have when we are on the road. At one point an elderly gentleman, seeing the strange bags of food we periodically brought up to the dining cabin, asked one of the people who always sat at our table, "What is the matter with the two young people at your table?"

"Nothing," our table friend replied.

"Why do they eat all that other stuff then?"

"Oh, that's because they think it is good for them."

"Ah, now I understand. They are just mentally ill," he said sincerely.

As we gradually awakened to how others were beginning to perceive our life's path and passion, being on the fringe, being seen as "crazy" was a theme we were becoming accustomed to dealing with. Even Bob's parents were concerned that we needed to be deprogrammed. With the growing number of huge natural food super markets that we have today, it is hard to believe just how threatening brown rice was to mainstream America in the 70's. It was a quiet revolution. As my British training in occupational therapy and Bob's degree and diploma in human relations meant nothing in the US, we threw the idea of being medical professionals to the wind and became cooks and workers in the new food co-op movement. We even started our own cooperative restaurant, Tecumseh's Beanery, in Columbus, Ohio and periodically taught classes on the theory and diet of macrobiotics. It was in this happy, care-free state that we had our first baby. Not easily, I might add. She was born upside down and backwards, posterior breech, at home. Her head got stuck and her neck was dislocated. She was not a happy newborn. And learning to treat and nurture a baby based on the principles we were learning added a whole new dimension to our understanding and flexibility.

With our daughter, Kai Ling, now eight weeks old, I took her back to England to visit my family. Home birth and breastfeeding were still so revolutionary in America that I was glad to be back in Europe where it is more commonplace. I felt I needed the help of my family and native culture. So Bob sold everything we had and joined me. It was at that time that Bob trained in Shiatsu with Rex. We were also some of the first of our macrobiotic friends to have children and so joined with other young families to start "The Growing Family Center" at London's East West center, a large old school building in east London. It was there that Bob studied and innovated a new form of Reflexology is now one of the main forms taught throughout Europe. It is featured in our PediKarma™ and Tibetan Blissful Sleep treatment rituals.

Ever footloose and always wanting to learn more, we came back to America at the end of 1979. This time the call was more from a spiritual yearning. We wanted to be part of a Tibetan Buddhist community in Woodstock, New York. As more holistic approaches were helping to answer the questions about physical health it was Buddha Dharma that seemed to us to have the answers about the nature of the mind and inner well being. After another year and being a few months pregnant, we left Woodstock and headed west. We thought we were heading to Boulder again, so that Bob could study at the Naropa Institute. But we didn't make it all the way. We stopped in Columbus, Ohio again. There I had our second "buckeye" baby, Harriet Christina. Bob worked at the local co-op, trained as a massage therapist at a very traditional school, started a line of natural food snacks called "Simple Delights", and I was a stay-at-home mom. By then, however, more people in the Midwest were hearing of the work we were doing. A local physician, Dr. Ernie Shearer, introduced us to another one of our revolutionary friends and teachers, Dr. Walt Stoll, one of the founding members of the American Holistic Medical Association, and the head of the Holistic Health Centre of Lexington, Kentucky.

Being deep in the Bible belt this very successful holistic clinic was viewed by some as the answer to all prayers and by others as straight from the devil. Bob was asked to join the staff. He worked with a great team: the holistic M.D.; a holistic dentist and electrical acupuncturist

(EAV); Vince and Charles, both chiropractors; Marty, a physician assistant with a brilliant knowledge of iridology; Janet, the nurse; Steve, her husband and clinical psychologist; and Banks, spiritual counselor. Bob offered his massage skills, gave dietary consultation, and taught relaxation and biofeedback based on his yoga training. I taught natural foods cooking while running after two little girls and being pregnant once again. We were once more on the fringe and loving it.

Our third daughter, Shamara Phillipa, was born in December of 1982. Walt came as our guest to the birthing. He had delivered many babies in the hospital but had never witnessed a home delivery. I can remember him sitting there quietly with tears streaming down his face. It was a magical time.

But all things are impermanent and life ends when it is time. Sadly, Shamara died seven weeks later of SIDS and all our lives changed. The youthful zealous exuberance we had for our studies was tempered with a deeper truth about the fragile nature of life and that eating, exercise, and meditation could change the quality of life, but not necessarily when it was to be over. Bob felt a call to go deeper into his original work in counseling and so trained as a social worker at University of Kentucky. It took me a while to feel any joy or interest in living. In fact, I developed cancer during this dark time. I was fortunate in receiving the loving support of Bob and our friend Rex, who came to stay with us a while. Gradually feeling more like my old self, a stirring to learn more began to well up within me. And it was at that time that I met my main teacher, Dr Vasant Lad. It was his extreme kindness that brought me back to life and got me hooked on Ayurveda.

While Bob was finishing his social work degree, I was studying Dr. Lad's correspondence course. I began to make "macro-vedic" food, using our macrobiotic understanding to cook Ayurvedic dishes that Dr. Lad recommended. Once Bob graduated from social work school, we moved to Albuquerque so I could study with Dr. Lad in person. I was getting more and more answers to those original questions from this beautiful, quiet man who had broken with tradition and moved to the west. He spoke the truth and practiced what he preached. He was the first to publish a book on Ayurveda and, in his own sweet way, was also a revolutionary, bringing east to meet west.

While I was studying with Dr. Lad, we met Dr. Rapgay. Then a monk, he was once the religious secretary to the Dalai Lama. Bob had met him once before as a translator for His Holiness' physician, Dr. Yeshe Donden. He and Bob had an immediate connection and Bob was able to visit and study with him in San Francisco, learning and practicing pancha karma under his guidance. The marma work in most of our protocol comes from his teachings. At that time Dr. Rapgay had hoped to introduce Tibetan medicine into psychiatric care in this country, but has since become the director of a behavioral medical clinic at UCLA, and committed himself to working towards incremental changes in the western model of psychology and mental well being.

During the mid 80's and early 90's, Albuquerque was a focus for Ayurveda. Many of Dr. Lad's first students still lived and worked in the area and I was pleased to get to study with and become friends to such members of the Ayurvedic community as Amadea Morningstar, Dr. David Frawley, Lenny and Ivy Blank, to name a few. These people attracted and invited other Ayurvedic teachers from India to come to the US. Through these connections we met and studied with Dr Sunil Joshi, a pancha karma specialist who, with his wife Shalmali, turned their back on the easy road to riches to rediscover the benefits of the ancient arts of rejuvenation. We are indebted to them both for teaching Bob more about pancha karma and showing us its potential with very ill individuals. We also met Drs Pankaj and Smita Naram. Dr. Pankaj Naram is a grand master of the art of pulse diagnosis and his wife, Dr. Smita Naram, is a brilliant pharmacist. Their specialty is fertility and our son, Jabeth, born in 1990, was actually their first Ayurvedic baby in America. This energetic couple now has centers all over the world. We are pleased to seek their advice and train with them whenever we can.

In the mid 90's, our friend, Rex, having gone through his own journey, and curious about my interest and success with Ayurveda in my own road to health, asked me if I would teach a spa in Finland on what I had learned about Ayurveda, particularly as it applied to women and wellness. This was the birth of my book, *Ayurvedic Beauty Care*, and the start of our long relationship with the spa and beauty industry. Our involvement with the spa industry has continued to be by invitation.

Thus it was that in 1995, Jane Wurwand, owner of Dermalogica and founder of the International Dermal Institute, another innovator in her field, asked me to teach at her growing number of schools and it was in these classes that I learned how to teach Ayurveda "spa-style". Much of the theory presented in this book was developed by formulating a jargon-free Ayurvedic language that could convey the essence of Ayurveda's timeless concepts of energy and healing and presenting it to her students and teachers. Once we moved to California, I traveled monthly mostly in America but also to Australia, England and Germany. As my teaching progressed an interest in product and equipment developed and Bob became my point person. Diamond Way Ayurveda was born.

During this same time, our Buddhist community connected us with an excellent essential oil company in Germany, Primavera Life. It was the faith that owner Ute Leube had in us and the energy of her partner, Kurt Nubling, that inspired the formulation of the vata, pitta, kapha oil blends that are the basis of our Ayurvedic face and body oils that continue to delight us. And we have Donald Trump to thank for our shirodhara equipment. His spa in Florida requested that we create a shirodhara set to match the copper tub in his all copper spa room. We never planned to be formulators, manufacturers, or distributors but here we are journeying forward waiting to see what will be next to unfold.

Bob and I felt compelled to tell you of our journey into Ayurveda for many reasons. We want you to understand that Ayurveda is not only to be learned, but to be lived and made real in your own life. This is what we have done and this is what we want to share.

It is also important for you to understand that Ayurveda teaches that roughly 95% of what causes us dis-ease is related to stress and poor lifestyle habits. Thus whilst Ayurveda is as deep as any other medical system in offering advice for serious chronic and acute diseases, so much of what it offers to us on a day to day basis—diet, exercise, relaxation, massage and various forms of detoxification—are those things that will improve the quality of our living and ease so much of what we suffer with in these uncertain times.

This is our experience. This is what we are offering here. We do not see *Ayurvedic Spa* as Ayurveda "light", something of lesser significance than the more medical aspects and miracles of Ayurveda. We see the techniques that we offer here in *Ayurvedic Spa* as the gateway to an Ayurvedic life, a life built on wisdom, compassion, joy, and vitality.

Thirty years down the road and with a current spa market clamoring for more genuine and transformative experiences for their clients, Ayurveda has emerged as the paradigm par excellence. What once looked crazy, or was thought to be just a fad is here to stay. And after all our globe trotting we have found a home with many others of heart who do the work of loving their clients and quietly making this world a better place. We invite you to join us.

CHAPTER 2

What is Ayurveda?

*A*yurveda is like my main teacher. It has the heart of an artist, the soul of a saint, and a body that is delicate, flexible and marvelously enduring. It is a feeling, an intention that whispers to me from the depths of space, wraps around me, supports and inspires me. It is the truth that was able to awaken a healing power within me and coax me back to a richer life. It is what I turn to when I feel hopeless, and it fills me up time and time again.

From the first day I met the man who was to become the teacher to lead me along the path in Ayurveda, I was hooked. Meeting him was like walking into the home of my dreams. He was like the per-fect mother—radiant, joyful, energetic and so very kind. He was present, open, patient, and wise. I immediately felt I could totally be myself and share everything with him—even things I had never put words to before. I could be me and he made me feel I could be the best me I had ever been. I felt honored and loved. I re-member asking as he took my pulse, "Do I have a problem?" He looked at me with a look of surprise on his face and said, "No, it is I who has a problem. It is for me to discover how it

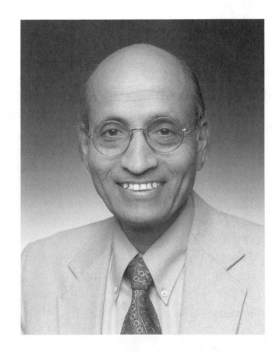

is I can help you." A heaviness was lifted from me and a spark was lit inside as hope was kindled. Here was someone that was willing to guide and support me to help me find whatever it was I needed to feel better, to be better.

Without this feeling, for me Ayurveda would be nothing—nothing more than an ancient and nearly forgotten science from half a world away. Ayurveda, as some of you may have learned or heard, is commonly translated as "knowledge of life" or the "study of longevity." It sounds profound but a little distanced from my everyday reality. In my experience to know life you have to be willing to connect with it, mingle with it, open up to it and love whatever life presents to you. It really doesn't matter to me where it comes from. Availability of air travel and electronic communications are making our world smaller everyday. And now more than ever the average person is more aware of the blessings and curses of many foreign cultures. I have been involved with Ayurveda for nearly 20 years and India, the traditional home of Ayurveda, has only very recently started to call to me. It doesn't matter to me that Ayurveda is ancient. I love modern arts and am awed by modern scientific discovery. But I am totally hooked on that loving energy I first encountered when I met Dr Vasant Lad. I am hooked on trying to understand, connect with, and love all living beings. For me that is Ayurveda. It is that energy that makes a treatment Ayurvedic and it is that artistic heart, saintly soul and enduring body that I want to share with you in this book.

So what is Ayurveda really? As the word itself implies, it *is* a study of longevity; a collection of information and hands-on techniques that have been gathered, refined and recorded for at least 2500 years. It is all the information you will ever need to discover how you are, who you are, and whatever it takes to reach your full potential. It is the perfect treasure map to help you discover your own personal path to wellbeing and happiness.

This notion of personal path is basic to Ayurveda. Ayurveda teaches that we are all beautiful, we are all unique, and just as there are myriad of paths we can take to find our own state of wellbeing, there must be different strokes for different folks. One of the biggest puzzles to solve, then, is finding a way we can sort out who needs what. This is the problem of the Ayurvedic doctor, the Ayurvedic therapist and—if you are interested in learning more about how to take care of yourself—it is the problem you will be working on.

Most of us in the west are spoiled for and confused by the almost endless choices available to us. Which ones are the best for us? What will work for us in the long run? Ayurveda says we have to start with question, "But for whom?". We have to start by knowing more about each of us individually. From one point of view, this task, like many puzzles in life, looks impossible—until we are shown the solution. So let's look at how the first masters of Ayurveda worked it all out.

Ayurvedic Energetics

Scientists and philosophers the world over have struggled throughout the ages to describe why things look the way they do and why they interact the way they do. For centuries the best minds in both the East and the West believed things were composed of four elements: *earth, fire, air,* and *water.* In the East a fifth was also considered: space, that in which the other four exist. Whether you decide to fully believe these ancient masters or not I suggest to you that this idea of five elements is worth entertaining because it is so helpful in solving the puzzle and is a wonderful tool for better understanding your clients and those close to you. If you like you can think of it as a very useful fiction and ultimately it is just that. It is, however, the best way I have yet discovered in how to understand, help and really love everyone.

Ayurveda explains that these elemental energies in nature combine in pairs to form what they call the *doshas.* You can think of them as the information carried on a computer chip that will make a program behave in a certain way. There are three doshas that go by the Sanskrit names of *vata, pitta,* and *kapha.* Vata dosha combines the energies of space and air or, as it is sometimes called, wind. Pitta dosha combines the energies of fire and water. And kapha dosha combine the energies of earth and water. So how does this help us with the puzzle? To start to really get know what this means and how it works, try this simple game.

Take a piece of paper and write the names of the five elements down the left hand side leaving an inch gap in between to fill. Start with space, then air, fire, water, and put earth near the bottom of the page. Now put your pen down, close your eyes, and take a few long slow deep breaths. As you rest comfortably, bring the word "space" to mind. Try and gently hold onto that idea. Notice what you associate with it. It may be a color, a smell, a sound, or an emotion. When you feel you have sense of where the notion of space takes you personally, open your eyes and write down the words that came to mind. Don't try to be clever and I assure you, there are no wrong answers. In your own time go onto the next element "air or wind" and do the same. Work at your own pace until you have words written down that you personally associate with all five elements.

Over the last ten years I've done this "test" with people from most of the states in the US, from Australia, Germany, Finland, and with people of all colors, ages, and both sexes. What is remarkable to me that the answers are always so similar. It is as if forever and for all time human beings everywhere know from deep inside what the elements are all about. If you take a look at the example page you will see I have given you some of the classic qualities in regular type that are usually given to the elements and some innovations from my classes in italics so you can get a better idea of what I mean.

Elemental Qualities

- SPACE—cold, formless, expansive, vast, open, all inclusive, dark, *freedom, floating, starry, dark blue, everywhere, peace, scary, weightless, stillness, magic, possibility, surprise*
- AIR—dry, cold, light, subtle, effects visible, changeable, *refreshing breeze, frightening hurricane, fear, easy to move, excitement inspiration, life giving, vital, clear, movement, penetrating, gusty*
- FIRE—heat, light, upward moving, intelligence, transformation, anger, *red, orange, yellow, blue, intense, passionate, destructive, warming, transformative, gives light, welcome, homey, devastating*
- WATER—cool, flowing, nourishing, lubricating, attachment, *wet, fluid, steamy, slippery, powerful, refreshing, life supporting, beautiful, glittering, clear, cleansing, sensuous, relaxed*
- EARTH—dense, cool, supporting, grounding, inert, stable, solid, *mother, round, giving, green, brown, strong smells, wholesome, slow to change, full of history, abundant*

The next step is to take these colors, sensations, feelings, or images and use them to begin to paint in your mind a particular way of being. Sometimes it helps to bring to mind phrases that use these elemental ideas.

Those that relate to space and air:
- *Blow hot, blow cold*
- *Light hearted*
- *Far out*
- *Spacey*
- *Like a breath of fresh air*
- *Freedom loving*
- *All over the place*
- *Wish upon a star*

Those that relate to fire and water:
- *Burning with passion*
- *Hot to trot*
- *Able to go with the flow*
- *Red with rage*
- *Fiery tempered*
- *Cool out*
- *A trail blazer*
- *Emotionally consuming*
- *Leaves you in the dust*
- *Warm hearted*
- *Floats your boat*

Earth and water:
- *A real brick*
- *Always there to lean on*
- *Goes with the flow*
- *Regular as the tide*
- *Stick in the mud*
- *One whose home is their castle*

We each have all five elemental energies and all three doshas at work making us look, act and feel the way we do. The amount of each dosha we have varies. Depending on different schools understanding, the three doshas come together and reveal and dominance in seven or ten permutations: dominant Vata, dominant Pitta, dominant Kapha, a mutual dominance of Vata and Pitta (and for some, also the distinction and slightly higher dominance of Pitta, then Vata), a mutual dominance of Vata and Kapha (or, similar to the above example, Kapha then Vata), a mutual dominance of Pitta and Kapha (or Kapha then Pitta), and then a tridoshic blend of Vata, Pitta, and Kapha, which means that the person has an equal amount of all three doshas.

Most people are Vata, Pitta, Kapha, Vata-Pitta (or Pitta-Vata), Vata-Kapha (or Kapha-Vata), Pitta-Kapha (or Kapha-Pitta). These 6 or 9 (however you want to number them) are what we find. Tridoshic prakrutis are the constitutions of saints. It means that the person is an alchemist and spiritual adept who can utilize their body and body energies however they see fit. Of course, many people take questionnaires and have reported to us that they come up equal amounts of Vata, Pitta, and

Kapha. Although we have no reason to doubt their sainthood, there is often a more reasonable explanation. More often even scores for vata, pitta, and kapha means we are actually experiencing ourselves in a great variety of ways or we are in a space of being very suggestible, which is more vata than perfectly balanced.

Each of the doshas has a job to do in the body. Vata rules all movement: movements under our control like moving our bodies to walk, movements that are spontaneous like blinking, movements we don't have to think about like our heart beating, even the movements of thoughts running through our minds. So if we have a lot of this vata energetic we will be a mover and shaker. We can either have our vata in balance or out of balance. Vata in balance will wake you early, and have you feeling fresh, vital, enthusiastic and creative all day long. Vata out of balance will make you feel like you cannot sit still, cannot concentrate for long, and it will make you feel both driven and directionless. In this state it easily becomes a habit to push yourself and forget to do even the most basic things to take care of yourself like eat regularly, get enough rest, and drink when you are thirsty.

Pitta dosha is the ruler of our metabolism. It is in charge of any process that involves chemical changes. The one most familiar to us is digestion. Pitta is involved in all hormonal processes and regulates heat in the body. Balanced pitta keeps us feeling warm and comfortable in an "all systems go" place. Mentally we feel clear and in touch with the flow of what is needed to makes things work. Organization comes easily to us and we feel naturally joyful and on purpose. If we have too much pitta we will feel hot and bothered, and become overly critical and easily angered.

Kapha dosha is the combination of elements that come together to form our structure, then stays plentiful enough to keep all of our joints and body parts well lubricated and helps to heal us when we are broken. When kapha is in balance we have a body and mind that has amazing stamina, strength, grace and loving quality. Too much kapha gives us the tendency to put on and keep on extra weight and feel mentally heavy too.

Each of us is a unique blend of these three doshas and we shall discuss this in due time. The important point to understand here is that each of us has all three and the primary goal of Ayurveda is the art of keeping all our doshas in balance so we can experience the perfections each of them has to offer rather than suffer the trials each will manifest if they are out of balance.

To achieve balance, Ayurveda offers many helpful methods. This book concentrates on some very effective forms of body work and offers the type of advice that is comfortable to share with a client or use for yourself at home. Our goal is to truly make this a book that is useful for massage therapists, aestheticians, spa directors and staff, and the average person who wants to experience the joys and benefits of Ayurveda. If you have been overwhelmed and confused by Ayurveda in the past, we have worked hard to keep the explanations simple and relevant so you can know and feel Ayurveda from the inside, from the heart, and you will be able to make it your life long friend.

Glossary of Terms

AYURVEDA—the ancient Indian art of holistic healing. Being at least 2500 years old it is the oldest and most complete teaching on how to be healthy, happy and feel inspired. Ayurveda is the key to beauty for your whole being.

PANCHAMAHABHUTA—the theory of the five elements space or akash, air or vayu, fire or agni, water or jala, and earth or prithvi.

DOSHA—the inherent intelligence within our body-mind system that is responsible for all physiological and psychological processes.

VATA DOSHA—the subtle energy that governs all movement in the body. That includes voluntary movement such as moving our arms and legs, involuntary movement such as blinking or our heart beating, even the movement of thoughts through our mind. It is also responsible for all transport within the body such as carrying nutrients in and wastes out, and delivering appropriate body messages. Vata means to move or enthuse.

PITTA DOSHA—the subtle energy that governs all metabolic and transformational processes which includes any type of chemical changes in the body and the activity of understanding in the mind. Obvious examples are our digestive processes and hormonal cycles but less obvious is the way we understand what we read, hear, or see. Pitta means to heat or transform.

KAPHA DOSHA—the subtle energy in the body that governs cohesion or holding together our body to give it form, liquidity or lubrication of all moving surfaces in the body, and growth and repair in all our tissues. Kapha means to embrace or keep together.

CHAPTER 3

"Long, long ago and far away..." A Brief Look at the Historical and Mythic Origins of Indian and Tibetan Ayurveda

*M*ost people who have either heard of or know something about Ayurveda think of it as being an Indian medical and healing system. But this science of living and longevity, although certainly with its roots and historical growth firmly established on the Indian subcontinent, has a history that pre-dates classical Indian culture, if not human culture in general.

The classic texts of Ayurveda make reference to Brahma, the supreme godhead of Hinduism, who is claimed to have passed the wisdom of healing on to the ascetics and yogis in the Indus Valley (now modern-day western Pakistan). What is curious about this reference to Brahma is that, for example, in the *Astanga Hridaya*, a classic of Ayurveda, it reads, "And Brahma remembered Ayurveda". What does this mean?

According to the Tibetan interpretation, it means that Brahma received teachings on healing from the source of healing, who they consider to be the Medicine Buddha. *Buddha* here is not meant to infer a religion, but rather a state of awareness; someone who has fully awakened to an understanding of what causes us suffering and the remedies to that suffering—on all levels of our existence. This transfer of knowledge between the Medicine Buddha and Brahma is said to have happened at a time that predates the existence of our physical universe; indeed, long ago and in a galaxy far away.

What this being, this Medicine Buddha, discovered is that each of us has the capacity to be a fully awakened, fully enlightened being. This is our birthright. What distinguishes an enlightened or fully awakened being from an ordinary being is that they have brought to fruition the potentials that are latent inside each one of us. These capacities can be classified as three qualities; a rainbow-like body, an unlimited mind, and precise, yet totally spontaneous action filled with joy. Our 'rainbow-like' body has to do with us fully realizing and experiencing the insubstantial nature of everything we consider three-dimensionally solid or real. When we fully grasp this, we attain a presence of mind and body that is limitlessly resourceful and fearless. Our unlimited mind is the elimination of all stiff ideas and addictions which in turn results in the blossoming of our capacity to know and understand things clearly as they are—from the most mundane to the subtly profound. This is the *natural* state of our mind. Finally, being limitlessly resourceful and knowing what needs to be known in any or all situations, we have the confidence and power to be and act in accordance with what is needed to benefit any or all beings in any situation. Freed from limitations and boundaries our interactions are fresh, full-bodied, and joyful. And what brings us the most joy is when we can share and contribute to the wellbeing of loved ones around us. What prevents us from experiencing life in this way?

The Medicine Buddha saw that while we possess the birthright of the Three Potentials as mentioned above, these Potentials are hidden from us by what he called the Three Poisons. Each and every one of us is gripped to greater or lesser degrees by the Three Poisons that are the causes for us not realizing our Potentials. These Three Poisons are Ignorance, Attachment, and Aggression. Simply put: We don't understand fully what is going on or what resources we have at our fingertips. With this restricted view, we develop stiff, restricted ideas about what we think is going on. And when someone challenges our world view or what we are doing based on our own stiff ideas, we get mad, indignant, or combative with them; seeing them as competition or a threat. What the Medicine Buddha could also see is that this way of thinking and acting effects us at every level of our being. The Three Poisons are the reasons we make choices the way we do, whether it is in our preference of friends, food, occupation, or religion. Thus these poisons are the source of all of our dramas, be they spiritual, emotional, or physical.

To remedy this situation, we need an antidote to the Three Poisons. To antidote them does not mean to eliminate them, but rather, in accordance with the tradition and teachings of the Medicine Buddha, to transform them. As we transform ignorance, we re-connect with our resourcefulness—our rainbow-like body. When we let go of our attachment to stiff ideas, our minds become open to their unlimited nature. When we give up our territorial perspective and see ourselves as intimately connected to each and every being, competition gives way to joy and everything we do becomes a spontaneous expression of our awakened being.

When Buddhas teach, they always give spiritual teachings and ways in which we can transform our everyday existence at the most ordinary levels. Spiritual practices, such as contemplations, prayers, and meditations are intended go directly to the source of the problem; in this case the Three Poisons. Ultimately it is our view that needs to be transformed. In the case of the Medicine Buddha, the spiritual practices that he gave specifically address and go head-to-head with the Three Poisons. For whether our discomfort or dis-ease with our world is spiritual, emotional, or physical, it is the transformation of our experience of living in and from perspectives based on the Three Poisons that needs to happen.

At the same time, the Medicine Buddha could see how caught up we as human beings are in our experience; that because of our emotional or physical pains and discomforts, we cannot step outside of our predicament and realize our full potentials. And so, to eradicate the symptoms and conditions that weigh us down, he gave teachings on medicine. These teachings were passed on from this Enlightened source through gods and human beings over the generations.

These are the teachings Brahma came to and learned. And, later on, when the time was right and the information was necessary in the world, he remembered and Ayurveda became a part of our human heritage. The Tibetans would even go as far to say that this knowledge was not only transmitted from Brahma to the masters of the Indus Valley, but that the great healing traditions all over the world, whether it is the Hellenic medical traditions of Greece, the corvendera tradition of Central America, or the healing practices of the Hopi and Navajo, have as their source the Medicine Buddha of so long ago.

Then Until Now

The earliest record of Ayurveda is from some five thousand years ago. Starting first as an oral tradition, it eventually became codified in such great works as the *Charak Samhita*. It is often assumed that because this healing system came from the Indus region of the world and that many healers and those who passed on this tradition are Hindu, that Ayurveda is connected to the religion of Hinduism. Indeed in many texts and when you listen to more classically trained Indian Ayurvedic doctors and their western students, descriptions of Ayurveda are peppered with a variety of Sanskrit terms and references to various Hindu gods.

What needs to be understood is that Ayurveda pre-dates Hinduism. It is not a part of a religious belief. It only stands to reason, as Ayurveda is introduced or imported to new cultures and is used to understand the psychological, emotional, and spiritual dimensions of healing, that the culture it finds itself in will include its own spiritual terminology, notion or pantheon of gods, and whatever is perceived as sound spiritual interpretations. But please bear in mind, **Ayurveda is for everyone**. For certain, over the next hundred years, as Ayurveda becomes interpreted more and more from our own western cultural perspective, ways of expressing and working with this amazing healing paradigm will seem less foreign and eminently attractive to more and more people.

Going back to our brief history, Ayurveda was not only practiced by Hindu healers and priests, but over time, attracted the interest of other groups and traditions. In particular the historical Buddha, Sakyamuni, saw the great potential in Ayurveda and encouraged his students who were healers and doctors to learn Ayurveda. Thus Ayurveda began to spread out from the Indian subcontinent and go to regions where Buddhism was becoming influential.

What also contributed to the spreading of Ayurveda was the growing conflict in what is now modern day Pakistan (but is, as we mentioned earlier, also the birthplace of Ayurveda) between Islam coming in from the Middle East and Hinduism. This began in the 8th century. As this conflict grew over the next seven centuries, culminating in the Mogul invasions and the succession of Mogul emperors, there was a dispersion of Hindu and Ayurvedic teachers and masters into the Himalayan regions where various religious and healing traditions were preserved.

As these conflicts were arising in India, the northern Himalayan kingdom of Tibet was coming under the influence of Buddhism, which brought with it Ayurveda. So intrigued by Ayurveda in particular and healing in general were the seventh century king Srongsten Gonpo, and then in the eighth century King Trisong Detsen, that the Tibetan court sponsored probably the first holistic health conferences ever to be held in the known world. Physicians and healers from along the Silk Road, from China, India, and Southeast Asia gathered in Tibet, discussing and sharing the various healing secrets each of their traditions possessed. The result was a form of medicine practiced in Tibet that is at its foundation Ayurveda, with a philosophical and cosmological umbrella of Buddhist morality, ethics, spiritual insights, and practices. Within this framework various forms of healing were included in a way that creates a unique and dynamic healing paradigm, the potential of which is yet to be fully understood in the west. This body of knowledge was codified and preserved in the eleventh century by the court physician, Yutok Yonten Gonpo, the Great Turquoise Physician, who produced the *Ambrosia Heart Tantra* or *Gyud Zhi*. It is this text, the *Gyud Zhi* that most succinctly carries this body of knowledge to us today.

In 1959, with the Chinese invasion of Tibet and the destruction of some 6000 monasteries, many teachers and their followers fled into India. With them they brought volumes of written texts and materials of their spiritual, cultural, and healing heritage.

As they settled into the various refugee camps that were established for them, they began to interact with the local Indian population. Many of them had become sick from going from high to low altitudes to quickly. As they consulted with the Indian doctors who were available, it soon came to the attention of the Indian doctors that there was material of their own Ayurvedic tradition contained in the Tibetan medical texts. In fact, whole bodies of information on the earliest practices of Ayurveda long lost in India were, in fact, preserved by the Tibetans. In a time of darkness for the Tibetan people, the richness of their spiritual and healing heritage has emerged to be available to us. And the full bloom of Ayurvedic practices has come together and enriched the lives of many people both in the east and the west.

Thus it is that we wish to offer you, the reader, knowledge and practices that come from both the classical Indian Ayurveda and also what has been preserved and transformed by the Tibetan tradition. Because of the way in which culture always influences medicine, there are some differences in practice and philosophy between the Indian and Tibetan forms. A few of these we would like to enumerate right from the start.

What Are the Differences?

In many respects, just as Ayurveda on the Indian subcontinent learned to understand and work with the various indigenous, shamanic, and imported healing sciences brought to India over the centuries, so Ayurveda in Tibet learned to assimilate and work along with similar influences that came to Tibet. With these factors there are the environmental circumstances that shaped what was emphasized in various locations with respect to climate, seasons, available flora and fauna, rural and urban environments, and so on. Thus, for example, the dietary practices that Ayurveda recommends in India with an emphasis on vegetarianism, does not work well in a climate where few vegetables were able to grow and, as a result, the populace is more dependent upon dairy and meat products. This is explained more fully in Robert's Tibetan Ayurveda.

Closely aligned with these environmental differences and the divergence of emphasis that each system of Ayurveda offers is what we consider to be the primary difference between the Ayurveda of Indian and the Ayurveda of Tibet. Simply put, Tibet has a harsh climate: twelve to eighteen thousand feet above sea level in general, cool to cold, very dry, and a rugged terrain. All of these facts contribute to what we call an extremely Vata-genic climate. Thus, to combat Vata-aggravating influences, Tibetan Ayurveda goes to an extreme degree in emphasizing the monitoring of and reduction or balancing of Vata—or, as it is called in Tibetan, LUNG (pronounced LOONG).

Indian Ayurveda also recognizes the importance of balancing the humor or dosha of Vata when it is aggravated. In fact, there is an entire approach to treatment that is devoted solely to reduction and balancing of Vata. However, by and large, the Indian subcontinent, whilst it certainly is varied in its climate, is hotter, lower in altitude, and moister. Such conditions help to mollify Vata in themselves. And herein lies the crux of the matter that we have observed over the years.

With respect to spa treatments or more medical interventions, such as the practice of Panchakarma, to be explained later on, Indian Ayurvedic physicians and their technicians seem to be more willing to bring a client to a catharsis, where detoxification occurs more rapidly, than are their Tibetan counterparts. Such catharsis, where there is a dramatic change in the body-mind system, may be Vata-aggravating or deranging. In a culture such as India, that understands cleansing and healing rituals and where the climate is more sub-tropical and mildly temperate for the most part, this Vata aggravation is less of a critical issue and is addressed not only in the course of treatment, but also within the support of the cultural and belief systems already in place.

However, here in the west, we do not have a system of medicine or way of thinking about health that at the most basic level supports energetic medicine and shifts that can create symptoms that some western doctors would tell you are dangerous, even bordering on malpractice. In a litigious culture, we have sadly seen Ayurvedic practitioners prosecuted because clients had little if any support for what they were going through in their Ayurvedic course of treatments. Beyond a lack of historical or cultural support for such ideas or eventualities, we also have additional Vata-aggravating stresses with the tremendous amount of over-stimulation with respect to ideas, cultures, and media influences in the form of thousands and thousands of impressions entering our minds at a phenomenal rate. Then there is electro-magnetic smog, petrochemical poisoning, and a food supply that for the most part is genetically engineered or contaminated with hormones, pesticides, and petro-chemical fertilizers. And we are so mobile, sometimes commuting to work two or three hours each day. There is little homogeneity or cultural consistency in our western existence. We have created a very Vata-aggravating environment.

One of the symptoms that arises from being influenced by a Vata-aggravating environment is to develop a body-mind dis-connect. In such state of disconnect, we become energy junkies, craving to solve the disconnect by adding more stimulation—an attempt to feel more. So we get involved with intense forms of exercise and drive ourselves to panting exhaustion and call that a workout. We eat things with super taste; high in salt, pepper, chili, garlic, sugar, caffeine, and so on. We stay intense, worked up, stressed out, caught in the whirlwind of high and low emotions until we collapse into a spiral of exhaustion, inactivity, depression, and the feeling that nothing we eat satisfies us or is being digested.

In such a chaotic lifestyle, if detoxification or the shift in the body-mind is too strong and creates a cathartic physical or emotional response, it becomes one more Vata-aggravating event. The person experiencing the catharsis may cry, even experience god, their angels, whatever. In this situation, it's all just a manifestation of aggravated Vata; nothing to get excited about because, in fact, over-excitement is just the problem.

Tibetan Ayurveda, having addressed this issue because of the Tibetan environment, coupled with the Buddhist philosophical canopy that emphasizes the importance of body-mind integration, contemplation, and meditative mindfulness, is most appropriately applicable to our western world. A Tibetan doctor doing panchakarma, another form of detoxification, or other treatment will always monitor the pulse to make sure that Vata is not being aggravated by the treatment. They may slow down, even stop treatment to let things calm down. For, if true healing is to occur, the mind needs to keep pace with the bodily changes and vice versa. Such a way of approaching healing ensures an integration of experience that creates a solid foundation upon which great healing and growth can take place. It is not that this point is lost on Indian Ayurvedic practitioners. It is just that we have seen that Tibetans and the approach they have to Ayurveda makes them more keenly aware of this fact.

Another dimension to this is that in the east, many who come to be treated through Ayurvedic therapies are more in need of physical healing than they seem to be in need of mental, emotional, or spiritual healing. When you live in a culture where survival is a critical issue, existential and psychotherapeutic issues are considered less important or an indulgence. We in the west, however, do not worry so much about survival and signs of our demise with respect to old age and death are kept more hermetically from the public here than on the streets of India. As such, western clients have issues that require an approach that allows for emotional exploration and expression, as well as spiritual searching. Here again, the Tibetan contemplative approach seems most suited.

Thus, what you will find presented in this volume are time-tested, traditional Indian and Tibetan Ayurvedic bodywork methods for home and spa environments with a Tibetan sensitivity to Vata and how to keep it balanced. This is how we have been trained. The result is stress-reduction, detoxification, and rejuvenation that leave you feeling clear, grounded, and alert.

This is the goal of our work.

A Wellness Model for the Future

It is hard to imagine that a healing system from such an ancient time would be applicable today. It surprises many to learn that Ayurveda includes every aspect of medicine we know of today: embryology, pre- and post-natal care, pediatrics, gerontology, medicine specific for women and men at all ages, psychiatry, surgery, spiritual issues, and so on. In the *Ambrosia Heart Tantra* or *Gyud Zhi*, Yutok Yonten Gonpo placed recommendations and treatments for all ages and conditions within four general categories or levels. In sequence, these levels range from least to most invasive, the idea being that we start simple and go deeper if the condition and suffering of the being demands a deeper level of attention. Of particular interest to the spa therapist are the first two levels, for this is where you will find that you do most of your work.

The first level of medicine taught in the *Gyud Zhi* has to do with **lifestyle changes**: diet, exercise, quality relaxation and rest, and hygiene. According to Tibetan Ayurveda, roughly ninety-five percent of the symptoms of distress and dis-ease that we experience would be eliminated if we were to just make lifestyle changes that were more in keeping with our particular constitution (prakruti in Sanskrit and *rang-zhin* in Tibetan) and our current condition.

Knowledge of our constitution is determined by a Tibetan or Ayurvedic healer/physician who would do pulse diagnosis, urinalysis, observation, palpation, and take a detailed medical history (which would include the medical history of one's parents and also astrological information). The result of such an examination is an understanding of the client's unique blend of three basic energies, called in Sanskrit *doshas* and in Tibetan *nyepas*. These three energies are *Kapha* (Tibetan—*bekan*), which has to do with the physical basis of the structures and tissues of our bodies, *Vata* (Tibetan—*lung*), which has to do with all movement we experience—from how our mind moves from one thing to another to how our blood moves through our bodies and even how we move from one place to another, and *Pitta* (Tibetan—*TrIPA*), which has to do with all the transformative processes in our body (such as metabolism). These three energies come together in a particular mix that determines our stature, how we process information, what emotions are more pronounced, even our spiritual inclinations and propensities. These can be reduced down to seven basic constitutional types. Knowing **our** unique blend will help us to better live a lifestyle that is less stressful and more conducive to accessing our deeper potentials. Being able to classify symptoms that the person is *currently* exhibiting, known as *vikruti* in Sanskrit, will help a healer to hone this information even more to reduce aggravating symptoms and lead a client back to living in balance with their constitution.

Although the pulse is crucial for making an accurate assessment of the constitution, to learn it proficiently takes years. However, it is possible get a rough estimate of what a person's constitution and the current condition is by familiarizing yourself with characteristics of Vata, Pitta, and Kapha, learning some simple palpation techniques, and using questionnaires. These will be provided shortly in the chapter entitled "Discovering Your Elemental Mandala". This information will give you enough to go on when it comes to making lifestyle recommendations and providing treatments for your clients.

Knowing that we often let things get out of hand before we are willing to admit that something isn't quite right, the Medicine Buddha saw that there are times when deeper levels of intervention are necessary; when we are too weak or sick to engage, practice, and possibly even see the benefits of lifestyle changes alone. Thus, the second and third levels become more relevant in the person's immediate situation, providing that in the long run, the client embraces a better lifestyle so that they need not get themselves into the same predicament again.

The second level of Tibetan Ayurveda has to do with processes of **detoxification and rejuvenation**. Sometimes we need to be rid of excess waste and other expressions of imbalance before we can gain the benefits of a better lifestyle. Thus, detoxification is necessary. To accomplish this one may use herbs, supplements, and other detoxifying medicines, massage, hydrotherapies, and methods known in both Indian and Tibetan Ayurveda as the Five Karmas (Sanskrit: Pancha Karma and in Tibetan: Len Nga). These include enemas, purgatives, emetics, nasal treatments, and blood letting or blood purification. It is only after proper detoxification that the second aspect of this level, rejuvenation, is effective. For rejuvenating the body, one may use herbs, supplements, essence extracts (examples being the various Chulens and Precious Pills in Tibetan tradition and what in Indian Ayurveda are called Rasayanas), massage and hydrotherapies with rejuvenating herbs, even herbal enemas. Rejuvenation, however, may also be practiced before detoxification in situations where people's energy is so depleted that in order for them to be able to benefit from an ongoing lifestyle change or to detoxify in the future, they need to be built up and strengthened initially. Such an approach to rejuvenation is of relevance in our own culture where people are often obsessed by fad or crash dieting and the need for detoxification and become so emaciated and depleted that in order for them to restore a proper balance, they need to be built back up.

As a spa therapist or individual health practitioner that does hands-on therapies and recommends supplements to clients, this is the primary level at which you work with your clients. This level is considered more invasive, and thus needs more expertise and understanding. Especially as one begins to physically interact with the client, doing massage and administering the various pancha karma cleanses, it is taught that one is beginning to influence the person at a deeper level. This has consequences for both the client and the health care practitioner and is why most healing professions are wise to have standards of practice and codes of ethics. And at this level it is said that the client must feel comfortable with and have confidence in the practitioner, both in terms of their expertise and their ethics. There is a definite bond that is established between client and therapist that is undeniable. It is an absolute fantasy on the part of spa owners to think that any two therapists with the same skills would be able to offer the same identical service for all clients with same level of satisfaction.

The third level of Tibetan Ayurveda is even more invasive and is usually not a part of client services in a spa setting, unless of course the spa is a medi-spa where more formally trained physicians are available. Here we are looking at emergency medicine and the treatment of deep-seated problems that need a more radical intervention. These interventions include **surgery, acupuncture, and moxabustion**—a form of acupuncture involving heat.

It may seem shocking to our modern-day notions of ancient times, but medicine as it was practiced in India, Tibet, and other areas of the world included surgical procedures which, although not having all the technology we now have surrounding it, was remarkably sophisticated. In the case of the Tibetan practice of surgery, it was banned at some point during the time of our Middle Ages due to the fact that the mother of a king died during one of the procedures.

Tibetans claim to have discovered acupuncture (the Golden Needle techniques) and that it was they who taught it to the Chinese. At the same time, there is an entire system of acupuncture that also existed in the Indian version of Ayurveda. So who was the first to use these techniques is a rather muddled issue. Nevertheless, the form of acupuncture most applicable to a high, dry, mountainous climate, moxabustion, has remained as the treatment of choice in this level of Tibetan Ayurveda.

Such methods were considered last resorts rather than initial interventions—unless of course the situation was an emergency. The Medicine Buddha taught of there being subtle energy systems; pathways and points within the body. Cutting on or through them or stimulating them in the wrong way could result in problems for the client later on. They could even be fatal. Here skill and timing were both necessary. For example, Tibetan Ayurveda teaches that such strong interventions as surgery will yield poor results if done on the New Moon. On the other hand, there are days of the month, like the 8th day of the Lunar Month, the Day of Medicine Buddha, that are quite beneficial. A person's astrological chart would also be taken into consideration. Even with the use of moxabustion, it is considered that certain times of day and seasons are better than others when addressing various complaints. Of course, in an emergency, things need to get done when they need to get done. Such action will have its own consequences that must be accepted when they present themselves. But if at all possible, to wait for the most auspicious time is what is preferred.

From the above description and caveats, it is clear that many of these energetic considerations and an understanding of consequences would well be heeded in our current uses of surgical and other invasive procedures. In the context of the medi-spa, where laser and cosmetic surgery may be a part of services offered, it behooves practitioners to investigate and take such precautions into consideration. By doing so, practitioners may see increased benefits, quicker recovery times, etc.

The last level of recommendations and healing in the *Gyud Zhi* is **spiritual medicine**. This is considered the deepest, most invasive level. Why?

If it is true that how we think and perceive our world will determine how we act in it, both for ourselves and in relation to others, it only stands to reason that a change of paradigm, a new or different belief about the world will have an impact on us at all levels. Does a new paradigm or new belief help to transform or just compound matters? This is a critical question, one we usually don't address well enough, especially in the west. Confused, negative, and uninformed perceptions and views can lead us to adopt habits that don't serve us. They can destroy close ties to family, friends, and loved ones. They can even alter how we view life and death itself and lead us down paths that have little to do with any real sense of purpose.

It is increasingly clear from observing the trends in both day and destination spas, that people want to go beyond just being pampered. They are looking for a nurturing that goes deeper, even to the roots of their stress, tension, and dis-ease. There is a call to re-connect with spirit at the most fundamental level of body and mind. It stands to reason, therefore, that such practices as yoga and meditation have made their way into the spa menu; services that facilitate relaxation, openness, and clarity. Without such qualities, changing our lifestyle and living in harmony with ourselves and those around us is not possible.

It is at this level, the level of spiritual medicine, that the *Gyud Zhi* teaches various methods that involve the client in practices of contemplation and meditation. Tibetan practices in the *Gyud Zhi* can be far-reaching and exotic. However, there are any number of methods from this tradition that are infinitely suitable for the spa environment and have been tested over the millennia as to their benefits. Some of these methods will be shared in the chapters that follow.

Therapist as Healer, Teacher, Role Model

When someone comes to see you at your business or in a spa and they allow you to touch them, you are operating at the second level of Tibetan Ayurveda. And because of the inherent intimacy that is created, more than likely you learn a lot more about your client than most other people they encounter do. With this openness comes vulnerability on their part and responsibility on yours. It puts you in a position of not only being a healer, but a counselor—even if you do not want to or feel incapable or unqualified to fill that role. And you become, as well, an unwitting role model for your client.

Thus, while you may have been hired to give a good massage, you are probably asked about what you do to stay healthy. Do you exercise, meditate, get a good massage? What do you eat? And what would you recommend to them?

Thus, knowledge of the first level of Tibetan Ayurveda is not only something you should consider with respect to taking care of yourself as a therapist so that you can provide quality service with minimal strain to your own body-mind type, which we shall address later on. It also behooves you to learn this information for your client.

This does not mean that you need to become an Ayurvedic doctor or counselor. Certainly as you work on their body, if you know Vata, Pitta, and Kapha, you will be able to direct them to types of exercise most suited to their needs. The same is true for relaxation and hygiene. With respect to diet, if your license or scope of practice does not allow you to talk about nutrition, you may refer your client to those who can offer such guidance. If you have or market products that relate to hygiene and beauty in particular, an understanding of Vata, Pitta, and Kapha and how they are present for your client will make it possible for you to direct them to the most effective product available for them. The result? Greater effectiveness and satisfaction for them.

Ayurvedic Therapies for the Spa and Holistic Medi-Spa

Ayurvedic therapies can be defined as those that come from the traditional Ayurvedic texts and medical tantras and also those practices done with an Ayurvedic perspective. Thus, while it often spices up a spa menu to include treatments that have an Indian or Tibetan flair, the most important aspect of these treatments is that they are coming from an Ayurvedic perspective. What this means is that above all, for treatment to be "Ayurvedic," it needs to be done from an Ayurvedic perspective or paradigm, regardless of whether or not they are "Indian" or "Tibetan." Thus, although here we shall mention the treatments that we think fit best into today's western spa menus, we want the reader to understand that there are many excellent therapies, hygiene practices, and exercise regimens, which (if offered to people on the basis of their Ayurvedic constitution and current condition) produce brilliant results and are just as Ayurvedic as those that are imported from India or Tibet. We shall address this more fully in the section entitled, "Customizing Treatments". **At this point, however, we want to spell out that the treatments that we shall elaborate on in this book are either very traditional Ayurvedic treatments—both from the Indian and Tibetan texts—made more spa-friendly, or hybrids that combine traditional Ayurvedic treatments with other spa and massage techniques common to the spa environment, but modified to conform with Ayurvedic principles.**

Before elaborating on the treatments that we recommend for the spa environment, we would first like to further elaborate on the role of such second level practices as massage, hydrotherapies, detoxification, and rejuvenation practices from an Ayurvedic perspective.

Massage is an integral part of Indian Ayurvedic tradition and Indian culture in general. Infants receive regular massage as it is considered to improve vitality, keep the baby strong, nourish the tissue and help with motor development, as well as keep the baby more relaxed and content. What a way to begin life!

In adulthood, massage has all the therapeutic values we ascribe to it: nourishing, detoxifying, stress and pain reducing, rejuvenating, etc. depending on what form is used. And there are a number of forms of massage and a number of variations on all of the forms, which include oleation or oil massage, dry brushing-style massage, marma and pressure point therapies, and polarity. Traditionally men would work with men and women work with women. This is to make sexuality or sexual arousal less of an issue, unless, of course, that is the goal as in the form of massage in the practice of Tantra. And there is a whole tradition of self-massage, used for all of the reasons given above. In general the practice of massage, whilst present in the Tibetan texts, was not as relied upon as in India. Some of this has to do with climate (Who wants to get naked at 15,000 feet above sea level?) and the fact that most of the healers were monks or nuns. Thus, Indian Ayurvedic practitioners are more familiar with and skilled in the massage techniques.

Hydrotherapies include such practices as saunas, localized and general steam bathing, baths themselves, and various fomentations, both hot and cold. They can be helpful in opening the body up and allowing massage oils and herbs to penetrate deeper, thus increasing their efficacy. This can be for both detoxifying and rejuvenating purposes. In combination with oil massages, general steams and herbal baths create the basis of what is called preparatory or *purva karma*. If steam is not available, Tibetans recommend herbal baths before a massage. If steam is available, then steam is done after the massage. This is what is done to prepare clients for panchakarma. However, such things as localized steam (*nadi swedana*), fomentations using hot and cold packs, and even stones, which may be included in the purva karma process, may be used at other times for specific conditions.

Beyond the stress and pain reducing aspects of massage and hydrotherapy, Ayurveda sees detoxification and rejuvenation as the primary functions of these therapies. Indeed, even the stress, strains, and pains that we experience from day to day are expressions of how our body accumulates imbalances that need to be cleansed so that our tissues can be re-nourished and/or rejuvenated if necessary for proper functioning. Such detoxification and rejuvenation finds its greatest, if not its most intense expression in the practice of pancha karma.

Pancha means five and karma means action. The five actions including enemas, purgatives and so on have been highlighted earlier. To perform these five actions, the body needs to be prepared, which is the purpose of *purva* karma, massage and hydrotherapy. The goal is to clean the client's body of toxins and then re-nutrify it with a better diet, herbs, adjunctive Ayurvedic treatments such as Shirodhara, and even rejuvenative preparations for such pancha karma treatments as nasal treatments and enemas.

Pancha karma is best monitored by an Ayurvedic physician or a healer well trained in pulse diagnosis. Hence, many spas are either misled, mis-informed, or misguided in claims to be offering this service. Most of them, in fact, offer *purva karma,* Ayurvedic massage and hydrotherapy. Even the ones that do have the sufficient Ayurvedic medical support will more than likely offer a generic form of pancha karma which will do a great deal to alleviate suffering and promote wellness, but may fall short in achieving the results pancha karma has the potential to achieve. This is something that still needs to be developed further in the west at this time, especially in the US.

This does not mean, however, that the techniques in pancha karma cannot be used outside of the context of systematic detoxification and rejuvenation. Nasal treatments (*nasya*) can be an excellent way to relieve head congestion and stiffness in the neck and upper body. Enemas (*bastis*) are an excellent adjunct to the colonic therapies that spas do offer. And such adjunctive therapies as *shirodhara* and *nadi swedana* definitely have a place as Ayurvedic treatments on a spa menu. These will be elaborated on later in the book.

The traditional Indian and Tibetan Ayurvedic treatments that are definitely practiced in today's spas and that we find most suitable for spa environments include:

- AYURVEDIC FACIAL MASSAGE SEQUENCE—a unique and comprehensive massage for the face, scalp, neck, shoulders, and upper chest using strokes and secret, vital point (marma) massage. These points have been used traditionally to bring balance to both body and mind. Now, for the first time in the west, these points have been organized into a massage sequence that is easily customized to the individual client to promote facial rejuvenation and an unparalleled sense of tranquility.
- ABHYANGA (pronounced AH-BIH-YAHN-GAH)—a full-body oleation massage using dosha-appropriate oils and touch, marmas, strokes, and cleansing procedures to promote proper hydration, circulation, and reduce stress.
- TIBETAN ACUPRESSURE—light to moderate rotational pressure applied to a specific series and order of marma and acupuncture meridian points. Tibetan acupressure (*Dzub Nyin*) offers simple but highly effective treatments for stress, insomnia, digestive complaints, sciatica, and eye strain to name a few.

- SHIRODHARA (pronounced SHI-ROH-DAH-RAH)—a luxurious and deeply calming experience of having a fine stream of warm oil poured on the middle of the forehead. This causes the release of serotonin, which deeply relaxes the body, melting tensions and thus helping to alleviate discomfort in the head, neck, and shoulder area, as well as engendering profound feelings of pleasure, inner balance, and mental clarity.

- SWEDANA—(pronounced SWAY-DAH-NAH)—This is the Ayurvedic version of a steam bath. Dosha-appropriate or tridoshic combinations of herbs are placed in the steaming water to better penetrate and work with the balance of the client's body. Such treatments are usually done only to the point where the client is perspiring freely. Generally, the head is kept out of the steam and if the client is more Pitta in nature, a cool cloth is placed on their head. This treatment is usually given following Abhyanga or other forms of Ayurvedic massage. Best results for this treatment are when the client is sitting up. However, many spas offer a lying down service. In lieu of this steam bath, if not available, Tibetan physicians recommend the use of baths with similar herbs prior to the massage.

- NADI SWEDANA (pronounced NAH-DEE SWAY-DAH-NAH)—is the application of a gentle jet of herbal steam to a specific area of the body that is especially tense or uncomfortable. This may be the whole or a specific area of the back, shoulder, knee or any joint. First, we apply warm oil, then we bathe the area thoroughly with the jet of steam. The skin becomes soft and warm, the tissues relax, pain and tensions are pleasantly melted away and the joint feels better able to move.

- KARNA PURANA (pronounced KAR-NAH POO-RAH-NAH)— filling the ear with warm sesame oil while applying warm compresses to the jaw. This is an excellent way to help resolve pain and discomfort due to TMJ and tinnitus.

- NASYA (pronounced NAH-SIH-YAH)- application of herbal drops to the nasal passages. This technique consistently banishes those dark rings under the eyes and miraculously helps to alleviate intractable neck tension. It brings a fullness and freshness to the face and eyes and can also assist in relieving sinus problems and insomnia.

- NETRA BASTI (pronounced NEH-TRAH BAH-STEE)—a means of bathing the eye and the surrounding area in warm clarified butter. This is refreshing for tired, strained eyes and especially excellent for those working with computers or under artificial lighting. As tensions are released, the eyes gain a lustrous glow, fine lines around the eye are reduced, the head clears, and seeing become a gentle pleasure.

- TIBETAN EYE REJUVENATION—a medicated butter is applied to the feet followed by warm heat delivered by textured terracotta stones. The 'lotion' and heat draw stress and tension away from the face, particularly from around the eyes, leaving them moist and clear.
- KANSA VATAKI (pronounced KAHN-SAH VAH-TAH-KEE)—A uniquely forged three-metal bowl is used to massage the feet. The effect is to balance all of the body energies (doshas) and especially to remove excess heat from the body. This treatment is usually done with an appropriate foot lotion or ghee (clarified butter).

Each of these treatments can be offered on their own or in combination with other Ayurvedic or spa services. Later on in the book we shall mention various 90-minute combinations or treatment rituals, which we have found to be extremely effective and enjoyable for clients.

Please bear in mind that what we offer here are the treatments we consider to be most suitable for the spa environment. There are some treatments that are so much like conventional spa treatments that we do not elaborate on them and others that are best practiced under Ayurvedic medical supervision. Also, for those wishing to perform self-treatments, the ones we mention and suggest are, with some modifications, quite safe and beneficial. These self-practices will be included in the chapter on "Treatment Rituals."

Glossary of Terms

BUDDHA—awakened one. It refers to this state of being but also to a historical figure, the central teacher in Buddhism, Siddhartha Gautama, a tall and graceful Indian prince who traveled widely and taught with wisdom, conviction, and deep caring of ideas that every man and women can use to succeed in life, and to make their lives meaningful.

CHARAK SAMHITA—the first and most authoritative commentary on the original Vedic texts by Charaka, who is considered the father of Ayurveda.

PANCHA KARMA—five actions that deeply cleanse and rejuvenate the body including enemas, laxatives, therapeutic vomiting, sinus cleansing, and blood purification.

PURVA KARMA—pacifying actions, usually a series of oil massages and steam treatments, that prepare the body for deeper cleansing.

A summary of points you may want to remember

- Ayurveda means 'life knowledge', also known as the Science of Longevity
- Ayurveda as a tradition was first an oral healing tradition that sprang up around the Indus River Valley in modern-day Pakistan
- Ayurveda is practiced not only in India and Pakistan, but in other parts of Southeast Asia *and* is the foundation of Tibetan Medicine
- Ayurveda is *not* associated with any religion, but its goals are to help people to become happy, healthy, and inspired
- The terms used in Ayurveda, whether they are referred here in their Sanskrit or Tibetan forms, are not religious terms. They are purely descriptive
- Ayurveda is tailored to the individual's needs based on their body-mind type
- There are Four Levels of Ayurveda as delineated in the Tibetan tradition. The first two levels deal with wellness and prevention. These are the two levels from which all the information in this book is found.

What Makes a Treatment Ayurvedic?

*W*hat is unique about an Ayurvedic treatment? Let's begin with the goals:

- To use simple, heartfelt, hands-on techniques to bring about a better integration of mind and body.
- To offer the perfect touch to release the free flow of subtle physical and mental energy to restore their natural balance and give a lasting sense of relaxation.
- To help clients experience the deep pleasure of a healthy body, a clear mind and a balanced life.
- To teach that lasting beauty comes from feeling inspired to show love and kindness as much as possible even in these difficult times.

Simply, through discovering each client's personal balance of energies and working with them, Ayurvedic treatments intend to help clients look good, feel well, and be willing to share the benefits of this state of renewal for the common good.

As the spa industry embraces Ayurveda and Ayurvedic services become increasingly popular, there is a real danger that many new treatments will be invented and called Ayurvedic this or that. We have all seen this happen to aromatherapy. We could be cynical and decide that it is just the American way to jump on the bandwagon and use the latest buzz words. However, we feel everyone involved in the spa industry wants to do the best job they know how and mistakes are made due to lack of information and inadequate education. As educators we feel we must offer our personal view of what makes a treatment Ayurvedic in the hopes that some wonderful spa experiences will be created that will both fully honor the tradition and serve the needs of the clients.

Ayurveda is recognized as the oldest source for so many of the complimentary therapies we use today, such as polarity therapy, foot reflexology, aromatherapy, color therapy and healing through sound. As the source from which so many modalities have sprung it has to be regarded as the mother of all healing. But another, more important reason why we feel that Ayurveda is called the "Mother of Healing" is that it embodies and demonstrates to clients the finest qualities of a mother: love and respect for each and every client free of judgment, with gentleness, understanding and support to the end. Ayurveda always keeps as its focus what makes human beings healthy, happy, and inspired. It never separates out the body from the mind and/or spirit of an individual, but always sees integration and wholeness and always works towards bringing us back to that integration and wholeness. Ayurveda works from the understanding that the wellness of any part is dependent on the wellness of the whole at all levels.

The obvious next question is, "so how is that done?" To answer this, we wish to first outline some basic philosophical or theoretical principles upon which Ayurveda and Ayurvedic treatments rely. Secondly, we shall discuss how these are practically applied in the offering of spa treatments.

The Principles

Below is a succinct list of the principles upon which Ayurveda inspired treatments rely.

- There is a total and intimate connection between human life and nature. The same forces that harmonize our universe work in our bodies. We are intimately connected to one another and everything else in the universe. Ayurveda recognizes five of these forces with distinct characteristics that it describes as being like space, air, fire, water and earth. These forces are always at work around us and in our bodies. They change and shape the ways things are and they control all functions in our world. In the orient, these are known as the Five Transformations; in Ayurveda, they are called the Five Great Elements or *Maha Panchabhutas*. We use these five elements always, sometimes in a balanced way, sometimes not. When we do not work with them in a balanced way within ourselves or the world around us, we experience stress and dis-ease. Thus, Ayurveda seeks to create a balanced use of the elements in healing and creating wellness. And, in the spa setting, we try to do just that in the environment and ambience we create and the treatments that are offered.

  Space is the stage we set for clients to have memorable experiences, the space we create so the client can feel uplifted, inspired, relaxed and motivated.

Air is the atmosphere of the treatment room and spa facility that should feel fresh, warm enough and filled with pleasant aroma, with a feeling of both vitality and support.

Fire is the heat of the sauna, hot tub, steam, wraps, the warmth of the oil, our passion for offering treatments, the depth of understanding we show our clients and the intelligence we bring to our work.

Water is the liquid for bathing, steaming, cleansing, relaxing in, and exercising in, and our adaptability in working with our clients to establish a flow and trust our intuition.

Earth is the mud wraps, clay masks, and our sense of confidence and reliability.

- The elements combine dynamically within the human body. Working together in pairs they organize all the bodily functions that are necessary to life. These are the *doshas* of *vata*, *pitta* and *kapha*. The way we look, think, behave, and feel is the result of a unique combination of these subtle energies. They influence our being on a physical, mental, and emotional level. They are responsible for our similarities and our differences and they are wonderfully helpful in customizing treatments to make the best fit possible for the needs of each individual client. **This point is of critical importance in the proper application of Ayurvedic treatments, be they traditional ones from India and Tibet, or the treatments that you already do applied in an Ayurvedically-appropriate way.** You can learn more about the doshas and how to recognize them in your clients in the chapter on Ayurvedic body-mind type assessment. Here we have listed some key points to remember that are of particular importance when thinking about working with your clients but may be not be mentioned in the assessment section.

VATA—sensitive to touch and sound

Often troubled by pain that moves around the body close to the surface

Sensitive to cold and changes in temperature

Poor circulation

Nervous, tense and easily fatigued

Fidgety

Talkative

Subject to mood swings

PITTA—sensitive to sights and tastes

Often troubled by chronic tension or sharp localized pain

Inflammation is common in muscles and joints

Touch can trigger the expression of volatile emotions

Intense work-hard-play-hard types; burn out easily

Controlling

Demanding

KAPHA—sensitive to tastes and smells

Prone to carry extra weight

Pains are deep and dull

Often experience swelling, congestion or water retention

Takes time to establish a relationship and trust

Hard to motivate

Internalize emotion

Grateful but quiet

- Each individual has their own unique combination of qualities, natural perfections, and inherent challenges so each journey toward beauty, balance and wellness is a very personal one of accentuating the positive and addressing the difficulties. Beyond the theoretical understanding of doshas and customizing treatments accordingly, treatments must always take into consideration the individual's client's needs and lifestyle. We should never assume we know the problems a client is seeking help with and we must always be sensitive to working out a personalized suitable solution.

- Going to a more subtle level with respect to our experience, our bodies are on the most basic level energy and light. This means that every sensation we experience effects how we feel on every level, down to the subatomic and throughout our thoughts and emotions. This principle is the basis for what we call a six-sense approach to spa therapy. Take for example:

  SOUND e.g. the voice on the phone at the front desk or answer machine, how much we talk, what we say, music we play during treatments and in the spa in general, inside noise of equipment and packaging, outside noise be it from the weather or the traffic.

  SIGHT e.g. the style of the exterior and interior design, colors of the walls and decor, organization/placement of furniture and decorations, cleanliness, effect of lighting, Feng Shui (flow or feel of a room).

  SMELL e.g. aroma of product, cleaning materials, paint and carpeting.

TOUCH e.g. the shake of a hand, a hug, treatment touch-being light or deep, slow or fast, vigorous or gentle, straight or circular massage strokes.

TASTE e.g. types of drinks and snacks, hot or cold, before or after treatment and the "taste" of oil or other product on the skin.

HEART FEELING e.g. how we love and connect with one another intuitively.

Each of our sense perceptions and what we offer each of those senses contributes to or can detract from a treatment or spa experience and thus be more or less balancing for our doshas.

• Following on from the previous point, we are an intricately integrated system of physical, mental and spiritual energy so treatments have the potential to touch us on all these levels. Mindful of this premise,

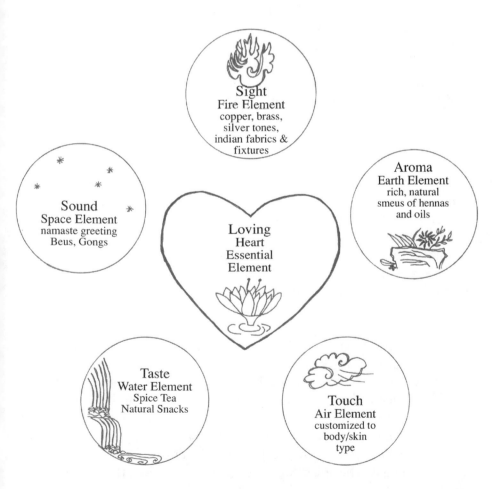

Ayurvedic treatments touch people deeply and in such a thorough way that it leads clients to feel qualitatively different afterwards.

- Each season and climate brings with it its own energy so treatments and treatment environments need to change with the seasons. We see this clearly in skin care. A client may easily have more oily skin in summer and experience more dryness in winter. Treatments and promotions should be seasonal to match climate and mood.
- All Ayurvedic personal care products must use vital, natural materials and ingredients that cause no harm to the body.
- Much of life is non-physical. Of course, we have our bodies and they move, grow and change. But the essence of our life, our life force, can only be experienced. To understand life then we have to use our intuition to gain knowledge about our clients. This goes far beyond a study of the doshas. Contemplation and meditation are recommended in developing this deeper perception and appreciation.
- We are the instruments and not the authors of the healing. Nature heals. It is the body itself that has a natural healing intelligence. Miracles can happen if we work to free the body of toxins, free the mind of useless habits, and train the emotion in a positive direction. One of the most precious elements of any treatment is the time to settle, relax and reflect. As the therapist works on the body our mind calms and our thoughts become more positive. We are setting the stage for the miracles to unfold.

These principles create a foundation of knowledge and understanding upon which Ayurveda and Ayurvedic treatments are practically applied. But probably the most important ingredient of all precedes these principles at the most basic of levels. The ingredient we speak of is having the right intention. We have to begin at the beginning with the right attitude. It is the only part of the treatment that is free and yet it is the most valuable. The right intention and attitude to begin with is LOVE!

Love

So often when we teach in spas the most sensitive and loving therapists will ask how they can continue to work without picking up the energy imbalances of their clients. Sometimes they mean physical ailments such as colds or headaches, sometimes mental struggles and difficulties, or just how can they avoid the feeling of being drained. Up until recently my response has been that only real saints can actually take on the suffering of others. If you begin to experience feeling the way you think your client is feeling it is because your energy is weaker than theirs is and their strong energy patterns are influencing yours. We have suggested that before every treatment try resting your left hand on the forehead and the right hand just below the belly button while resting the tip of the tongue behind the front teeth. Take a few deep breaths and imagine that you are surrounded by a deep blue light. This technique is designed to strengthen the aura and shield us from outside influences. It is a helpful technique but still does not go far enough in overcoming the view that all clients can be draining and that feeling tired and a little empty at the end of the day is just the way spa life is. It may make the therapist feel better at the end of the day. Some of this is the energetic benefits of the exercise, but some of it is also the result of magical thinking, which, in the final analysis does not hold up, for it encourages us to distance ourselves out a sense of fear and at best is not really nourishing to either party.

We were very excited when we came across an approach that better embodies the spirit of our company Diamond Way Ayurveda in a wonderful book called *The Tibetan Book of Yoga* by Geshe Michael Roach. He has a beautiful technique for cultivating love and overcoming that need to distance ourselves. This kind of love is the essential ingredient if a treatment is to be called Ayurvedic in our view. Here is a version of the technique that we feel is quite powerful and useful for anyone who offers help or service to another. Once you are familiar with it, it can take just a minute and is a powerful beginning to any treatment.

1. Focus on *ajna marma*, the point half an inch above your eyebrows in the middle of your forehead. Rest your attention an inch inside your skull at this point.
2. Without rushing bring your attention down inside your chest to rest at the heart level one to two inches in front of your spine.
3. In that space visualize the most beautiful rose you can imagine. It can be any color, any size, with a smell that is heavenly to you. Resting in the middle of the rose, see the biggest, brightest diamond you can imagine.
4. As you feel good inside bring to mind your client and imagine they are right in front of you and looking at you face to face.
5. Imagine now that all their pains and problems come together and form a dark pool or smoky little cloud about the size of a coin at their heart center.
6. Imagine how wonderful it would be if you could take away all these troubles, then decide that you will try.
7. With your next in breath imagine that the pool or cloud is moving up and out of their body and towards you.

8. Try to feel as brave as you can, believing that it would be better to hurt than see another suffering.

9. Focus on the rose and jewel inside your chest, remember the wonderful smell of the rose and brightness of the jewel. Know that this kind of beauty and brilliance can destroy all forms of darkness. Remember that you want and are willing to destroy it.

10. With your next breath, breathe in the darkness and let it touch the diamond in your chest. As it touches the diamond it explodes into golden light like the intense flash of a hundred cameras and is completely gone without trace.

11. Visualize the rose and diamond in your chest again. As you look at your client feel that all pains and mental disturbances have gone and they are perfectly happy.

12. Feel their happiness, be proud of how brave you were and notice how good you feel. (Footnote: *The Tibetan Book of Yoga,* Geshe Michael Roach, pp 34–36, Doubleday)

Ayurveda is about learning how to love one another, understand each other, and help each other as we are here and now. All Ayurvedic treatments should be done from a place of no judgment remembering that none of us are perfect, our doshas are somewhat disturbed, our minds not totally tamed, and our life choices not perfect, yet we are doing the best we know how. If you can work with this attitude, extend love, and work without judgment you will be amazed at how even the most difficult client can become the most beautiful angel and give you so much in return.

Oils

Harish Johari, in his book *Ancient Indian Massage*, declares that of all massages, those involving oil have the greatest benefit. Oil—and often plenty of it—is a central feature of most Ayurvedic treatments. Why? Because oil is the perfect antidote to vata, the wind energy in the body, that when whipped up into a storm is responsible for all disturbances in the body that cause stress, strain, pain and premature aging.

Ayurveda teaches that all oil is good but some oils are better than others for specific people, in particular climates, or to help ease different complaints. We have to remember that these classic recommendations were recorded hundreds of years ago so today I feel that we must mention the exceptions to that rule. Then, all oils were cold pressed and organic. Today, the picture is very different. Many oils are made from crops that have been heavily sprayed with pesticides, watered with chemical fertilizers, and even genetically engineered. Then, cold pressing was the only method of extraction. Today, heat and chemical solvents are used to increase yields. In ancient times petroleum products were not available. Today, together with synthetic fragrances and emulsifiers, they find there way into many products—even those described as natural. We can debate just how damaging these modern processes and additives may be to the body. At the very least we have to say that unless an oil is cold pressed and organic it is not the same thing as that which is being praised in our ancient texts. You should especially stay away from mineral and baby oils. Mineral oil blocks the pores and stops the skin from breathing. Interesting to reflect now on how sleepy you feel after using this oil in your suntan lotion and how you don't wake up until you have had a shower. Your skin is a major organ of respiration. Could it be that by using this oil you are oxygen deprived and so feel sleepy? Baby oil contains paraffin, emulsifiers, and synthetic scents. Never use it on a baby or on anyone else, for that matter. These chemicals can be toxic and are absorbed by the skin.

Massage with cold pressed organic oils has so many great benefits. If the list below doesn't inspire you to take up the Ayurvedic recommendation of a daily oil or at least weekly oil massage, nothing will. Oil is fire in liquid form, pure calorific energy that can transform body and mind.

Applying warmed oil to the body will
- help balance all the doshas, subtle body energies that when out of balance eventually causes all forms of discomfort and disease, by pacifying vata dosha—the force that has a controlling influence on pitta and kapha doshas.
- help relieve pain and swelling in the body by warming the subtle winds of the body which then expand to open subtle energy channels, thereby clearing the obstructions that cause the problem and mobilizing toxins.
- lubricate against friction so that the heat produced by rubbing during massage is evenly distributed throughout the skin tissue and is not allowed to build up and cause a disturbance in the doshas.
- protect the body against extremes of climate, environmental pollutants, even sudden changes in air pressure which is why oil massage is great before air travel and is the perfect antidote to jet lag.
- soften the skin, prevent dryness, combat the effects of aging, and create a healthy glow in the whole body.
- increase suppleness and durability and help maintain a youthful posture as some oils, such as sesame, can penetrate into the deepest parts of the joints within 20 minutes after application.

- help the body feel light and vital and build immune response.
- calm the nervous system that is constantly under assault from modern living.
- improve physical stamina and virility.
- improve intelligence, wit, and memory and build confidence.
- improve the circulation of blood and lymph.
- provide a source of nutrients that support a healthy skin and nervous system and balance the hormonal system.
- banish fatigue.

Oils can be used alone, infused with herbs and spices, or blended with essential oils to achieve specific results. In India oils are custom made for clients. Here in the west, there are fewer oils commercially available. I have listed those that are easiest to find in alphabetical order for ease of reference and I look forward to more being available one day. Some of the more commonly available and used oils in the western cultures are listed and classified later.

- ALMOND OIL: Rich and nourishing but must be avoided by those with a nut allergy. Helpful for Vata and Kapha constitutions.
- AMLA OIL: Rich in vitamin C, good for hair and for vata and pitta constitutions.
- AQUILARIA R OIL: A Tibetan blend that is very vata reducing. Use on the temples for headaches and on the belly for anxiety and upset stomach.
- ASHWAGHANDA/BALA OIL: A vata-reducing oil that is nourishing and strengthening to the body, especially the muscles.
- BHRINGARAJ OIL: A tridoshic oil used traditionally on the scalp to encourage hair growth and deter premature graying. It nourishes the brain and if applied on the feet helps gain a better quality of sleep. Reduces pitta.
- BRAHMI OIL: A pitta-soothing oil that helps balance heat in the body, calms and clears the mind, relieves insomnia, nourishes the nervous system and deepens meditative experiences.
- CALAMUS OIL: Excellent for helping to relieve nervous tension and anxiety.
- CASTOR OIL: Check for purity as this oil is often blended with cheaper synthetic oils. Castor oil on the belly with a warm compress will reduce vata and relieve pain and constipation. It is alkalizing and has been found to increase T cell counts making it a deeply healing

oil. Used in a warm compress it is amazing for healing knotty scar tissue and remobilizing joints after injury.

- CHANDA OIL: Helpful for relieving inflammation and headaches caused by too much heat.
- COCONUT OIL: A light soothing oil that is calming and cooling to the body. It is helpful for pitta clients and/or pitta conditions such as rashes, burns and infections.
- GHEE: Clarified butter, excellent for pitta and used in combination with a number of herbs for specific therapeutic benefits (i.e. Shatavari Ghee for breast massage and vaginal dryness).
- MAHANARAYAN OIL: A blend of over thirty herbs that is designed for soothing sore muscles and joints. One of the few oils recommended for rheumatic joints. Be aware that its red color will stain sheets.
- MUSTARD OIL: Warms the body, opens the pores, and cleanses the blood. Helpful in winter and for those with vata or kapha constitutions.
- NEEM OIL: A strong-smelling oil that is very antibacterial and anti fungal—very helpful for chronic skin conditions.
- OLIVE OIL: More warming than mustard or sesame oils, this oil captures the energy of the sun so our bodies can use it. It is particularly helpful for small children, the elderly, and others of vata and kapha constitutions.
- POMEGRANATE OIL: An herbal oil made from pomegranate rind in a mustard oil base used in small quantities for breast massage.
- SESAME OIL: Balancing for all constitutions. Black sesame is particularly nutritious and useful for the hair and nails. It can be used year round except by very pitta clients in hot humid weather.
- SHIKAKAI OIL: Favored for promoting healthy hair growth.
- VACHA OIL: Calming and balancing for the mind.

Just like foods, if you want to match oils, herbs, or essential oils to balance a specific dosha, you have to match the quality of the product to the balancing qualities for that dosha. The skin "tastes" the oils just as the tongue does, so

VATA is balanced by sweet, sour and salty oils that warm and calm.

PITTA is balanced by sweet, astringent and bitter oils that cool and soothe.

KAPHA is balanced by pungent, astringent and bitter oils that heat and stimulate.

Here are some guidelines for oils for specific dosha imbalances. Both herbal and essential oil blends are now commercially available. Check the resource section for information.

Below is a summary of the use of oils for the different doshas. We include here the essential oils, as well. Their inclusion not only speaks to their effects with respect to aromatherapy, but also to their use in face and body oils. Ayurvedic expert Dr. David Frawley has, in fact, stated that had the Vaidyas of India had the technical means of creating essential oils, they would have used them rather than the decocted and brewed oils that so characterize traditional Ayurveda. We expect that over time, the Ayurvedic market will have more and more oils that are infused with essential oils.

VATA

Oils: Sesame, almond, olive, castor, ghee, mustard
Herbal additions: Ashwaghanda, bala, calamus, passion flower, jasmine
Essential oils: Basil, bergamot, cardamom, cinnamon, geranium, ginger, orange, nutmeg, musk, rose, sandalwood

PITTA

Oils: Coconut, sesame, sunflower, olive, ghee
Herbal additions: Brahmi, coriander, gota kola. guduchi, jatamansi, licorice, manjista, sandalwood
Essential oils: Chamomile, fennel, jasmine, lavender, lemon, mint, melissa, neroli, rose, sandalwood

KAPHA

Oils: Mustard, sesame, sunflower, corn
Herbal additions: Bala, purnava, chitrak, calamus, juniper, rosemary
Essential oils: Cinnamon, clove, clary sage, eucalyptus, frankincense, ginger, juniper, rosemary.

Traditional Treatments

We believe that with the right education and the best intention, all spa treatments can be made more effective and enjoyable by embracing Ayurvedic principles. Could you then call these Ayurvedic treatments? We feel they embody the spirit of Ayurveda and find the idea of integrating old and new techniques to best serve today's clients exciting. At the same time we want to honor the tradition and make the spa market aware of as many truly traditional Ayurvedic treatments as we can. Not all the treatments mentioned here will be elaborated on in this book. The three reasons for not including some of them are that they 1) are more medical in their application, 2) are best administered under close clinical supervision, or 3) are too time consuming or messy to be offered effectively in today's spas. For now, the fuller descriptions we have chosen to share have to do only with the treatments that we personally have worked with and taught for the last ten years. This is a book about our experience and what we have so far discovered to work. We are thrilled that more and varied techniques are gradually working their way west and will eventually be more widely practiced. There are so many techniques with multiple variations. Rest assured, there are many more that will make their way into the spa and beauty industries over time. Be open when you encounter a treatment that is being called Ayurvedic; it may well stand on a long history and indeed be a traditional approach. As Ayurveda is becoming more and more popular and more widely practiced and accepted, I'm sure we will see even more varied and amazing treatment styles.

Here is a list of the more common traditional ayurvedic therapies.

- ABHYANGA: Full-body massage with warm oil that is designed to improve circulation, decrease dryness and combat the problems associated with aging, given on a regular basis by one, two, or more massage therapists.
- CHAMPISSAGE: Modern term invented for traditional head massage techniques.
- BASHPA SWEDANA: Steam bath for the full body keeping the head, heart and genitals cool with cool damp towels. Designed to mobilize toxins in the skin and deeper tissues.
- CHAKRA BALANCING: Working with seven energy centers to rebalance the mind/body system by clearing subtle energy blocks.
- DINACHARYA: Daily lifestyle guidelines for maintaining health.
- DRAVA SWEDANA: Hot baths given before full-body massage.
- INFANT MASSAGE: Regular full-body massage given from birth to two years. Traditionally done only by family members.
- KANSA VATAKI: Massage of the soles of the feet with a small bowl made of three metals.
- KAYA KALPA: Ancient rejuvenation procedures that are given in solitary retreat for varying periods of time.
- KARNA PURANA: Application of warm oil in the ears to help relieve jaw tension and tinnitus. Used in pancha karma therapy.*
- GARSHANA: Dry brushing with raw silk gloves or wool gloves or mittens that is given before full-body massage which stimulates circulation and helps balance acidity in the body.
- GEM THERAPY: Use of precious and semi-precious stones on the face and body to enhance energy balance and mental clarity.

- LEPANA: Application of herbal compresses.
- MARMA: Touching, gently rubbing, or pressing specific points on the body where there is the greatest concentration of vital energy to help the body get better in touch with its own natural healing processes.
- MUD: Application of fine clay and herbs to cleanse and re-energize the body. Akin to lepanas.
- NADI SWEDENA: Means "tube steaming"—application of a gentle jet of herbal steam to specific parts of the body such as the larger joints, hips, shoulders, or back to help melt always tension and pain and improve range of motion. Given as part of purva karma therapies.
- NASYA: Application of herbal oil or drops to the nose to clear the sinus and banish dark rings under the eyes. Used in pancha karma therapy.*
- NETRA BASTI: Bathing the eyes in clarified butter, or ghee, to help relieve eye strain and redness. Herbally infused ghees are used for various eye complaints. Just with plain organic ghee is very helpful for anyone that has to spend numbers of hours in front of a computer screen. Used in Pancha Karma therapy.*
- PANCHA KARMA: Five major purification treatments for purifying and rejuvenating the body that includes enemas, laxatives, therapeutic vomiting, nasal cleansing and blood purifying.*
- PISHINCHHALI: Vigorous herbal massage using a cloth bag full of cooked rice and a large amount of warm oil to deeply mobilize the muscles and ligaments.
- PURVA KARMA: Oil massages over a period of consecutive days to prepare the body for pancha karma.
- POST-NATAL MASSAGE: Special oil massage sequence that is given daily for forty days after delivery.
- TAPA SWEDANA: Application of dry heat to help reduce inflammation and congestion in the joints.
- SHIRODHARA: Applying a continuous stream of warm oil onto the head, usually the middle of the forehead. The stream may or may not be moved back and forth slowly to match the needs of the client. This is a deep relaxation treatment that is very helpful in reducing mental stress.
- UDVARTANA: Massage with herbal paste or powder that cleanses through stimulating lymphatic circulation.
- VISHESH: Deep tissue massage.

---

*Practiced only under the care of a licensed physician or by invoking the California or National Health Freedom Act.

Where do we go if we want to look beyond tradition and try to bring the core principles into the spa experience? Where do we even find these principles that have guided the creation of so many modalities? The spirit of Ayurveda is laid out clearly as principles outlined in the Vedas, the great texts of Indian wisdom. Modern science is just beginning to recognize these principles as verifiable truth, not just based on faith or superstition. These basic principles have not changed over the thousands of years that Ayurveda has been used. That is because they are based on universal laws of nature that are eternally true. We don't have to believe them. If we just reflect on them for a few moments we will begin to realize their truth. For the most part, we humans remember and use what we find to be useful. Over time, what has limited use we discard. This is the way of fads and if you are older than ten you will have seen many come and go in your life. Ayurveda, aligned to those truths that persist over time, is not like that. Consequently, that it has survived for over five thousand years and is now a part of the spa and beauty industries mean that Ayurveda is here to stay. That you can count on.

Customizing Treatments

Whenever my teacher, Dr Lad, would be asked if a particular diet, form of exercise, or type of treatment was "good or bad" his answer was always the same: "But for whom?"

A major part of the skill of giving any Ayurvedic treatment is in creating the optimal environment, applying the perfect touch and selecting the most balancing treatment and product. An experienced therapist will do this subconsciously but even they will have a certain style that they feel is optimal. Again we have to ask: "Optimal for whom?"

It is so tempting to believe that what we personally find comfortable, relaxing, inspiring or exotic must be what works in that way for our client as well. But customizing treatments means putting ourselves aside and discovering what really works for someone else. Here, Ayurveda is a great help because it offers what we call *our first best guess*. In other words, it gives us insight so we can make a better-informed choice about how to work with a particular client.

To accomplish this, Ayurveda offers various methods of assessing the client's balance of body-mind energies; again, *vata, pitta,* and *kapha.* Knowing this information about your client, whether it is to gain an in-depth understanding of their constitution (known as *prakruti*) or their daily condition (known as *vikruti*), will help you to properly apply a traditional Ayurvedic Indian or Tibetan treatment or, for that matter, any treatment. The chapter entitled "Discovering Your Elemental Mandala" will address assessment.

What we address here are the technical considerations one needs to keep in mind in honoring and working with the person's constitution or condition. Of the two and in the spa setting, knowing the person's *vikruti* or condition matters most when observing the following considerations.

Although not set in stone, the aspects of a treatment that we mention in customizing your treatment to meet the client's body-mind type needs are the ones we have found to work best with our clients over the years. And while they do rely on a therapist having a reasonable ability to recognize the dominant dosha of a client from learning assessment methods, it is important to be open-minded and flexible. Discovering what really works can be a very enjoyable and instructive game where everyone wins.

Lighting

Vata—These clients are happy to be treated like a baby. They are comfortable in womb-like spaces where the lights are dim and the atmosphere is safe and inviting.

Pitta—These clients need to see that the room is spotlessly clean and tidy but they have eyes that are very light sensitive. Any client that arrives in sunglasses or wears glasses or contacts is more or less pitta. Lights that are bright initially and then dimmed work, or use overhead lights that can be switched off leaving a small side light. Overhead lights, even very dim ones, can feel like torturous interrogation, so use eye pads or eye pillows when you can. Be aware that changes in light are particularly jarring so make these transitions gentle.

Kapha—They often like things delicate and pretty, so think of this when you select light fixtures. They fall asleep most easily so if you don't want them to miss the whole experience keep the lights a bit brighter than you would normally consider.

Temperature

Vata—These are the clients that feel the cold the most and find it very hard to relax if there is the slightest draft or change in temperature. Keep the room warm and cozy amd the table pre-warmed, but turn off electric blankets before the treatment begins. Warm your hands before you touch and warn your client if a product or piece of equipment is going to feel cool.

Pitta—These clients have a need for the air to feel clean and fresh. Of course you don't want your client to freeze, but they may be happiest with a window open a crack and a small fan moving the air. Too much heat will make them irritable and uncomfortable.

Kapha—Such clients behave like a cat always seeking the perfectly comfortable spot in a sheltered sunny corner. The middle range of temperature is perfect.

Linens And Bed Covers

Vata—Flannel sheets and down comforters covered in soft or raw silk are best for these clients.

Pitta—These clients will be most comfortable in crisp white cotton sheets, the best quality available, with cotton blankets.

Kapha—Interesting colors or designs such as flowers or paisley with mohair wool or chenille blankets will help these clients feel most comfortable.

Colors

Vata—Warm soft shades and darker blue like glass bottles often are most appreciated by these clients.

Pitta—These clients are most comfortable with white, cream, or colors found in nature—sea green, sky blue, etc.

Kapha—Strong rich color and bold designs keep these clients happy and comfortable.

Touch

Vata—Slow, even, long, nourishing strokes or gentle circles offered in a consistent, even predictable manner. Beware of very thin clients demanding deep work; they are feeling the need for a quick energy boost. Encourage them to experience the feel of a deeper renewal that comes from more subtle work. Those who are constitutionally or conditionally more Vata can feel, in a very tangible way, even the subtlest work that doesn't even involve touching the body such as Reiki or palm healing.

Pitta—Precise, well-educated, even work that encourages the body tissues to fill out into space by emphasizing movements that come away from the body rather than just pushing in. They may ask why you are doing what you are doing. Give them a good sound reason (they are not impressed if you tell them that your spirit guide or their totem animals are guiding you). Then they can relax, knowing that you know what you are doing.

Kapha—Firm, energetic, and a variety of styles. You want to keep them energized and interested in the treatment, so be lively and creative. Gentle movements that mobilize lymph are very useful too.

Music

Vata—Use calming gentle sounds of wind instruments such as flute. Vocals are too distracting.

Pitta—Soothing sounds of nature, intricate strings, or piano are most relaxing for these clients.

Kapha—Inspiring up-beat music such as light jazz will keep these clients interested and awake.

Talking

Vata—Encourage silence and communication on a more subtle level. Don't initiate conversation, and answer questions briefly. Some clients need permission to be quiet or have the value of silence pointed out to them. Asking, "Can we be quiet together for a few moments?" often works.

Pitta—Be ready for precise questions and well-meant critique. If you don't know the answer to the question do not bluff; you will be found out. It is perfectly respectable to say you'll find out and let them know; do remember to follow through. If too much detail is being asked for, suggest time for discussion at the end of the treatment, reading a brochure or book, or making a separate consultation time in order to answer fully.

Kapha—A few words from the therapist so the client does not sink into deep sleep and wake feeling groggy is a good thing. Don't take their silence to mean they don't like or appreciate the treatment; they will express themselves in other ways.

Aroma

Vata—Use sweet floral smells for these clients.

Pitta—Light fresh scents work well for these clients.

Kapha—Rich, exotic, even woody aromas help these clients maintain interest and focus.

Section Two

Welcome to the Spa!

To create an Ayurvedic Spa, you do not have to make your facility look like the Taj Mahal or fill it with Indian or Tibetan décor or paraphernalia. What matters most is that you are mindful of and try to apply the universal principles that Ayurveda considers important for creating a safe, nurturing, aesthetically pleasing, and inspiring oasis for your client.

CHAPTER 5

Ambience

*T*hese days, most spa staff, whether from the standpoint of the managerial positions or the therapists, will probably agree that people want more from their spa experience. Sure, pampering is fine, but many clients want to go deeper than that. In uncertain times when life may seem more convenient but more stressful, people are looking for meaning and purpose. Of course few—if any—spas hold the keys to these answers. But in their ambience, and in the services they offer, they can create a nurturing and safe space to facilitate self-exploration and a flowering that begins from within.

Life out of balance is where we become over-stimulated in some areas of our lives while being under-stimulated in others. In a serene, undistracted atmosphere, much of our mental clutter and excessive chatter becomes more silent. In an aesthetic and balanced setting, our vision is less burdened by what is harsh and unpleasant and joy begins to naturally arise. Pleasing scents of pristine and aromatic places that we associate with nature and our connection with it eases the tension in our breathing and slows the rhythm of our life. Through cleansing, nourishing, and re-hydrating the body's tissues, we are brought back to our sense of presence and inhabiting rather than feeling burdened by our body. Providing the body and mind with nourishing, tasty snacks that revive the body to once more meet the outside world completes the sensorial appreciation of being alive and capable. If a spa can fulfill all of these requirements for its clients, it has fulfilled the task for which spas of antiquity were renowned. To become "spiritual beings having a human experience", first and foremost we have to come back to our senses. And the Ayurvedic spa accomplishes this by addressing all of the physical senses, both in the treatment room and in the spa as a whole.

In this and the next two chapters of the book, we shall address these physical and environmental considerations to making your spa's ambience and physical environment more in line with Ayurvedic principles. In conjunction with this, we suggest you read the chapter on assessment, "Discovering Your Elemental Mandala", as it will greatly facilitate your understanding of what each of your clients notices and expects from the spa environment.

Setting the Tone and Intention

At this juncture, however, we wish to address what we feel is one of the most critical aspects for a successful and happily functioning spa. This dimension is by and large invisible, yet it can permeate every facet of what you offer. We are speaking of your spa's ambience and, in particular, the actual working environment and the relations and understanding between and amongst staff and management. This is the space, the 'vibe', into which you are inviting your clients. Each of you as a staff person spends hours a day putting your time and energy into a collective endeavor. The atmosphere is saturated with your hopes, wishes, intentions, etc. If there are a lot of communication and relationship problems amongst the staff, if there is a 'behind-the-scenes' tension between management and spa technicians, you may find that clients have a harder time relaxing and when they do, they get exhausted not by the great detoxification that they experienced, but rather by being over-burdened by the stress and tension they feel from the hands of their therapist or in the hallways. It is more than just a metaphor when someone says "You could have cut the atmosphere with a knife". Such an atmosphere can have an adverse effect on client satisfaction, repeat business, and sales.

Basics for Clearing the Air

To start with, we should first understand that, in keeping with Ayurveda's intention, each of us wants to be happy, healthy, and feel inspired. Few of us enjoy being miserable and making those around us miserable, at least intentionally. It stands to reason, therefore, that each person who works in a spa wants their work environment to feel happy, to be healthy for them as well as their clients, and to be a place it is a joy to come to day in and day out. How do you accomplish a task at which so many businesses fail?

Understand that there are few businesses where the ambience and the mood of the therapist and staff are such a dramatic feature of client satisfaction. You can buy a television from a miserable salesperson, but it is another thing to receive a massage from a disgruntled therapist. Your TV is not going to get cooties from the salesman, whereas a client can feel burdened, irritated or worse from the hands of someone who is distracted, worried, or indifferent. Thus, for the sake of your clients and business, it is vital for spas to achieve harmony amongst those who contribute to it.

To break the ice in a non-judgmental, non-threatening way, we suggest that every staff member study our chapter on assessment. Each person has their own work and management style and although there are universal principles with respect to courtesy, respect, confidentiality, etc., how people communicate, their daily needs, how they relate to time and space with respect to clients and scheduling has more to do with their *prakruti*, or Ayurvedically-determined individual body-mind type than you could possibly imagine. Why are some managers sticklers for forms and time? Why do some therapists have difficulty keeping on time? Why do some therapists get cranky if they can't have their lunch break? You can make this study a wonderful exercise in getting to know each other in an interesting and playful way.

There are also some general comments that we would like to make after having been witness to and a part of the spa and beauty industries for over the last decade. These comments could apply to businesses in general, but are even more important to a spa. When I was in Social Work graduate school, one of my main studies was looking at management styles and studying the styles that existed in the most successful companies. What I learned was that the most successful companies have management whose primary focus is the success and happiness of the workers. If workers feel valued, are appreciated for what they do, and are rewarded accordingly, their happiness will be felt by the clients they are serving. In a business where 'energy' and 'vibes' are important ingredients in whether a client likes a service or not, management needs to grasp this fact and honor it almost over and above all other truths about business and management they may have studied. One of the ways in which some businesses accomplish this is by letting all staff members contribute to the mission statement upon which the business runs. An overall philosophical statement of goals and intent created by each person in a spa has a very powerful effect of bringing people together at the level of core values. It also sets the tone upon which all other decisions are made.

In accordance with this, the "bottom line" cannot be the primary determinant of a spa and/or its atmosphere. Too often, time and money pressures make the atmosphere of a spa charged with tension and anxiety. Especially if spa work is effective, clients want or need more. Maybe they need to emote and it is hard to just get them off the table and out the door. If scheduling does not account for these 'human' experiences, mechanistic efficiency soon becomes a tyranny that creates rushed services, therapists who have no time to eat or go to the bathroom, etc. The result is a higher level of burnout (in this context, we taught a class where a very fancy and reputable spa had five of its therapists receiving disability because of tight schedules and excessive client bookings).

Spa management and auxiliary staff should all experience every treatment that a spa has to offer. Perhaps they know what a massage feels like, and therefore draw the erroneous conclusion that all the other treatments feel similarly. But it is very difficult to communicate the effects of a marma treatment or shirodhara without first-hand experience. By trying every treatment, they can better empathize with therapists and can more effectively communicate with clientele as to what they will experience once they step into a treatment room and the door is closed.

Spa therapists need to be given adequate time to train. This is especially true of energetically based therapies, such as those of Ayurveda. Such therapies need space and time for therapists to focus and feel their effects. Too often we have been asked to train therapists who have had to run out of the training to treat scheduled clients. Of course, this is a dilemma if a therapist is not on salary and every hour in training is an hour not making money. And some spas see training as expensive, cutting into profits by taking therapists away from clients. The simple truth is that unless a spa therapist is adequately trained, they will do a treatment poorly and will more than likely discourage clients from booking them for that treatment in the future. If spas treat staff well and train them well, perhaps the rates at which staff members burn out or leave will decrease.

The High Road

The final point we wish to make here has to do with *karma*. In the west we have the saying, "What you sow, so shall you reap". This is what karma is about.

If your spa focuses on the bottom line, if money goes into the décor, but not into staff training or staff benefits, if corners are cut environmentally, then why would you not expect to have cash-flow problems, wage disputes with staff, and various problems with plumbing, electricity, unwanted noise, smells, and so on?

Of course, no one in business wants to run at a loss. It is important to make money. In a spa, where aesthetics do matter, you had better make the first appearance a great one. And you can't always be as environmentally conscious as you would like, sometimes for very practical reasons. The thing is that often, the solution to these problems is not found by attacking the problems head on, but from adjusting our attitude towards the problems. In this instance I am not speaking about having more information per se, but looking at these situations from the level of ethical and moral considerations.

More often than we would like to admit, we are morally remiss. We know better, but cut a corner here or there, either because it is more convenient or think that if no one is looking, we can get away with it. But we are looking. And because we do, because we always really know what is going on even if we don't want to admit it to ourselves, it weakens us, weakens our judgment, makes us reactive, increases our stress, on and on.

The first level of Tibetan Ayurveda has to do with lifestyle changes. What is generally addressed here are things like diet, exercise, relaxation, and hygiene. What is not mentioned, but is included at this level, is morality. For turning a blind eye *can* lead to eye problems. Skimping on basic necessities, finding cheap but poor quality options, can leave us feeling hungry and malnourished. Having a big mouth (gossiping, bullying) *can* lead to dental and mouth related problems. Beyond the physical connection, however, there are also social repercussions that can affect our livelihood and business.

Of course, there is no way to adequately address the topic of personal morality in this text. It is also not the place. However, the lessons of personal morality can be translated into how we conduct business. And how a business is conducted based on moral principles will affect its bottom line, staff retention, client satisfaction, and so on.

Towards this end, we strongly recommend for staff managers to read and study Geshe Michael Roach's *the Diamond Cutter: The Buddha on Strategies for Managing Your Business and Your Life*. The text is based on an ancient Tibet text called "The Wheel of Sharp Weapons", by Dharmarakshita. "The Wheel of Sharp Weapons" looks at problems we have in our lives and how we have contributed to them. Geshe Michael Roach translates this wisdom into business terms. I would like to offer the reader a cogent sample of the wisdom this book contains.

Business Problem #1: *Company finances are unstable, in a state of constant flux.*

Solution: *Be more willing to share your profits with those who have helped you produce them, and be very strict about never making a single penny through any improper action. Remember, the* amount *you share with those around you is not what determines the strength of the imprint, it is your* willingness *to share whatever you have made, even if it's not a lot. (Page 88,* The Diamond Cutter, *Doubleday)*

Understanding each other on your staff team based on Ayurvedic body-mind type awareness, practicing a more transparent and clear morality, and honoring what you each contribute to a healing, vital, and transformative service for your clients will create an atmosphere that is magnetizing and healing in itself.

Having set the tone and intention upon the high road of serving your clients for everyone's benefit, let us explore further how we can make your spa radiate these intentions.

CHAPTER 6

Creating Harmony in Your Spa Using Vastu Shastra

This quote is from Michael Borden's teacher and on his site and we have permission to use it:

> "In the heart cave of the body there is space
> and in that inner-space there is the vibrant thread of consciousness.
> It is this thread of consciousness that functions as the
> string of the sarira-vina (bodily instrument).
>
> The structure of the vaastu inspired building vibrates with
> cosmic energy and bodily instrument resonates with this vibration.
>
> To create and offer the house of supreme bliss, and to enable us
> to experience that supreme bliss here in this mundane house
> itself—these are the prime motives of the Vaastu science"

BY DR. V. GANAPATI STHAPATI
TRANSLATED BY ALTAVISTA'S BABELFISH

Having good intentions, running your spa ethically, creating harmonious relations within your staff, and all the other considerations we have mentioned to create a healing and vibrant spirit that will also attract clients to your spa are essential ingredients to your success. As a human caring service, our human relations have to remain a primary focus.

But what if you could create a physical, material environment in and around your spa that would support, even encourage such a spirit of healing? For we all know that some environments are more uplifting than others to live or work in, or come to for health and healing. Some environments can make you feel that in maintaining a positive outlook, not getting bogged down is more challenging. Working in a cubicle facilitates less creativity than being able to look through a window and see a beautiful forest. Lying down in a warm, beautiful room, with sweet scents and music is more conducive to relaxation than a room that looks more like a medical examination room. There is common sense in this. With this in mind, if you look into the chapter on assessment, you will gain more insight into the senses, colors, and textures to which each of your clients is attracted. An Ayurvedic elemental sensibility is invaluable in creating a spa that is truly uplifting to the greatest number of people, regardless of whether your spa offers Ayurvedic services. At the same time, Ayurveda has a sister science associated with it that utilizes the same universal principles to address other factors that will improve and enhance the quality and intentions that we set or aspire to in our living and working spaces. This is the focus of the Indian tradition of Vastu Shastra.

Vastu Shastra is the Indian equivalent of what many in the west have come to know as Feng Shui. Vastu in Sanskrit means nature, our surroundings, immediate environment, or that which lives forever. The word "Vaasthu" comes from this root word Vasthu, and means a place, house, shelter, or building. Shastra in Sanskrit means 'systems'. Vastu Shastra is then understood to mean the ancient art and science or the principles and practices of designing and constructing buildings that bring a strong and harmonious balance between human beings and nature. Such buildings, when brought to life with the power of ceremony and kept alive by the pure intention of the occupants, have such a life force of their own that they bring happiness, health, wealth and prosperity to all who enter in. Imagine standing in a spa that, like some of the great cathedrals and temples of the world, would heal and inspire you just by being under the roof!

How is this done? The ancient sages of India worked with many forces of nature including the Pancha Bhutas (five elements) namely earth, space, air, fire and water; gravitational and magnetic effects; and rotational influences of Sun, Moon, Earth and the other planets in our solar system to help make this connection between man and the healing power of our universe. Working with these forces Vastu Shastra seeks to design buildings that would be the perfect residence for the spirit of health, harmony and ultimately enlightenment. Just as we try to prepare for everything in the spa environment to attract and embrace our clients, Vastu Shastra aims to create a space that is so perfect that the divine balancing energy of the universe enters and does not want to leave. The building then becomes a vibrant living form, an instrument that harmonizes us, body and soul, just by our being in the space. We think using Vastu Shastra to design a spa, especially a spa focused on Ayurvedic treatments, would be ideal, but this takes more that hanging chimes in the doorway or putting a plant by your cash register. Vastu Shastra starts literally from the ground up. So here we shall focus on some ideals for you to consider.

To attain this kind of perfection the site for such a building is chosen with care, the floor plan is laid out to be in harmony with the magnetic forces of the planet, and every section of the building is designed to accommodate traditional use. The outer form may be designed to embrace traditional styles. Just as examples we have chosen two designs from the work of Vastu Shastra teacher Michael Borden; one design is found in the eastern United States whilst the second is more western in style.

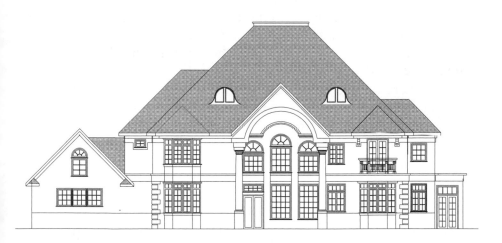

Mallidi Residence   South Elevation

New England Style Building Using Vastu Design
Drawing by Michael Borden

We maybe lucky enough to custom build our home but few get to custom build their spa from the ground up. The question then naturally arises: How practical is Vastu Shastra to the spa owner and developer? For Michael Borden commented that, unlike the modern practices of Feng Shui, to date he has found nothing in the traditional texts on Vaastu architecture that documents any cures that work to improve the energy in an existing structure.

Borden's research has lead him to conclude that, like traditional Feng Shui, Vaastu architecture principles are founded on the premise that one constructs a new structure that follows the geometric patterns of resonance with cosmic energies. You just have to work from the ground up. Because of the expense and labor involved, these refined esoteric sciences were reserved for the private use of kings, emperors, and the wealthy. But, as with Feng Shui, Vastu Shastra has now become of interest and availability to those of more modest means who want to live and work in more harmonious environments and there is a demand to somehow apply Vaastu principles to existing structures. And just as many Feng Shui 'cures' are innovations to accommodate modern times, Borden has developed some Vastu protocols that he calls 'rectifications'. The most important point to understand regarding rectification is that the results are not really predictable. In rectification, we take some of the basic principles of the science and work with the building as best we can. Unlike classical Vaastu this "tweaking" does not stand on thousands of years of tradition. It is a modern use of the principles that seem to be beneficial but we have to call the results anecdotal at this point. And the same is true for those of you who swear by the Feng Shui cures you have been advised to make.

If you were to read a book on Vastu Shastra or consult with a Vastu Shastra practitioner, Borden suggests that these would be the considerations for rectification using Vastu Shastra principles:

- Orientation of the building.
- Direction the main door is facing.
- Which rooms are being used for what function such as storage areas, eating areas, prep rooms, retail space etc.
- Geometry and mandalic frequency of the building with regard to the application of Ayadi calculation analysis.
- The creation of a Brahmastan or sacred open space in the center of the building.

His latest ideas for a solution to existing buildings is to either to

- create a space within the building that has a perfect orientation and resonance for good influences; i.e. an ideal treatment room, or
- create a small structure within the boundaries of the property that is a perfect with regard to Vaastu principles and rely on it to spread a positive influence. This is not an uncommon practice in many of the world's geomantic traditions, whereby a powerful and beneficial structure, shrine or monument is created to cast an aura of good energy all around it.

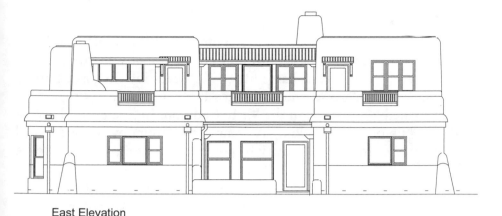

East Elevation

Adobe Style Building Using Vastu Design
Drawing by Michael Borden

Like Feng Shui, Vastu Shastra takes into consideration not only the structure and shape of the building, the arrangement of the rooms, the plumbing, power lines, and so on, it also considers the whole property including the grounds or outer environment of the structure as well. Vastu pays particular attention to what can be influenced in the immediate outer environment, such as gardens, etc. Plants and the landscapes they occupy are not left to chance in Vastu design. A holy basil plant, known in India as tulsi, is thought to be a very positive influence inside or outside as it is said to naturally make ozone. Palm trees on the north and west sides are beneficial, coconut or banana trees are thought to bring health and peace of mind, and ponds with lotus flowers or water lilies are also favored, especially in the north or east sections of the property. Obviously, such advice is limited to climates that can support such flora. As such, plants recommended by Feng Shui practitioners accustomed to more temperate climates may be more suitable, but arranged according to the energetic principles of Vastu. Whereas Vastu differs from Feng Shui in its opinion about the value, use, and placement of bamboo, both agree that cacti or other plants with thorns should never be grown, either inside or outside, they create tension. Gardens inside a building should not have fountains and statues of deities are best in the south and west. The point here is that if you have grounds around your spa, there should be some thought and consideration in how it is laid out. Aesthetics do matter, but why not add to this the energetic benefits of knowing what plants will bring healing energy, promote wealth, and guard against negative influences?

Ceremonies

Space clearing, calling upon elemental and positive energies, and performing ceremonies to consecrate and create stability in the positive energies gathered are also a part of the Vastu tradition. Just as a baby is welcomed into the world when it takes its first breath, a property is bought to life by ceremony in the Vastu tradition. Before ground is broken and again once the building is complete a ceremony is done to call helpful energies from the main eight points of the compass. According to Vastu Shastra, if we revere and respect the powers of the eight cardinal directions, they will shower on us their blessings and benefits. There are similar beliefs in many traditions around the world. These are the attributes of each direction from this Indian system.

- Esshan ie Ishwar (North-east)—grants us wisdom and knowledge, serves all comforts, and relieves us from sufferings.
- Indra (East)—gives wealth and all pleasures of life.
- Agni/Fire (South-east)—gives us beautiful personality and all the best of life.
- Yamaa or Yamaha (South)—eradicates evils and grants all good things.
- Nissan or Niruti (South-west)—banishes fear about our enemies.
- Varun (West)—showers blessings through rain and brings all-around prosperity and pleasure in life.
- Vayu/Wind (North-west)—bestows on us long life, health, and strength.
- Kuber (North)—grants us wealth and all comforts of life.

Of course there are traditional ceremonies with beautiful chants, prayers and music but as with many things that are of the spirit it is the thought that really counts. When it comes to space clearing, opening your spa up for the first time, or resetting a new intention and focus for your spa or business, you might consider contacting a spiritual guide, a Feng Shui or Vastu Shastra practitioner to do a traditional ceremony. Or, as you know what intention you want to set for your space, you may consider choosing elements from various cultures or ceremonies that are meaningful to you and designing your own ceremony. I think all businesses feel more alive if the staff feel connected to a sense of a greater good and feel blessed to do the work and help others. We can all benefit from divine blessing so go ahead call it in and "may all beings benefit".

As you can appreciate, there is a lot to this system. So much, in fact, that we can only give it the briefest mention in the hope that you will be inspired to delve further yourself. The internet is a great resource and Mr. Borden has one of the clearest sites and a great home study program. If you are interested in working with these ideas, or have the ambition to build one of the first Ayurvedic spas that would be designed using Vaastu, we urge you to connect with a qualified professional. You can find more information in the resource section.

Clarification of Terms Used in This Chapter

As spellings vary, and sometimes the words mean the same and sometimes the meanings are just slightly different, you might find these definitions helpful.

- Vaastu Purusha—the energy contained in the Earth.
- Vastu—derived from the word "to dwell, live": That which lives forever. If you take the universe and crush it into a drop—that is Vastu: the substance of the universe. It is eternally living. Also: vasthu
- Vaastu—what has issued out of Vastu is Vaastu. Vaastu is the manifest Universe: every "thing" in it. Vastu becomes Vaastu. $E=mc^2$ Energy becomes matter: this is the Divine formula. Also: vaasthu
- Vastu Purusha Mandala—The plan of the layout of a temple or a residential building. Also: mandala purusha vastu, mandal purush vaastu
- Vastu sastra—science of energy, of energy applied in a vastu. Also: vaastu shastra, vasthu saastra, vaastu shaastra and other spellings
- Vastudevata (vastupurush)—the energy, or deity, of the premises.
- Vasthu Vidya—knowledge of vasthu.

CHAPTER 7

How Environmentally Friendly Is Your Spa?

*B*ecause Ayurveda is such an ancient science there are a host of modern inventions that, of course, are not mentioned in the traditional text. The beauty of Ayurveda is that it is not a dogma. Ayurveda is a set of principles that are based on ultimate truths. When these truths are properly understood they can be used at all times and in all places. As students of Ayurveda we believe it is our responsibility to strive to understand the principles and apply them in our modern world. One very basic principle is that in order for a product to be acceptable for use in an Ayurvedic spa and creating an Ayurvedic lifestyle it must cause no unwanted side effects. To us this means not only that there should be no negative impact on human health from using the product, but also that producing the product must create no negative impact on either human health or on the environment and the life of the very planet that supports us. This includes social dimensions as well; i.e. no negative karma produced by unfair trade practices. We know this is raising the bar for all. Nevertheless, there are companies that either have adopted these ideals from the start or are aspiring to include them in the way they produce products and conduct their business—and they are being honored. In the 2004 alone, we have seen major skin and spa product trade journals honoring those companies going 'organic'. Some do this to catch the next wave. However, a growing number of people understand the link between individual health and the health of our planet and our more immediate environment and are willing to pay a little extra to do the right thing. I don't want to get into particulars or argue here about just how toxic certain glues may be, the financial benefits of purchasing from sweatshops or the problems of using old growth woods. I simply want to say that if you are embracing the spirit of Ayurveda, think about all your choices. Your actions speak louder than words. Here are just a few ideas to ponder. They are not in an order of importance, but rather considerations we have put together with the hopes that where you can, within the context of your own spa, you can adopt the ones that work best for you and your clientele.

- Use bamboo floor covering. It is beautiful, very hard wearing and comes from a resource that grows very quickly.
- Where carpeting is needed, use pure wool carpeting. It feels luxurious and has a very life-supporting energy to it.
- Choose environmentally friendly paints and varnishes. It does make a difference. Treatment rooms are often small and enclosed, and the less gas the paints let out the more fresh and alive the room feels.
- Use a negative ion generator and air purifier overnight, regardless of whether your room has standard or eco-friendly varnishes and paints. These devices help to also cleanse the germs and bacteria that naturally accumulate where people are sweating and discharging fluids, gases, etc. If you want to take this even further, you can use diffusers with essential oils of eucalyptus, tea tree, or manuka.
- Consider using organically produced fabrics such as cotton, hemp, wool and silk in your décor as well as on your treatment tables. Ask about natural dyes. Generally they are not as stable as the chemical alternatives, but for rooms that get no sunlight anyway they are beautiful. The more we create a demand for organic everything the more will be produced and eventually our ground water will become cleaner and healthier.
- Serve organically grown foods and teas whenever possible. Support local farmers or organic project in other parts of the world.
- Serve filtered or spring water to clients and your staff. It makes little sense to cleanse the tissues only to re-hydrate with water full of chlorine. In that regard, with respect to your thalassotherapy tubs and steam baths and unit, try to get filtration onto the taps into these units so that clients do not have chlorine around their bodies for these treatments.
- Support local craftsmen and artists; your spa could be a great showcase for their work. Tell the story of your community of helpers.
- Support local welfare-to-work programs, sheltered workshops and international cooperative projects.
- Re-use and recycle as much as possible.
- Choose environmentally friendly cleaning products whenever possible. Web sites for people with environmental sensitivities have great sug-

gestions for cheap and effective homemade cleaners. Do make sure to keep the rules in your state for sterilizing equipment and tools of the trade etc.

Sometimes it's the availability, sometimes the cost, sometimes it's the lack of effectiveness of the product that puts us off. All we are asking is that you think about it and do what you can. It is all part of acting in line with the core story of *Ayurvedic Spa*. We asked a friend who has worked with environmentally friendly building material and house-hold products to give us a list of companies she has worked with successfully. Check our resource guide for these tried and true products that really work well.

Section Three

Treatments: Polishing Your Client's Mandala

You are a Rainbow Body
Your mind is Limitless
Your true nature's expression is Spontaneous Joy
DIAMOND WAY AYURVEDA SLOGANS

CHAPTER 8

Discovering Your
Elemental Mandala

*I*n Tibet, one beautiful morning greeting translates as, "How is your mandala shining today?" In this next chapter we will be introducing ways you or your clients can discover their own personal elemental mandala or dosha balance. In our opening comments about Ayurveda we talked about how the way we look, what we feel and the style in which we act depends on our own personal blend of elemental qualities that are like space, air, fire, water or earth. Now we want to take the next step and invite you on a journey to discover more about how these elemental qualities express themselves in our bodies, minds and emotions.

The traditional assessment of one's true Ayurvedic body-mind type (prakruti) is a very deep and complex matter. Traditionally, to get the best assessment possible, clients had to eat very simple vegetarian food for at least one week, not engage in any extra-curricular or out-of-the-ordinary events, and come early in the morning for an appointment. The physician would prepare himself in the same way. He would also pray and meditate so as to be extra clear before he would read the pulse, look at a sample of urine, touch the pulses, take a medical history (which include information on one's family of origin), and check out astrological data. With all of this preparation and then synthesizing the information gathered and provided, the physician would be able to tell the constitution, the basic energetic, or *prakruti,* of their client and also their present energetic, or *vikruti.*

Learning to read the pulse accurately takes time, patience and good teachers, none of which are easily found in our busy western lives. Then, even the great masters of pulse do not claim to be 100% accurate though they have proven their amazing skills to me personally many times. Of course in a spa setting we are not likely to be testing urine or asking intrusive medical questions, but we can learn a lot if we train our eyes to see, cars to hear, hands and hearts to feel and even our noses to smell our clients. We can learn so much by quietly and lovingly observing. The best therapists do this already. It comes naturally to them. Here we want to show the connection between what you observe with the elements and doshas. We also offer questionnaires and some of the simple hands-on assessment tools that we find are extremely useful in helping to see basic energetic patterns or tendencies. These tools will provide you with enough information to guide you with lifestyle choices, and help you give appropriate suggestions to your clients. Most importantly for the work at hand, they will help you to be better able to work with clients in a massage, aesthetic, and spa environment by perfectly customizing their treatment so they have an experience that is a treasured memory.

Your Outer Mandala—or What You Can See With Your Eyes

Ayurveda teaches that each of us is a combination of energetic qualities, a dance, an ever-changing design. When you look at yourself or your client remember you are looking at the whole outer mandala, the complete picture. In this totality of their form and physique, some parts will be more *vata*, some more *pitta*, and some more *kapha* in quality. It is the unique combination of these qualities or *doshas* that give each of us our own special beauty, our personal way to shine. Taking a moment to appreciate the body that we have and smiling at the whole person that we are, let us now look at the parts.

Remember, we have three *doshas*. One way to get familiar with each of them is to decide to take a day to feel *vata* body qualities, another day to observe *pitta* body characteristics and a separate day to be with the kapha body qualities around. Don't try to put anyone in a vata, pitta or kapha box. Just notice their vata-, pitta-, or kapha-ness if you will. When you have a better grasp of the parts, you can then put it all together and see what the whole looks like again. In this loving and thoughtful way you will appreciate more of who they are and really see their outer mandala shining.

Let's take **Vata** qualities first. Vata dosha combines the qualities of the elements Space and Air. Some of the properties associated with each of these elements are

SPACE—dry, cold, formless, vast, expansive, open, all-inclusive, peace, and dark.

AIR—cold, light, subtle, changeable, fear, excitement, and inspiration.

Together they give us the classic qualities of *VATA* starting with *vata's* unique properties of:

DRY, COLD, LIGHT, IRREGULAR, MOBILE, SUBTLE, QUICK

Think of these qualities. Now consider how they would manifest in our bodies. Try to imagine what a body would look like if these qualities were a strong influence. Consider each of the following categories and write down your ideas using these headings. Our answers are in italics.

Archetypal Image—*fairies and goblins, butterflies, bees, hummingbirds*

Build—*fine bones, light muscles, thin, easily can feel the bones under the skin, fragile bones, irregular proportions, small breasts, weight can fluctuate-harder to gain*

Face—*smaller, thinner, longer*

Movement—*fidgety, restless, chaotic, needs extra support to be comfortable, flits like a humming bird, joints click and pop easily*

Speech—*very talkative, expresses emotion, talks about changes, sensations and travel*

Skin—*cold, especially hands and feet, dry especially over joints and in winter time*

Hands—*cold, bony, long fingers, and dry*

Feet—*long and thin or rather short*

Nails—*dry, bitten, broken, ridged, irregular shape*

General features—*irregular size and arrangement*

Hair—*dry, brittle, wiry, dry scalp*

Eyes—*dry, blinky, darting, twitchy, small, short eye lashes*

Mouth—*uneven top and bottom lips, dry lips, receding gums, crooked teeth*

Voice—*higher tone*

Now let's look at **Pitta** dosha in the same way. Pitta is a combination of the elements of Fire, Water, and some aspects of Air according to Tibetan understanding. Some of the qualities associated with each of these elements are

FIRE—heat, light, upward moving, bright, intelligent, transforming, anger.

WATER—cool, flowing, refreshing, nourishing, lubricating, attachment.

Together they give us the classic qualities of *PITTA* starting with *pitta's* unique properties:

HEAT, OILY, LIGHT, REGULAR, INTENSE, FLUID, SHARP

Again, think of these qualities mentioned in relation to the elements and the qualities of the dosha they form. Think of the human body and try to imagine what a body would look like if these qualities and properties were dominant. Be precise and think of as many details as you can. Consider each of the following categories and write down your ideas. Ours, again, are in italics.

Archetypal Image—*warriors, wolves, foxes, eagles*

Build—*well proportioned, muscular, athletic, even proportions, more angular frame, disciplined about weight and fitness, medium breasts*

Face—*average size, more triangular*

Movement—*good posture, precise, measured, purposeful, energy efficient, assertive, in command like a bird of prey*

Speech—*precise, concise, good vocabulary, asks detailed questions about results, timing and ingredients*

Hands—*warm, strong, capable*

Feet—*warm, prone to strong smell*

Nails—*evenly almond shaped*

Skin—*warm, soft, rosy, glowing, can flare up in rashes and breakouts*

General Features—*even, sharper shapes*

Hair—*lighter colors, straighter, shiny, oily, grays early, hair thinning*

Eyes—*bright, sparkly, penetrating, expressive, engaging, easily stressed by light*

Mouth—*even lips, red gums, yellowish teeth, prone to fever blisters*

Voice—*medium, sharper tone*

Now last, but never least, let's think how **Kapha** manifests in our being. Kapha is a combination of the elements of Earth and Water. Some of the qualities associated with each of these elements are

EARTH—dense, cool, supporting, grounding, inert, stable, solid.

WATER—cool, flowing, nourishing, lubricating, attachment.

Together they give the classic qualities of KAPHA starting with kapha's unique properties:

DENSE, AMPLE, COOL, OILY, STABLE, STICKY, THICK, SMOOTH, DULL

Now, once again, think of the qualities mentioned in relation to the elements and the qualities that they create. Try to build a picture in your mind how a body would look if these qualities were dominant. Go through the same categories once again and check if you agree with our offerings that appear in italics.

Archetypal Image—*benevolent rulers, kings and queens, bears, swans*

Build—*solid, full figured, curvy, busty, even proportions, heavy bones and thick muscles, gains weight easily especially around the hips*

Face—*large, round, or square*

Movement—*slower, flowing, unhurried, luxuriates, graceful like a swan*

Speech—*soft, quiet, ponderous, deep, speaks only when spoken to*

Hands—*strong, square, fleshy, clammy*

Feet—*strong and heavy*

Nails—*strong, square*

Skin—*thick, rich, full, cool, prone to congestion*

General Features—*round, square and full*

Hair—*heavy, full of body*

Eyes—*moist and deep like pools, tranquil, heavy eyelashes*

Mouth—*full lips, thicker saliva, strong, white teeth*

Voice—*lower soft tone*

With a little practice you will be able to recognize these qualities and begin to get a feel for which one or two of the *doshas* seem to have the strongest influence.

Although our unique blend of *doshas*, our prakruti, does not change, lifestyle, circumstances, and age can affect our doshas. Thus over the course of life, depending on how attuned we are to our constitution and the needs of the time, they can either be in balance, meaning we look great and all is well, or they are out of balance, which causes all sorts of problems. Theoretically speaking, our doshas get out of balance when they are allowed to accumulate in our tissues. What "out of balance" almost always means is extra vata, pitta or kapha. This means then that whatever quality the balanced dosha gave to the body, for example dryness, when the doshas is unbalanced that quality is exaggerated becoming, in this case, extra dryness. Keeping with purely physical appearance let's think about now extra *vata*, *pitta* and *kapha* would change how we look.

Extra Vata

Build—*very thin and unable to gain weight, osteoporosis, spinal deformities, huge weight gain after shock or trauma, curvatures in the spine*

Face—*very small, thin or long*

Movement—*very fidgety, hyperactive, unable to sleep even when tired, very pain-sensitive so great difficulty staying comfortable, difficult to get into the room to start the treatment because so easily distracted, joints painful and stiff, cramps, tremors, giddiness and feeling weak or faint*

Speech—*cannot stop talking or extra slow, stuttering*

Skin—*icy cold and shivering, teeth chattering, slightest breeze stops relaxation, very dry*

Hands—*cannot get warm, very dry, numbness, stiffness*

Feet—*fallen arches, turned strongly in or out, numbness, stiffness*

Nails—*badly bitten, very ridged, cracked, painful hang nails*

General features—*disfiguring irregularities*

Hair—*bad split ends, very flaky scalp, very wiry*

Eyes—*very dry, sunken eyeballs, constant twitching, cannot focus for long, drooping eyelids, cataracts, pain in the eyes*

Mouth—*very uneven top and bottom lips, very dry cracked lips, badly receding gums, loose teeth, crooked teeth, dry mouth and yawning a lot, loss of taste*

Voice—*very high or hoarse*

Extra *Pitta*

Build—*very muscular, overly disciplined about weight and fitness*

Face—*very sharp and angular, hot, flushed, red, excessive perspiration*

Movement—*braced posture, overbearing posture*

Speech—*hurtfully accurate*

Hands—*burning, red, grasping*

Feet—*burning hot and itching, smelly*

Nails—*prone to infection or inflammations around the nail*

Skin—*hot or feverish, constant flare-up in rashes and persistent breakouts*

General Features—*very angular, strangely even*

Hair—*premature gray or bald*

Eyes—*red, inflamed conjunctivitis, infected, very light-sensitive, bothered by all oils and makeup*

Mouth—*fever blisters, bad breath, metallic or sour taste in the mouth, excessive thirst, inflammation in the mouth, sore throat*

Voice—*piercing or grating*

Extra *Kapha*

Build—*extra weight that only changes with exercise not diet alone, clients that have had breast reductions or weight reduction surgery*

Face—*full and puffy, very heavy bones*
Movement—*difficulty moving due to weight*
Speech—*silent, will not talk*
Hands—*very clammy*
Feet—*very thick especially around the heel, clammy*
Nails—*strong, square*
Skin—*badly or deeply congested*
General Features—*extra round and full, double chins*
Hair—*oily, heavy on the body and face*
Eyes—*puffy, sticky, watery, cloudy, heavy lids*
Mouth—*sticky mouth especially at the corners of the lips, sweet taste in mouth, mucus in the throat*
Voice—*low rumble*

While we are focusing on the physical body I want to give more particular attention to the skin. For aestheticians, this additional information is essential to help them with selecting particular and appropriate products. It is also key for massage therapists who have to select appropriate oils and body products. Just as *vata*, *pitta* and *kapha dosha* can be in balance or out of balance in the body the doshas can be in or out of balance in the skin. Here instead of separate lists we've given the in balance quality first and the out-of-balance qualities in italics.

Vata Skin Qualities

My skin is

- dry—especially when I travel, in winter or windy weather
- *very dry, I have cracked heels, flaky forehead, chapped lips, dandruff, dry eczema*
- fine—I can easily feel my bone structure
- *paper thin and my blood vessels are clearly visible*
- cold to touch
- *icy cold especially on my hands and feet and even with blankets I feel cold*
- tans deeply and easily—I love the sun
- *never burns and I feel I have no energy without the sunshine*
- enjoys oils and rich creams
- *dehydrated and needs moisturizers all over year round*
- finely lined especially around my eyes

- *wrinkled around my eyes and on my forehead, even in high school*
- drier and sometimes cracked on my lips and around my mouth
- *in need of chap stick on my lips all the time*
- looks lively and energetic
- *lifeless, tired and has poor tone*
- rarely has breakouts
- *rarely breaks into a rash with nervousness*
- Darker tones
- *Grey especially under the eyes or ashen when stressed*

Pitta Skin Qualities

- generally more sensitive
- *almost all soaps and cosmetics easily give me itchiness or rashes*
- medium thickness
- *very well defined by muscle and more angular bone structure, warts*
- warm and soft to the touch
- *hot, flushed, or sweaty*
- fairly easily burned and has a few freckles and moles
- *very easily burned, covered in freckles, has many multicolored moles or has uneven pigmentation*
- prefers light lotions or gels
- *intolerant of even talk about using oil, especially in the face*
- has a some high skin tones
- *has visible blood vessel especially on my nose and cheeks—rosacea*
- my gums bleed occasionally when I brush
- *lips are prone to bleeding and I get recurrent fever blisters*
- more golden in tone
- *yellowish, sallow, or flushed when stressed*
- occasionally inflamed or itchy from heat
- *prone to inflammation, rashes, reactive to insect bites*
- prone to acne or congestion in the "T" zone
- *troubled by acne or breakouts in the"T" zone*

Kapha Skin Qualities

- thicker—I feel full flesh when I touch my face
- *puffy and prone to fluid accumulation*

- cool and moist to touch
- *sticky and clammy to touch*
- slow to tan
- *content and comfortable in the shade with a breeze*
- easily congested by heavy or oily cosmetics
- *congested, has white- and blackheads*
- generally larger pored
- *especially large pored on my nose and chin*
- moist and full in the lips and around the mouth
- *sticky and accumulates mucus at the corners of my eyes and mouth*
- paler skin tones
- *very pale*
- full
- *edematous or swollen*
- rich
- *flabby, cellulite*
- prone to scarring
- *troubled with bumps, deep congestion or deep cysts*

In both the body and skin type sections we have chosen qualities that would apply to all races. We have avoided mentioning specific hair or eye colors for this reason. Some skin tones maybe more evident in particular ethnic groups. Redness shows more on a fair skin, for example, but the darkest black skin can have rashes. **Terms such as lighter, darker, paler, straighter should be viewed as comparative as measured against someone of the same ethnic background.**

Using Aroma as Your Guide for Skin Care— Scent Strip Test

In the spa industry, a significant element of any treatment is enjoyment and so it is essential that a client love the smell of the products. You can recommend a particular blend of oil, lotion, cleanser, mask, or whatever, and you can educate the client as to why you think it is the best choice for them, but they have the final say and considering that most products look the same from the standpoint of what is in the bottle, more than likely smell is going to be the clincher.

Most Ayurvedic companies have products that are designed to help balance the *doshas*, with smell being one of the chief components. At the same time, smell is more or less a culturally acquired sense and we have seen that even with the best Ayurvedic products, if people are not used to Indian or Tibetan types of smells, they cannot relate to them. But as we have said time and again, Ayurveda is about principles. And, as our sense of smell is also basic to our enjoyment, an herbal blend or essential oil from Europe or one's own heritage may be more Ayurvedically correct for a client than any other.

To help make the best choice with your client, we suggest using a scent strip. We use this test with our blends but it can be used with any single essential or herbal oil.

1. Put a drop of each of the product on a scent strip or tissue. Mark each scent strip so you can quickly and accurately identify the aroma.
2. Instruct your client to wave each scent strip under their nose without sniffing strongly.
3. Ask which aroma is their favorite. Often we find that one is not liked and a second "smelling" is needed to choose between the ones most preferred.

Interestingly, most often clients choose the aroma that is best suited to their skin type. Our sense of smell is very primordial and not easily fooled, unlike our sense of taste. If the client cannot decide, use the questionnaire and your skills of observation to help with the selection process. Both the questionnaire and the Scent Strip Test are useful, but keep in mind that the client's personal choice of an aroma that appeals to them is very important. A major part of any aromatherapy and using aromas as part of a treatment is enjoying the aroma.

Most often our skin type and body type are the same, but not always. For example, clients with *vata* body type may have *vata* skin qualities, but they may have *pitta* or even *kapha* problems at times, and so on. Working to understand the doshas is not a means to put your client in a *vata*, *pitta*, or *kapha* box, but a way to understand how their subtle energy is dancing today. Be open, be flexible, and enjoy the whole beautiful picture.

Your Inner Mandala—What Comes from Your Mind

Just as the energies of *vata*, *pitta*, and *kapha doshas* determine what we look like, they also influence how our minds work. When a *dosha* is in balance, we experience all the positive qualities that make life pleasant and enjoyable. When a *dosha* is out of balance we experience all kinds of mental suffering.

The perfection of *Vata* or the times at which *vata* is in balance is known in the Tibetan tradition as being in a space where we can experience our Unlimited Mind. The qualities of an Unlimited Mind are shown here in the left column. When *vata* becomes unbalanced, we will experience the mental/emotional problems in the right column.

Mentally energetic	Mentally exhausted
Enthusiastic	Undiscriminating
Open-minded	Indecisive or weak willed
Optimistic	Feels "the grass is always greener"
Pleasantly objective	Distracted
In tune and in touch	Overly sensitive
At peace and centered	Spaced out
Content	Flighty
Understanding	Fearful
Easy with oneself	Furtive, nervous
Creative, an original thinker	Scattered and eccentric
Multi-talented	Disorganized
Able to multi-track	Easily overwhelmed
Endlessly capable	Stupidly impulsive
Even tempered	Feels life is meaningless
Accommodating	Flustered
Flexible	Awkward or clumsy
Great mediator	Confuses issues
Artistic	Non-productive
Free spirited	Unaware
Embraces change	Jittery, no confidence
Inspirational	Confusing or distant
Magical	Inappropriate
Sensitive	Moody
Intuitive	Suspicious

The perfection of *Pitta* is when a person exhibits a Spontaneous Joy; they are passionate about life and their actions are precise and unencumbered. Even if they do not possess this entirely, the positive qualities you will observe when a person's *Pitta* is balanced are listed in the left column and the qualities of imbalance in the right column.

Well organized	Obsessive
Discriminating	Prejudiced

Compassionate	Cruelly critical
Nurturing	Dogmatic
Visionary	Blinkered, narrow
Natural leader	Dictator
Ethical	Tyrannical
Risk taker	Addicted to danger
Charismatic	Proud
Unconventional	Overly responsible
Passionate	Irritable
Warm	Intense, hot tempered
Enjoys their body	Overly intellectual
Sensual	Indulgent
Flamboyant	Theatrical
Clear communicator	Sharp tongued
Smart	Opinionated
Purposeful	Driven
Accomplishes a lot	Hindered by being perfectionist
Powerful	Dominating
Appearance-conscious	Fashion-obsessed
Appreciative of life	High level of assumption
Accepting	Very confrontational
Able to go with the flow	Frozen, stiff, tight
Joyful	Unable to take a joke

The perfection of *Kapha* is when a person exhibits what in Tibetan tradition is called a Rainbow Body; they are in touch with and act from a strong sense of their unlimited potentials. Even if they do not possess this entirely, the positive qualities you will observe when a person's *Kapha* is balanced are in the left column and those when out of balance in the right column again.

Enduring mental energy	Mental lethargy
Good concentration	Mentally dull
Stable	Inert
Grounded	Conservative
Generous	Neediness
Loyal	Clinging
Sincere	Cool liar or silent

Learns thoroughly	Learns slowly
Not easily swayed	Lacking in creativity
Compassionate	Insensitive
Independent	Lonely
Patient Inflexible	
Honest	Quietly sneaky
Responsible	Carries the weight of the world
Ease in dealing with money and possessions	Hording
Confident, secure	Resigned
Reliable Inert	
Prioritizes well	Stuck
Loves routine	Works only by the book
Home loving	Low in energy
Patient	Stubborn
Romantic	Dogmatic
Accepting	Hates challenge
Selfless	Self pitying
Moral	Humorless

Just as your skin type may or may not match your body type so your emotional or inner type may or may nor not be the same as your body type. For example, you can have a body that shows all the qualities of *pitta* but a mind that is more *vata* or *kapha* and so on. Our emotional state changes more quickly than our body type so as the *doshas* dance through us day and night their fluctuations influence our mood. But, as in accordance with Tibetan Ayurveda where it is emphasized that mind always proceeds body, if the mental-emotional patterns of one *dosha* becomes a dominant pattern, this will eventually influence and change our body's condition or *vikruti* to manifest imbalance in that direction. We have all probably felt these fluctuations. Remember the last time you felt great just because the sun came out, or how miserable you felt when you last had a head cold.

When is comes to attributes of the mind we do not say these are positive and those are negative. We say some ways of being are more balanced than others and seem to produce more positive outcomes and others the opposite. However it is interesting to notice just how much is in the mind of the beholder, or simply depends on time, place, sex, and situation. As an illustration I offer a quote from Barbara Streisand as this male/female contrast comes up a lot with my students and so may be interesting to you readers.

A man is commanding—a woman is demanding

A man is forceful—a woman is pushy

A man is uncompromising—a woman is a ball breaker

A man is a perfectionist—a woman is a pain in the ass

He is assertive—she's aggressive

He strategies—she manipulates

He shows leadership—she's controlling

He's committed—she's obsessed

He's persevering—she's relentless

He sticks to his guns—she is stubborn

If a man wants to get it right, he's looked up to and respected

If a woman wants to get it right, she's difficult and impossible

If he acts, produces and directs, he's multitalented

If she does the same thing she's called vain and egotistical

I don't agree with all of it and hopefully for all womankind these attitudes are changing. As the industry is so female dominant I hope we can all contribute to the change.

Your Worldly Mandala

If all these are feeling a bit too academic or heady for you, then you might get a better feel for what we are trying to put across by reading through these lists and checking how many "ah hahs" you get.

Here is a list of things you will hear or might observe with yourself or your client that would clue you in to there being more *Vata* energy at play:

- I love to travel anytime.
- I am easily bored by routine.
- I tend to "shop till I drop".
- I don't bounce back like I used to.
- I love new ideas quickly but get forgetful about details.
- I think, speak, and act more quickly than most.
- I never have problems with weight.
- I have difficulty about making any sort of decision.
- I have a sensitive body, my digestion is easily upset by food or emotion.
- I suffer in cold or changeable weather.
- I am easily overwhelmed or worried.
- I am energized by heat and sunshine.

- I do things quickly and like quick results.
- I am sensitive to atmosphere and subject to strong changes of mood.
- I have difficulty sleeping or waking rested especially when I travel or feel under stress.
- I often have bad hair days.
- I am creative but not always practical.
- Naturally I like to snack on crunchy things rather than settle for meals.
- My credit card is my best friend.
- I have big dreams but few plans.

Here is a list of things you will hear or might observe with yourself or your client that would let you know more *Pitta* is about:
- I enjoy challenges in all aspects of my life.
- I am not cheap but appreciate quality and value for money.
- I think, speak, move and look at others in a focused fashion.
- I am disciplined about my weight and many things in my life.
- I can be critical and I'm my own strongest critic.
- I much prefer to lead than follow.
- My body is resilient but heavy fatty, spicy foods and alcohol bother me.
- Hunger, inefficiency and lack of punctuality bother me.
- I consider myself intelligent, focused and direct.
- I love to plan—thriving on details, order and practicality.
- Heat and sun makes me feel irritable and fatigued.
- Anger is an emotion I am familiar with.
- I am competitive and like to work hard and play hard.
- I can function efficiently on little sleep.
- I love my computer and all types of clever gadgets.
- I hate to admit I perspire easily and my sweat smells strong .
- I am naturally athletic and love the ocean or getting out into nature.
- I have lots of sunglasses or one expensive pair.
- I appreciate efficiency, precision and knowledge.
- I am passionate by nature and need loving support.

Here is a list of things you will hear or might observe with yourself or your client that would let you know *Kapha dosha* is at work:
- I thrive on comfort and making a home.
- I enjoy doing things methodically, following instructions, or having a routine.

- Regular rest is essential for me to be alert, I am not a morning person.
- I am viewed as a calm, stabilizing influence.
- I have to take time to understand new ideas but my memory is excellent.
- Cold damp weather makes me feel lethargic and depressed.
- People trust me and find me a reliable friend.
- I tend to bear grudges and hold onto the past.
- I am a surprisingly good dancer and have great natural rhythm and grace.
- I have steady and enduring energy.
- I am a devoted supporter and life-long friend.
- I am not easily upset or influenced but hurts tend to go deep and linger.
- My body easily accumulates mucus, fat and water weight.
- My features are large, even and exotic.
- I enjoy sweet creamy treat foods.
- I have a kind and giving nature.
- I feel light and energized by eating less and less often.
- I have to exercise and diet to lose weight.
- I sleep easily and deeply, naps leave me groggy.
- I easily accumulate material goods and money.

Questionnaire for Your Clients

Vata—If the shoe fits, buy one in every color.
Pitta—Life shrinks or expands in proportion to one's courage.
Kapha—How beautiful it is to do nothing, and then rest.
PROVERBS

Besides your direct observation and questioning, you may also want to offer your client a simple questionnaire.

After many years of working in the spa and skin care industry, I have determinbed that such questionnaires need to be

1. Short enough that it would take a maximum of ten minutes to fill out
2. Only asking questions that are comfortable to answer in a spa setting i.e. not about the type or frequency of bowel movements and menses
3. Fun to answer and relevant to modern living.

Like all of the other assessment material, feel free to copy and/or format this material any way you wish to serve your clients.

Check the qualities in each list that best describes you, then total your answers. Before each statement think either I, I am or I have . . .

Vata Dosha	Pitta Dosha	Kapha Dosha
Slim, fine boned	Medium, athletic build	Heavy boned, curvy
Have lively darting eyes	Have intense, sparkly eyes	Have a calm soft gaze
Talk a lot	Ask a lot of precise questions	Say little but think deeply
Have a poor memory	Remember dates and figures	Great memory
Prone to worry and fear	Prone to angry outbursts	Prone to depression
Hate cold	Hate heat with humidity	Hate cloud and damp
Energized by sunshine	Thrive by being out in nature	Enjoy medium heat
Spend easily, love sales	Only buy top of the line items	Save money easily
Easily over-extend myself	Work hard and play hard	Enjoy rest and quiet
Often late	Always early or on time	Prefer regular time schedules
Carry hand lotion or Chap Stick	Wear sunglasses, glasses or contacts	Carry a large purse full of useful things and pictures
Am attracted to touch, feel and hold things	Aware of cleanliness, colors and design	Sensitive to aromas and comforts
Love to travel	Need to be in charge	Prefer to be left alone
Creative and sensitive	Intelligent and courageous	Strong willed and caring
Often forget to eat meals	Love gourmet foods	Comfort food eater
Dry, coarser hair	Silky, straight hair	Thick, heavy hair
Sleep poorly	Have colorful dreams	Sleep easily

continued

Vata Dosha	Pitta Dosha	Kapha Dosha
Like fine and soft fabrics	Like expensive jewelry	Like homey accessories
Behave like a humming-bird	Behave like a eagle	Behave like a swan
Shop for fun, especially shoes	Enjoy reading, movies, and outdoor sports	Have no problem relaxing at home
Total:	**Total:**	**Total:**
		Vata Dosha _____ Pitta Dosha _____ Kapha Dosha _____

Dominant Dosha Today: A Touch Technique

We have now given you tools to observe, questions to ask, and question-naires you can give your clients to come to general sense as to what your client's constitution is.

More than likely, because of the fact that most people have a dual-*dosha* dominance, you may find that the questionnaires and questioning leave you with two categories that are equal in number. And if, for example, they are a combination of *Vata* and *Pitta*, should you try to heat your client up with suitable products and treatments or cool them down in order to bring them to balance?

This brings us to the issue of **Vikruti** or condition right now just to-day. Age, circumstance, climate, season, and lifestyle can each influence what manifests balance and imbalance in our *doshas*. Thus, at one point, our *Vata-Pitta* client may be more *Vata* imbalanced and at other times more *Pitta* imbalanced. The questionnaires will be of help somewhat. But here is an excellent and very simple test you can do with your client to decide how you are going to approach them *today* using a simple touch technique from the Tibetan tradition.

Diagnostic Points

There are three diagnostic points on the back that are useful for all treatments or protocols where knowing which dosha (Tib. *nyepa*) is dominant will determine what product and/or type of *touch* will be employed.

These three points are located on the spinous processes of the 7th cervical and 1st and 2nd thoracic vertebrae. These spinous processes represent:

C7—Vata (Tib. Lung)
T1—Pitta (Tib. TrIPA)
T2—Kapha (Tib. Bekan)

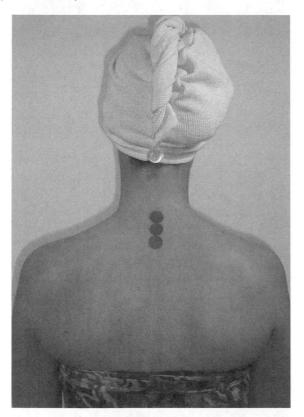

PALPATION:

To locate these points on the back of your client, start with trying to locate the spinous process of the 7th cervical vertebra. This is *usually* the first noticeably big bump on the center of the spine at the base of the neck. However, because of injury and how we have grown accustomed to sitting, this large bump can also be the spinous process of the 1st thoracic vertebra.

To eliminate doubt, have your client bend their neck forward and trace with your fingers along the cervical vertebrae from the base of the skull until you reach a spinous process that feels more prominent.

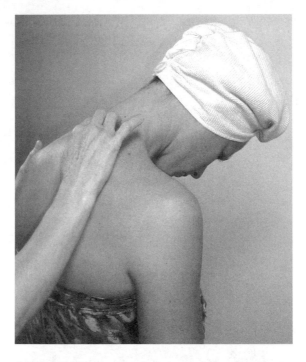

Place your middle finger on this bump—the actual spinous process—
and instruct the client to turn their head from side to side.

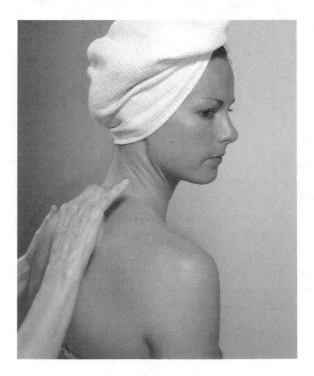

If the bone moves underneath one's finger, shifting slightly from side to side, then this is the 7th cervical vertebra spinous process. If the bone remains stationary, then this is the spinous process of the 1st thoracic. Thus, to palpate for the 7th cervical, you will have to move one spinous process up the neck. This spinous process will still be relatively larger than the ones above it.

Once you have determined the 7th cervical vertebra spinous process, the two below this one will be the 1st, then 2nd thoracic spinous processes.

TESTING THE POINTS:

You will use either your thumb or a three-pronged Tibetan method where you bring the tips of your index and ring fingers together and allow the tip of the middle finger to rest over the other two. The pressure to use for diagnostic purposes is relatively firm.

Begin with the 7th cervical spinous process. Rub it in a clockwise direction for about five (5) seconds. Ask the person to notice how the point feels. Then proceed to the next two points and follow the same procedure.

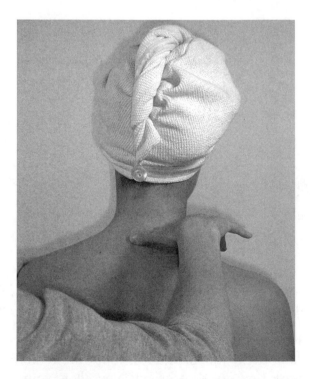

Have the person report to you which of the three points feels most tender. More than likely one the points will be. Usually this is in keeping with the client's constitutional mix of doshas. If they are *Vata*, then the 7th cervical vertebra will probably be sensitive. If they are a two-*dosha* constitution (which most people are), this will let you know which dosha needs to be addressed for today's treatment. **If *none* of these points feel tender *or* they *all* feel the same, then treat for *Vata* and use the *Vata*-pacifying products and style of touch for the given protocol to be performed.**

WHAT IF TWO OF THE POINTS FEEL SENSITIVE?
With some clients, you may find that they report that two of the points feel equally sensitive. If this I the case, you need perform one further test.

Have your client get on the table on their back with their knees drawn up. You will then be palpating three points on their abdomen. A point approximately three-quarters of an inch below the xyphoid process of the sternum is the *kapha* point. The *vata* point is just above the navel. Equidistant between these two spots is the *pitta* point.

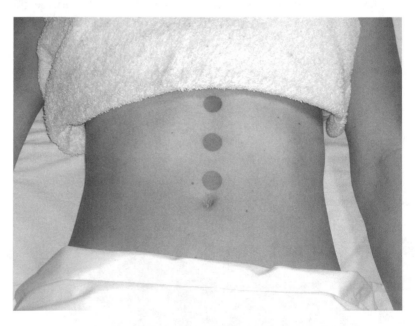

You will *only* palpate the two points that represent the two dosha points that you found sensitive on the spine. So if, for example, there was sensitivity on C7 and T1, you will only focus your attention on the point just above the navel (*vata*) and the one above that (*pitta*).

Ask your client to breathe in and rest your thumb on the appropriate point. As you ask them to breathe out, you allow your thumb to sink down on to the point with some pressure. Do the same thing for the other appropriate point. Whichever they report as being most sensitive is the *dosha* that needs to be balanced for today.

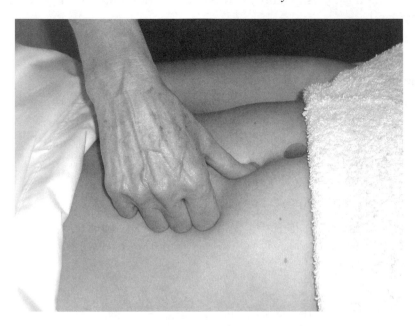

What Unbalances Our Elemental Mandala?

As we keep journeying to discover just which *dosha* is dominant in our body-mind system and we keep checking qualities of balance and imbalance it becomes obvious that balance is the preferable way to be. Why isn't that so for us all the time then? The short answer is that if you were perfect you wouldn't be here; you would be in a heavenly realm focusing on something else. Planet Earth is for Life 101 and Ayurveda is the Cliff notes. We are all here to learn and to try to bring ourselves and our planet into balance. So what sorts of things keep throwing us off course? We invite you to look at these lists and identify for yourselves what grabs you, where you get stuck, or what throws you off. Such lists can also be offered to clients, giving them their own "ah hah" or "that's why I've been feeling so lousy lately" revelations.

My *VATA* is thrown out of balance when

My BODY is

- not getting enough rest
- not getting enough supportive loving touch
- skipping meals or not eating well—especially leftovers and deli items

- forgetting to drink plenty of fresh water
- drinking iced drinks and sodas
- traveling a lot—especially air travel and when change of time zone is involved
- running around too much doing long commutes
- exercising excessively
- feeling extra dry to the touch—flaky or rough skin
- living in places that have dry or very changeable climates
- sitting in cold draughty places or in air conditioning
- working where there is a lot of electrical smog or continuous or especially loud noise
- making a lot of long distance phone calls
- having my period or giving birth
- experiencing gassy indigestion whatever I eat
- in intense pain

My MIND is sensing I am
- worried or fearful
- having to make numbers of decisions
- hurried and don't have time for myself
- having to respond to a great variety of demands
- going through changes—even positive ones
- feeling unsupported
- needing deeper relationships

My SPIRIT is moving me to believe
- my deepest beliefs and values are being questioned
- I am no longer sure who I am
- I don't feel I have the space to express myself
- I am out of touch with my body and inner being

My *PITTA* is thrown out of balance when
My BODY is
- working too intensely
- eating foods that give me heartburn—especially oily or spicy foods late at night
- getting very hungry
- not drinking enough pure water

- living on coffee and/or cigarettes
- drinking too much alcohol—especially spirits
- in front of my computer screen too many hours a day
- never away from my mobile phone
- being competitive even in my leisure time
- getting very hot when I exercise and not cooling down
- feeling my skin is extra oily or sensitive
- living in hot and/or humid climates
- sitting in the sun or working in intense heat
- breathing any type of fumes such as those from cars exhaust and cleaning agents
- not getting outdoors enough
- feeling my hormones are in turmoil

My mind is sensing I am
- oppressed by deadlines
- needing things to be more perfect than they can be
- unreasonably jealous
- not loved or appreciated
- being overly sexual
- easily moved to anger

My spirit is moving me to believe
- I have become dogmatic and intolerant
- I have lost my passion
- my heart is not singing
- I feel disillusioned

My *KAPHA* is thrown out of balance when

My BODY is
- not getting enough exercise and feeling sluggish
- sleeping or sitting home too much
- comfort eating—especially heavy or sweet foods
- gaining weight
- eating late at night
- drinking a lot of beer
- feeling my skin is extra sticky or congested
- living in a cold damp climate

My MIND is sensing I am
- depressed
- unable to let go of negative feelings
- loving and not being loved
- not feeling sensual-not loving my body
- living in the past
- apathetic
- stuck in a mundane routine
- my loyalty is being abused

My SPIRIT is moving me to believe
- I am not acting on my intuition
- I feel alone in my devotion
- I am distant from the light
- I am not living up to my potential
- I am unimportant

My last offering in this assessment section isn't about assessing ourselves or our clients. It is a game you can play in a staff meeting that might help staff get a real grasp of the feel of vata, pitta and kapha qualities while have some fun, as well. I stumbled across this approach when one sweet student, after three days of class, came up to me and said, "I think I finally get this vata, pitta, kapha thing. If kapha were a horse would it be a Clydesdale?" "Yes," I said, "so what would be a pitta style horse?" "A racer or show jumper," came the reply. "And a vata horse maybe an Arab?" She had done it after three days of confusion. In her own way she had made the knowledge her own. So let's try a few more. By the way, we are not saying all race horses are only pitta. What we are trying to get at is that the race horse style has a lot of pitta qualities. So give it a try. Whatever the category, think to your self what style would embody qualities of each dosha.

You can choose anything so long as you have some idea of the options and their qualities. I have tried to choose things here that would be understood internationally but you could try movie characters, TV shows, politicians or styles of yoga.

It is interesting when you observe people's choices to know that a traditional ayurvedic slogan says "Like increases like". So all the vata choices above will bring more vata energy around you. The same applies for pitta and kapha. We do shape our world and our choices with what vibrantionally makes sense to us so in that way even these choices can guide us to better understand our dosha balance.

Category	Vata	Pitta	Kapha
Dessert	Meringue, sorbet	Selection of fresh fruits and raspberry sauce, Death by Chocolate Cake	Ice cream sundae, fudge brownie and whipped cream
Bedding	Silk sheets and multiple pillows	Crisp cotton duvet cover and buckwheat hull pillows	Family quilt and mothers feather pillows
Seating	Wicker porch swing	Leather love seat	Overstuffed sofa
Vacation	Quick weekend get-away	Educational or romantic cruise	Return to family cottage or favorite spot
Dog	Terrier, whippet	Chocolate Labrador, German Shepherd	Great Dane, Saint Bernard
Vegetable	Lettuce, endive	Peas, peppers	Pumpkin, cucumber
Flowers	Babies breath	Rose	Lily
Political Party	Green party	Democrats	Republicans
Choices At A Sport Club	Spin bikes and steam room	Weights and sauna	Walking track and shower
Outside Sport	Rock climbing, running, X bikes	Surfing, snowboarding, the "no fear" sports	Walks with the Sierra Club
Jewelry Choices	Quartz crystals or amethyst droplets on a delicate chain	String of pearls or a single precious stone in custom setting	String of larger amber or turquoise
Trees	Japanese maple	Pine	Oak
Cheese	Parmesan	Gouda	Ripe brie
Sandwich	Crisp bread or crackers and low fat cream cheese	Tuna melt	Fried peanut butter and jelly
Cups	Porcelain tea cup	Stainless steel coffee cup	Pottery mug

Additional Food For Thought

We decided to offer the following brief descriptions of *vata*, *pitta*, and *kapha* clients, co-workers, and bosses so you can see the doshas dancing all around you in not only your clients but in those you work with and work for, as well. Some of the following material comes from an article that Melanie wrote in January of 2001 for Les Nouvelles Esthetique. We hope it will help you flesh out the *vata*, *pitta*, *kapha* mandala we have tried to paint for you so it shines beautifully and clearly for you every day at work.

The *Vata* Client

The perfection of *vata* energy is an unlimited mind. The *vata* client is very open-minded, excited, and interested in any new services. They are the 'touchy-feely' types, lovers of sensual pleasures and always up for new experiences. They know that to run at the speed they love to live at requires down time to refuel on all levels. They are very appreciative clients who visibly enjoy every second of being pampered. They spend freely and love a sale.

The *Vata* Co-worker

Working with someone with strong *vata* dominance can be inspiring. *Vata* gives one a zest and bubbling enthusiasm for life, knowledge, and new experiences. It is the *vata* that fuels the creative and artistic side of our nature. It also makes them sensitive and responsive. Giving that extra bit of care or attention to their client can sometimes throw off the time schedule, but is usually well appreciated by whoever the client was they were so intent upon serving.

The *Vata* Boss

Energetic, enthusiastic, and innovative are the key gifts of a boss with more *vata* energy. This boss is an independent, original thinker who is not afraid of change and is always ready to embrace new trends. Looking deeper, you will find a highly attuned individual that is charged by a sense of higher purpose.

The *Pitta* Client

The perfection of *pitta* is spontaneous joy. This is deep joy that is released when we feel in harmony with the worlds around us, when we sense a steady hum of things feeling right. The *pitta* client is very punctual, is precise, and always follows instructions. They want results and have a genuine interest in both your products and your services. They especially love refreshing wet treatments and the intensity of both hot and cold applications. If you demonstrate a professionalism and precision with what you do and offer them, you will see this client's heart open up and shine. Looks are very important to these clients and they always buy 'top of the line.'

The *Pitta* Co-worker

This co-worker has a passion to keep learning and the thirst for responsibility. They are the practical 'just do it' types. Punctuality and precision work is their forte. *Pitta* nature affords them a strong appreciation for visible surroundings and light and as a result they have a great sense of color and design and love to create elegant surroundings or displays. They take pride in being clean and well organized.

The *Pitta* Boss

Pitta is a fiery quality. Just as we are always drawn to look at a cozy fireplace or a glowing candle, *pitta* people are naturally looked to for leadership. Hence, they are very comfortable in leading. Although very practical and have an allegiance to the 'bottom line,' they are often visionary and like the challenge of a gamble. The *pitta* boss sets high standards for himself or herself as well as for others and are very goal oriented. Often highly educated themselves, they also realize the value of education and new levels of training for their staff. Underneath that strong self-assured persona beats a tender heart of gold.

The *Kapha* Client

The perfection of *kapha* is called rainbow body. This is a resourceful person who is gentle and at peace with themselves. Quiet, loyal, and regular as the tides, *kapha* clients keep coming back. Being natural givers they also appreciate being given to. They like to be lulled by routine, but even more than that appreciate stimulation of the new or unexpected. *Kapha* clients are charmed by small or little extra luxuries and are generous tippers and gift certificate buyers.

The *Kapha* Co-worker

This co-worker's quiet, kind, and consistent temperament makes them the obvious shoulder to cry on or the person to confide in. Abundant in every way, the *kapha* co-worker is naturally giving, thoroughly reliable, resilient, and totally trustworthy. Their patience allows them to handle with ease even the most difficult of clients.

The *Kapha* Boss

The *kapha* boss will have a business built on tradition and solid business practices. It will often be a venture that has started small and grown slowly, but steadily. *Kapha* bosses are interested in long-term relationships with staff, suppliers, and customers. Loyalty is very important to them. If you stick around and demonstrate your loyalty in return, you will find that the *kapha* boss is more than willing to consider your new ideas. They are truly generous and very understanding. We all can learn a lot from this unfashionably cautious and deep-thinking type.

Accentuate the Positive

When it comes to hearing about or looking at ourselves for some strange reason most of us are conditioned to hear the worst. Our perfections and what is possible to bring out as our inner, outer, and secret beauty—the true goal of Ayurveda—often get over-shadowed. Most Ayurvedic literature, because it has been written for those pursuing medicine and healing, emphasize the maladies that result from an imbalance of the *doshas*. However, here we would like to focus on the positive and beautiful qualities each of the *doshas* offer us. For it is our firm conviction that if we accentuate the positive and look for the beauty in each of us, then not only do these qualities shine through, but we are affirming their balance—which can go a long way toward promoting a healthy, radiant being. Of course, we recognize fully that in order to do a proper assessment, to offer treatments that truly benefit each client, one has to investigate imbalances. But in a space of valuing what each of the *doshas* offers us and in a space of non-judgment and love, we shall be able to more effectively assess and uplift our client through what we say and offer to them.

With this in mind, we ask each and every reader to look at themselves, their clients, their co-workers, and their bosses in a new and positive light. Appreciating the gifts each *dosha* brings the people we live and work with and work on everyday and approaching ourselves, those who we work with, and those who we work on with a more positive perspective will inevitably bring greater clarity and balance to our being, our relationships, our work. Everyone benefits.

The "Diamond Way" of Ayurveda is to hold to the truth that we are the rainbow body, that we possess an unlimited mind, and that our true expression is spontaneous joy. If we look for these qualities in everyone around us, then we no longer focus on the clouds, we bask in the glorious sunshine of all that all that is created.

"But for Whom?"

Once we know which of our *doshas* seems to be the most dominant or out of balance and we have some idea of what may be causing the problem, then we have to choose to do something about it—or not. All Ayurvedic body work and especially work with marmas seems to help open the mind to new possibilities, new ways of doing or seeing things. But just as we are not in the business to diagnose in a spa setting, we also cannot insist that our clients change. We can suggest, we can educate, we can offer anecdotal stories and that is our limit.

That being said, here are some of our suggestions that we leave up to you to apply to your own life or offer to your clients as you see fit. Like all Level One lifestyle suggestions, they look simple but we feel that they get to the heart of the matter. And suggesting them will not make you sound too threatening or medical.

It is easy for me to get frustrated with the seemingly foolish choices clients make so before I ever give advice I always try and remind myself that we are all trying to do our best with what we've learned thus far in life. If we were all perfectly balanced at birth or knew how to live to keep our life in balance we would be born as fully realized beings. We are all born as ordinary beings each with our own unique imbalances. Life is a journey of working toward balance. Ayurveda is an excellent guide. May we all become older and more balanced.

To Help Balance *Vata Dosha*

Everyone's *vata* increases when it is cold or windy, in changeable weather, when traveling especially by air, at times of change (even positive change), with aging, after giving birth, or when under stress. Beyond the treatment and products that you are recommending for your client, encourage the following . . .

- get to bed at a regular time, before 10pm
- keep warm, especially your feet, lower back and ears; hats help
- eat fresh food regularly—three meals plus nourishing snacks
- give yourself or get a warm oil massage often, daily or weekly
- take quiet time for yourself
- drink warm drinks only, nothing with ice in it
- avoid caffeine, cigarettes, and liquor
- try and keep a routine going of nurturing activities

To Help Balance *Pitta Dosha*

Pitta dosha increases when the weather is hot and humid, when working under tight time schedules, when passion or anger is high, and when working with computers. Beyond services and products you offer, encourage your client to . . .

- try to go with the flow more
- rent funny movies and laugh more
- accept loving care
- keep cool physically and mentally
- eat plenty of greens and fresh fruits
- drink plenty of water
- spend time near lakes, rivers or the ocean
- avoid red meat, shellfish, alcohol—especially spirits, and drugs

To Help Balance *Kapha Dosha*

Kapha will accumulate when the weather is cool and damp, when we sleep a lot in the day, overeat, forget to exercise, or feel stuck. Beyond the services and products you offer, encourage your client to . . .

- find a type of exercise you enjoy
- take juice for breakfast, eat your main meal at midday, and have dinner before six
- get out, get involved
- brush your hair a lot and dry brush the body
- avoid heavy, sweet, cold foods

As time is often short at the end of a treatment it is useful to have these suggestions in written form. You might like to use an introductory statement such as the one below as a means of inviting clients to take a more active role in working toward personal balance and personal best.

I, _____, promise to focus my energy toward creating a happy, healthy and inspired life. From now on I shall take full responsibility for learning about the many needs of my body, mind and spirit, and how these needs can realistically be met. In addition, I promise to nurture myself with the people, places and things that bring me the most joy. In so doing, I acknowledge that I am developing a deeper knowing of myself so I can care for myself fully and with renewed strength, bringing care and knowledge to others.

—MELANIE SACHS

And add these words at the end as encouragement and a reminder to be patient with your progress. Remember to be gentle to yourself and others,

We are all children of chance,
And none can say why some fields blossom
and others lay brown
(Kent Nerburn, *Letters to my Son*)

CHAPTER 9

The Treatment Rituals

*A*nd now we come to the central focus of this book: spa treatments that relax, rejuvenate, and inspire. For those of you who are therapists and spa technicians, each spa treatment ritual that is offered has modular components. What this means is that while we present them in a certain sequence for what we consider a luxurious and deep spa experience, you will be able to take components out and use them with other treatments or by themselves—mix and match them if you will. In this respect, we shall provide you with suggestions and contra-indications. With each full protocol we offer a list of all of the products and equipment you will need to perform the ritual (descriptions of specific Ayurvedic items will be found in the Glossary towards the end of the book), marketing tips, and descriptions that you are free to use or modify in your spa menus. In the final section of the book, "Taking it Home," therapists and those of you who pick up this book for self-care and spa treatments at home will find modified self-treatments. These 'home' versions can be a nice touch that you share with clients before they leave. They can then take the spa experience home with them and get even deeper, more lasting results. For it is our experience that educating your client by giving them something they can take home and do has little impact on whether they return or not. On the contrary, by offering a little extra to your client in this way, you have entered into their home with them and every time they do the home ritual, they will be reminded of the spa and the experience they had there.

The first five treatment rituals we offer are a blend of both Tibetan and Indian Ayurvedic techniques. They have been modified to suit western home and spa environments. Following these we shall look at more medically-oriented Ayurvedic services that can be done on their own or used to enhance other treatments. What distinguishes these special treatments is that they are best done with or under medical supervision. At the same time, they can also be done in modified home versions with excellent results.

We would also like to make a point here that we feel compelled to for the benefit of our previous students. After years of teaching, we know that our methods have changed, some because of intuitions and insights, especially for bringing these treatments into the spa and beauty industries. And then there have been times when more personal idiosyncrasies have entered into our protocols without us going back to the original texts from the master who taught us. Please be assured that what you have been doing has never been a danger to your client. It's just that they could have been better. Thus, when you read along and follow the protocols, you will notice some changes that will make your work even more dynamic.

Liability: Who Can and Cannot Offer These Treatments?

Regrettably, in a litigation-crazed society, the question as to who can and cannot practice various treatments goes far beyond the matter of training and expertise. So, based on the current information we have, let us spell out what you need to take into consideration to do the different Ayurvedic treatment rituals outlines here.

First, let us look at the five major treatment rituals described.

- Ayurvedic Face Rejuvenation—This treatment ritual can be done by aestheticians, cosmetologists, massage therapists, and anyone who is licensed to therapeutically touch another person.
- Himalayan Mountain Abhyanga—As this is a full-body massage, only those who have a license to give massage should do this protocol. This excludes aestheticians and cosmetologists unless they have been cross-trained.
- Tibetan Shirodhara—Shirodhara is now an insured service according to the American Massage Therapy Association. And because of the fact that during the pouring of the oil in the shirodhara practice there is no contact, this practice is acceptable for aestheticians as well. There are some aspects of the treatment ritual that are more massage than is accepted by aesthetic or cosmetology licenses. Licenses vary from state to state; in some places aestheticians cannot touch below the shoulders or above the knees. Thus, these may need to be modified or eliminated, thus only doing the actual pouring of the oil from this treatment.

- Marmas and Mud Magic—Similar to Ayurvedic Face Rejuvenation. The reason is that even though the marma series covers the entire body, as oils are being applied to specific points, it can be defined as an aromatherapy treatment, which in some states, is covered under an aesthetician's license. However, where a state says that aestheticians can only do face, neck, and declote, we advise caution to aestheticians and cosmetologists. Obviously, again if they are cross-trained, then no problem.

- Tibetan Blissful Sleep—The issue that comes up here has to do with the reflexology portion of the treatment. Obviously for massage therapists and those who have a license to do massage, there is no problem here. Again, some states have reflexology as part of their training for aestheticians. If not, then the same considerations come up as for the Marmas and Mud Magic ritual.

- PediKarma™—Same considerations as for the Tibetan Blissful Sleep.

When it comes to the Special Treatments, other issues arise.

- Nadi Swedana—As facial steaming is acceptable for aestheticians, and most massage therapists are licensed for hydrotherapies, this treatment should not be a problem for anyone who is trained to perform it.

- Netra Basti, Nasya, and Karna Purana—The liability here has to do with the fact that each of these treatments works within an orifice of the body; netra basti in the eye socket, nasya in the nasal cavities, and karna purana in the ear canals. Even though we feel that each of these treatments is completely safe to administer once one is properly trained, the insurers for the spa and beauty industries cannot insure or approve of these services. Thus, we recommend that you do these under medical supervision or in a facility where there is a licensed medical practitioner available.

Beyond these considerations, however, we want to direct therapists to current California legislation, SB-577, the California Health Freedom Act. What this legislation spells out is that if you describe to your client what it is that you are going to do to them during a treatment session, and if they sign a waiver, then you are—more than likely—legally protected from prosecution. I say, "more than likely," only because there can always be accidents and the possibility that if you are not properly trained or are not competent to offer a treatment properly, you may harm the client in a way that has nothing to do with the treatment itself. An example of this is if you have someone sign a waiver for receiving netra basti, but don't cool the ghee down to the right temperature, hence burning their eyes.

The California Health Freedom Act is an important step for consumers and clinicians, especially as there is no standardization for what constitutes a licensed Ayurvedic practitioner and there are currently few states that license Ayurveda as a limited or alternative health care practice. However, with the monopolization of health care and a cry from the public for access to the health care providers they want, there is a national movement to allow clients to seek holistic and alternative health care practices without undo government interference. We encourage practitioners and clients to go to www.nationalhealthfreedom.org to see which states are creating state regulations similar to The California Health Freedom Act.

Preparing to Offer a Treatment Ritual

The reason we speak of treatment "rituals" is to honor the seriousness and sacredness with which Ayurveda views the offering of bodywork.

As mentioned in our overview of the four levels classified in Tibetan Ayurveda, massage, the touch of another for healing purposes, is considered a second-level practice. The moment you put your hands on another person to make some kind of change, you are entwined in a karmic dance. And, as they have come to you, you are the one who takes the lead. Consequently, you should feel centered, relaxed, and intently focused on offering your client a service that will benefit them in the short or long term. As you do this work day in and day out, you may view what you do as protocols, routines, or treatment processes. What we would like to suggest is that if you recognize the sacredness of the charge you take when working with another, the word "ritual" will elevate what you do and create a focus and rhythm from which both of you will benefit.

Towards this end, we would like to offer some guidelines and advice in preparation for bringing your client into your treatment space and some useful points to pay attention to throughout.

1. First, focus on yourself with respect to appearance and influences on your body energetics. See the section on ergonomics. Beyond what is suggested, have your **hair tied back** if it is long. Ayurvedic treatments tend to be very oily and product intensive. If you have to constantly get your hair out of the way, you will end up looking like a greasy mess by the end of the treatment. The same applies for clothing. Flowing fabrics will get ruined within a relatively short period of time. **Have toweling or aprons around** so you can drape those areas that risk being covered in oil.

It is also good to **remove as much unnecessary jewelry as possible**. Quartz watches should generally be removed, but this goes doubly for Vata body-mind types as their body energetics are more affected by the electromagnetics of such devices. Most jewelry made of precious or semi-precious metals and stones can be beneficial. But if they are bulky around the hands and wrists, their jangling and surfaces may interfere with strokes and thus irritate your client. Especially when you do any treatment that uses vital energy points (marmas), acupuncture points, or subtle energy lines, following this step is essential for good results.

2. **Have your space prepared for welcoming your client.** Pay attention to the guidelines we mentioned earlier with respect to customizing your space for their body-mind type. At the same time, each treatment has its specific products and equipment. Have it all handy and easy to get to so as to not interfere with the flow of the treatment ritual. **Refer to the lists we provide with each of the rituals offered here.** At the same time, do the same for each and every treatment you do. If you work in a spa and switch from room to room, this may take some time. A simple thing that is often overlooked but can cause discomfort for you later on is to **see whether the table height is right for you**. Be sure that it works for you ergonomically; that is easy for you to work over. More about ergonomics will follow later. **If you have a heating pad on your bed or table, turn it off before your client gets onto it.** This has to do with EMF (electro-magnetic frequencies) which can interfere with the treatment and actually leave your client feeling more tired or agitated by the end of the treatment. Having your space organized and free of clutter actually eliminates a lot of mental distraction that can interfere with your rhythm and the client's experience. Some of these details will happen somewhat at the last moment, once you have done your Client Assessments and palpations to determine which oils you are going to use, what music you are going to select, etc.

3. Regardless of whether your client is new or a regular, spend a short time **explaining what it is that you will be doing with them** for the time they are with you. This will go a long way toward calming the client, setting the mood, and eliminating unnecessary questions about the treatment as it unfolds.

4. **Take a few moments for quiet.** Close your eyes, place your open hands over your belly just below your navel. This is the area of the chakra *svadhisthana*, the great ocean, or what in Japanese is called *hara* and in Chinese *tan tien*.

Let your tongue rest behind your top front teeth and breathe through your nose, both the inhalation and exhalation (**try to observe this throughout the treatment**). As you breathe in, feel the breath travel down your body to the area that you are holding below your navel. As you breathe out, feel the energy of the exhalation move up through your body into your arms and down into the palms of your hands. Feel the warmth in the palms of your hands and allow this warmth to move into your belly. Do this for three, five, or seven repetitions. While you are breathing you may say to yourself some positive affirmation, a focusing thought to bring attention to your client for their benefit, or a prayer. In other words, prepare yourself for making a deeper connection with the person you are about to transform through your touch.

You are now ready to approach and touch your client to begin the treatment ritual.

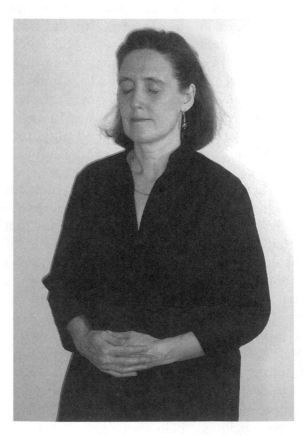

5. As you approach your client, step slowly and mindfully into proximity with them. The average human aura extends out about one hand

span from the surface of our body. So when you get within this range, the person is already feeling your presence and their tissues are beginning a dialogue with you. This accounts for why you can even do some strokes within the aura and create noticeable physical effects.

6. **Squeeze, pour, or dab whatever product you are going to use on your client into your own hands first.** Do not pour anything directly onto your client. In this way you are warming and charging the product with life through your hands. A nice technique on the limbs and back if you are using oil in a squeezable bottle is to squeeze the oil into your palm and kind of squeegee it onto the limb or back as it flows down off of your palm. See the photos on the Himalayan Mountain Abhyanga.

7. **Try to keep both hands on your client when performing any stroke or hold.** One hand may be just resting while the other hand is doing the work. That is fine, so long as both hands make contact with the client. This has to do with the energetic polarity of our bodies. If you have one hand on your client and the other somewhere else, your touch will feel unbalanced. (Unconsciously, they'll wonder where your other hand is.)

8. In general, Ayurvedic techniques use massage strokes that are universal to almost all systems of massage throughout the world; forms of friction, kneading, pressure, and tapotment. Types of touch for the various body-mind constitutions and conditions has been discussed previously. Here what we want to emphasize is that when doing kneading strokes or applying pressure, try to perform this action using **clockwise, circular motions**. This motion helps to nourish Vata, calm Pitta, and is enjoyable for Kapha. Counterclockwise motions can be used to provide more stimulation, but in general have more of an agitating quality. In this regard, our teacher Dr. Rapgay suggests that the therapist develop their intuition to better understand the needs of their client. This is more important than getting too parochial about this matter. Thus, while I shall mention clockwise throughout the texts with respect to general massage strokes, use your sense of feel to guide you.

When it comes to acupressure and marma points, however, the preferred form of point stimulation is with pressure combined with a clockwise circular motion. Here, Tibetan Ayurveda emphasizes two different methods, both of which can be used interchangeably, depending upon the ease of offering the stroke to a given portion of the body; one using thumb pressure and the other, a three finger "prong" approach where the index and fourth finger are connected at the tips with the middle finger lying on top of them. This "prong" posture is especially useful on bony processes (such as on the spinous processes that are touched in many of the Tibetan marma point series). In both cases, the contact need not be vigorous to be effective. We have found that the emphasis should be on "making contact". If the points are in deep or fleshy areas, you may lean into them, but stop where you meet resistance.

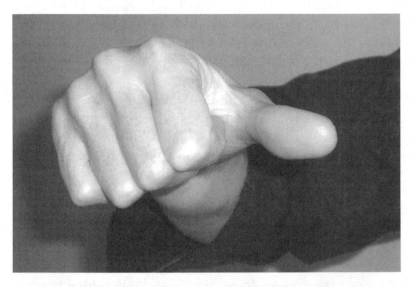

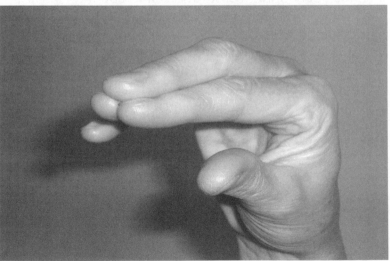

Another point to keep in mind comes from our work with right-left brain exercises.

Try to avoid bi-lateral, symmetrical stimulation on points or areas.

Note that there are many times in many massage techniques when you use your hands on both sides of the body on the same points or areas at the same time. In some systems, like oriental styles of shiatsu as well as when one is trying to mechanically effect a specific area, such as when chucking a particular muscle or muscle group or doing deep abdominal work. This point is even taken to an extreme in two-person abhyanga, where practitioners will do identical strokes on both sides of the body at once. In this latter case, Dr. John Douillard, says that this is to overload the brain and thus coax the body into letting go to a more profound level.

Sometimes the body does need bilateral stimulation to a region or area to create a mechanical effect. And there are times when overwhelming your client to allow them to 'let go' is also warranted. Thus, we do not discourage you from either of these approaches outright, provided you know that overwhelming is what you are doing.

But here, because we are focusing on making each treatment ritual an experience where the body is relaxed and refreshed and the mind is open, clear, and radiantly alert, we encourage you to use alternating hand techniques as often as possible. For example, you will notice that in all protocols where marmas are touched, they are done on the right, then on the left. If they are being touched simultaneously, the stroking is done in a clockwise fashion on both sides, which means that the strokes are going in opposite directions as clockwise on the right side of the body looks and is performed differently than on the left side. The only times this rule is not followed is when points are just being held, as in a polarity style of holding.

Such a mindfulness will take some getting use to. However, what you will notice is that you will tire less and your client will not be so 'out of it' at the end of the session. For we contend that much of this 'out of it' sensation has to do with system overload as a result of doing things on both sides of the body that activate the right and left side of the brain and nervous system.

9. **When you complete working on an area or point, breathe in as you come away from the point or area.** What this does is leave your energetic impression on the client as you move to another area. In general, breathe in as you move away from or lift your hands off of an area and when you go to touch and begin your stroke, breathe out.

Meridian Energy Flows Front and Back

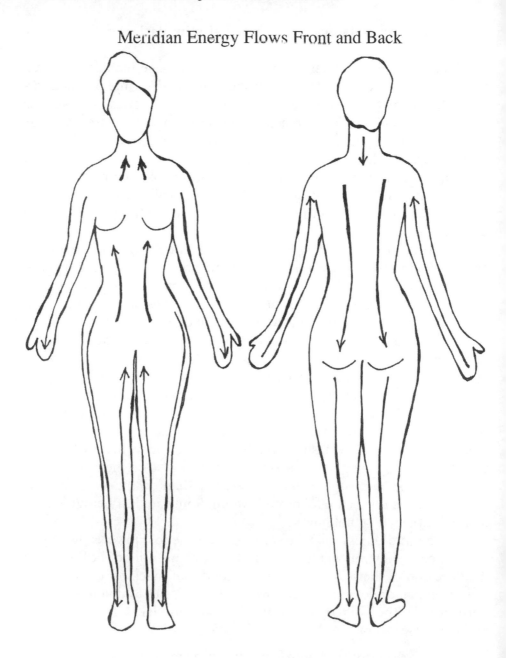

10. A traditional form of acupuncture meridian stroking is done as part
of most of the treatment rituals offered here. Although this is not
classically Ayurvedic per se, it is a simplified means of addressing
what some call the "flows" in the body. Basically, the meridians that
charge our organs and the elements of which they are a part move up

the front of the body and down the sides and back of the body. By finishing the work on an area with stroking in the direction these meridians flow, you are moving from the mechanical to the energetic and thus, helping to calm and rebalance the area. The diagram below shows how to stroke every area in the body. This alone can be quite powerful, especially in the case of the very young, the elderly, and the convalescing. In the context of the Treatment Rituals, the stroking is done on the area you are focusing on as "finishing" strokes.

11. When you are finished with one part or area of the body and are moving to another area, **move around the table in a clockwise direction**. At an energetic level, what you are doing is placing your client in the center of a vortex that is calming, as the clockwise direction has a more calming influence. At the level of ritual, it is like viewing the body as a sacred temple. In the east, devotees will often circumambulate clockwise around temples, stupas, and other holy sites. So we create a greater level of reverence in the entire process by moving in this way.

Keeping the Client at a Comfortable Temperature

Keeping the Client Warm Enough

Many clients find it very difficult to relax unless they are really cozy. Of course the room should be a pleasant temperature, but sometimes a little extra warmth is needed. We feel that all electric powered pads or pillows interfere with the body's subtle energy and create a certain level of tension. They can be useful to warm the bed or blankets initially but should be turned off and unplugged during the treatment.

Usually the quickest way we have found to get someone warm is to get warmth to their belly, around the navel. This area, the region of the large intestine, is called the seat of Vata. Clients that are especially more Vata in their body-mind type or in their condition (vikruti) tend to feel colder than most others. But others may experience this as well. To remedy this situation, we use a special tummy warmer we designed that is a small organic cotton bag filled with white rice, rock salt and fennel seeds. It can be heated in the microwave for 4–5 minutes or more gradually warmed in a hot towel cabinet. The rice keeps pleasantly warm for a full hour. The salt helps the pillow to hold heat and the fennel benefits digestion. The pillow is usually used on the lower abdomen, resting just below the navel and the just above the pubic bone. This not only warms the client but helps them feel more relaxed and secure. The pillow can also be used under the ankles to warm the feet or under the neck to provide support and ease tension.

The tummy warmer or any other form of hot pad should not be used directly on the head, over the eyes, on the heart area, or genitals. Heat on the belly is not advised if the client has a digestive upset as it tends to cause diarrhea, during a menstrual period as it can increase the flow dramatically (though it is great for cramps), if ovarian cysts are suspected, or unusual abdominal pain is being experienced. You may also notice that those who are more Pitta will want a towel or padding between them and the tummy warmer or may even ask to have it taken off sooner than most. Trust your client. Their comfort is what matters.

Try to use natural fibers on the massage table. Oil comes out of them more easily and they do not interfere with natural energy flows. Providing a choice of extra covers is a special way to customize treatments. You might offer down comforters, far-infrared comforters (which keep the body warm if the person gets cold and cool if the person gets hot), cotton woven or knitted blankets, heavy wool blankets, or lighter mohair throws. Heat lamps are also useful, but be careful where they are shining as they are hot enough to scorch surfaces and skin if you are not careful.

Always remember it is the client that must feel comfortable. Lying down drops everyone blood pressure so we all feel cooler when we are horizontal for a period of time.

Keeping the Client Cool Enough

Yes, it is possible to get uncomfortably warm in some heat treatments or even in stuffy treatment rooms. During any heat treatment you should keep the client's head, middle chest and a man's genitals cool. A cool damp towel is usually enough. This protects the brain, heart and reproductive tissues from getting too hot and causing harm. Also have a cool drink on hand that is in a container easy for the client to drink from without moving much.

During regular treatments a spritz to the face, wrists, and ankles is very refreshing. Use bottled spring water as tap water can smell of chemicals and be harsh on the skin. You may even choose rose or other herbal waters. Cool fennel seed tea is pleasant in a spray and even soothes heat rash. White sage, melissa or lemon verbena teas are also wonderfully refreshing.

Heat tends to gather around our eyes, one of the sites of Pitta. When we get tired or stressed, extra cooling here is an excellent way to help someone to "cool out". We have noticed this to be especially true for those in the tech industries who work around a lot of computer terminals, and classic Pitta-style type-A personalities. There are many kinds of cool packs for the eyes. We use an organic cotton eye pillow that is filled with flax and psyllium seed. We use cotton because it is naturally cooling. We find silk eye pillows are great for texture but can be heating, something you don't want to do with the eyes. The psyllium also keeps the eye pillow light. We find many eye pillows to be too heavy and make the eyes bleary for a time after they are removed. We don't use herbs in the pillows. Lavender is often used because the aroma is so relaxing but we find that for long term use in the spa the herb breaks down and goes powdery and can become irritating to the eyes.

Of course damp gauze pads do a great job. Use rose water for a richer experience. Slices of cucumber or cool wet tea bags are soothing and also help relieve puffiness. My all-time favorite for cooling the eyes has to be fresh rose petals that have been dipped in milk. They are unbeatable for smell and texture and also, by the way, do an amazing job of gently removing eye makeup.

If more air and breeze is needed, a small fan to move the air is a must if you have no access to a window or means of regulating your room's temperature. The quieter the room is, the better. A small ozone generator helps to clear the air in between treatments. A number of air purifiers on the market now double for these two.

Mudras for Your Client

A mudra (pronounced moo-drah) is an energetic seal whereby energy in the body is channeled back into the body to create a certain effect. Mudras are done in meditation and yoga to bring control to the body and awaken the heart and mind to a particular focus in awareness. Thus there are mudras for cultivating compassion, wisdom, peace, and so on.

Generally speaking, when we offer Ayurvedic or any other treatments, that relies on the flow of subtle energy, we encourage clients to not cross their legs or clasp or hold their hands in any manner. In that way, you as the therapist can make an energetic impact on the client and get the energy moving the way you want it to. However, there are times when people are in a state of uncertainty or anxiety and need some additional help beyond soothing words or your touch. This is where two mudras can be quite useful. They come from a Tibetan bodywork tradition called Rang Drol. We thank Eva Boss of Germany for sharing these with us.

The first mudra we offer is to help your client with anxiety and feeling antsy on the table. Its effect is to help someone feel settled, comfortable, and at home no matter where they are. Consequently, it is even useful when they are at home, in stressful circumstances, etc.

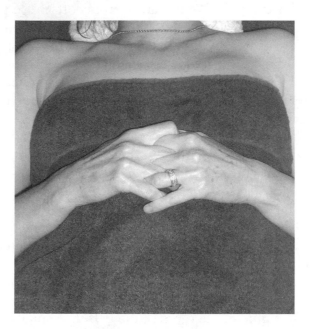

The second mudra is designed to facilitate a sense of joy for the client. It opens them up and helps the energy in the body flow smoothly.

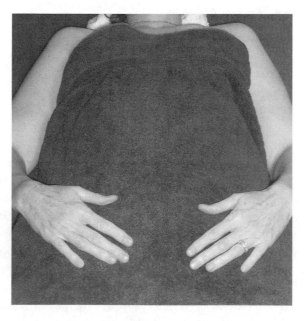

Either of these mudras can be done above or under the sheet.

Mudras for Helping Breathing

Sometimes people find it difficult to relax their breathing while on the table. Here are a series of mudras that Melanie was taught by her teacher, Dr. Vasant Lad. They are not only helpful to clients while on your table. They are also an excellent take-home series of exercises for those who suffer periodically from lung congestion, as well as asthma and emphysema. They can be done in bed or in a chair, or even while standing.

Our thumbs are associated more with the subtle aspect of Vata or prana than the other fingers. This is why they are used as the primary digit for offering massage to vital energy points, be they acupuncture points or marmas. In Chinese medicine, the thumbs are associated with the lungs. Consequently, when the thumbs are placed in relation to the other fingers in various positions, changes happen in the energy to the lungs. If you have a hard time believing this, we suggest you try this exercise for yourself.

Levels of Breath

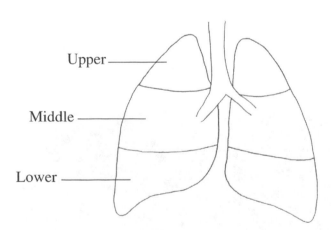

The diagram is not referring to the
anatomical lobes of the lungs but the
level to which the breath travels

Each one of the four positions presented will stimulate different lobes of the lungs. Allow yourself or encourage your client to hold each of the presented hand mudras for two to three minutes. And, while doing this exercise, try not to force the breath. Just allow your breath to move in and out naturally.

POSITION ONE: Place the thumbs so that they are touching the tips of the index fingers. This will open the energy into the lower lobes of the lungs. It will also relax the diaphragm.

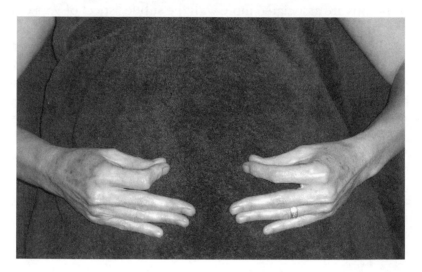

POSITION TWO: While the thumbs remain touching the tips of the index fingers, gently curl the remaining three fingers up into a loose fist. This opens the energy in the middle lobes of the lungs. You will feel your rib cage actually expand outwards.

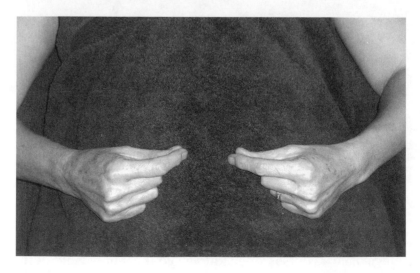

POSITION THREE: Now place the thumbs at the base of the fourth (ring) fingers and wrap the other fingers over the thumbs. This opens the energy in the upper lungs. You may notice that you feel your shoulders rising.

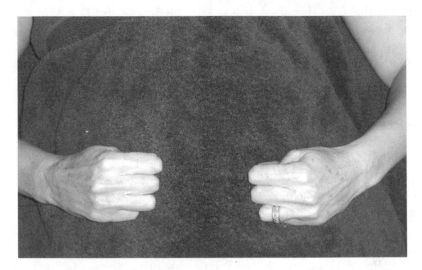

POSITION FOUR: With your hands in POSITION THREE, press the backs of the knuckles against each other. This position may cause you to feel a bit of a stretch in the backs of your wrists. This position helps to revitalize the entire lung.

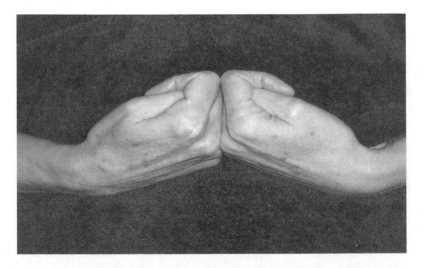

To finish, after POSITION FOUR, do POSITION THREE, TWO, then ONE to the count of five breaths. Then relax and watch your breathing for a few minutes.

A Few Words about Hydrotherapy

Ayurveda has a great reverence for the power of water in therapy, both internally and externally. With respect to its internal use, we only wish to emphasize that as a therapist, it is extremely important that you stay well hydrated while offering treatments. For one thing, **standing for any length of time has a wearing effect on the energy of the kidneys**. With respect to your client, especially if you are doing any treatments that heat the body to encourage sweating or if the treatment is intended to detoxify, it is essential to offer a client water at the end of the treatment. In both cases the water should be room temperature or warm.

The two most common forms of hydrotherapy in the spa are baths and steams. This is true for Ayurveda. There are also herbal wraps and mud treatments. Our "Marma and Mud Magic" treatment ritual discusses the use of mud. As we do not use herbal wraps, we shall not discuss them here.

In the July 2000 issue of Skin Inc. magazine, Ayurvedic physician Dr. Rama Kant Mishra extols the benefits of baths, but makes a caveat with respect to using tap water. Most of the water that comes from the tap in this country is highly chlorinated. Not only will this damage the skin, but it will also nullify some of the effects of the herbs as well as being a toxin that the body will absorb. Thus, **if you are doing *any* form of hydrotherapy, it is best to use purified water or have a filtration system on the tap that you fill your tub or load your steamers with**. (Pages 67–68, Skin Inc., July 2000)

In both baths and steams, herbs are used. These herbs can be in the form of the physical herbs themselves or essential oils. For practical purpose in the modern spa, unless you have access to organic herbs, it may be easier to find quality essential oils. Some companies are recommended in our Resource Guide. Although specific herbs can be used for different conditions, there is one tridoshic blend that we find pleasant for all body types. This is a combination of **bay, eucalyptus, and ginger**. This combination is balancing and detoxifying in either a bath or a steam.

In Ayurveda, baths are generally done before a treatment rather than after and steams are done towards the end of a treatment rather than before. Baths are used to warm the body, open up the pores, relax the body and prepare it for absorbing whatever oil, lotion, or other substance that is going to be applied. If they are done at the end, they tend to be exhausting and leave the client feeling lethargic and dull. The exception would be cold plunges, which would not be recommended for either Vata or Kapha body-mind types. Even in the case of some Pitta body-mind types, a cold plunge can be overly taxing—even if the person claims that it feels great! (Being a Vata-Pitta type, my own experience with cold water relates to swimming and body surfing in the Pacific Ocean on the US West Coast. My Pitta loved the cold, but what I found a few months later was that the cold had penetrated deep into my joints, causing a deep, lasting aching. It has taken several years to overcome this effect.) Steams, on the other hand, gradually relax the client and encourage whatever product you are using to be driven in more effectively. As steam penetrates quickly, the oil or lotion being used is somewhat protective of its invasive quality. Also, it does not warm the body as deeply as does a bath. For these two reasons, it is best to leave steaming towards the end.

If neither of these is available, wrapping the body at the end of the treatment is an excellent form of hydrotherapy. In our Himalayan Mountain Abhyanga treatment ritual, the body is kept warm by wrapping it well after the massage. In this way, the perspiration created drives the product deeper and facilitates detoxification.

With these guidelines in mind, let us now focus on the Treatment Rituals themselves.

■ *Ayurvedic Face Rejuvenation*

Understanding that beauty is the reflection of inner balance, this treatment works with the body from head to toe, then concentrates on the face, scalp, head, neck, and shoulders to refresh and renew your whole being. Techniques from the Ayurvedic tradition of polarity therapy are used to balance the subtle energies of the body, gentle massage of the joints helps make the client feel relaxed and comfortable, and work with specific marmas takes the treatment to a deeper level. The end result is a joyful glow and renewed twinkle.

The massage works locally and reflexively; locally it improves the skin and energizes the face, and reflexively it relaxes and deeply nourishes the whole body. Natural cleansers are used to prepare the face and customized organic essential oil blends are used to enhance the effectiveness and pleasure of the massage treatment. The Ayurvedic Face Rejuvenation can be offered alone as a 60 minute treatment with great results or it can be integrated into a longer 90 minute treatment that may include facial steam, compress, exfoliation, and mask, etc. The face massage section can also be shortened by doing each stroke just once so it will fit into a more traditional facial. The opening sequence can be used on its own to quickly and deeply relax even the most tense client prior to any treatment.

What are the Benefits of the Ayurvedic Facial Massage Sequence?

- Enhances nourishment and cleansing of tissues, which makes for a glowing complexion
- Maintains good tone and elasticity in all skin layers, which helps to hold youthful contours
- Melts away facial tension
- Re-directs subtle energies, relieving stiffness throughout the entire body
- Deeply nourishes and strengthens the body
- Gives rise to a sensual feeling of joyful excitement that re-energizes the whole body
- Develops a depth of being that cultivates a willingness to care for others; an inner richness that develops lasting beauty

---

Suggested Description for Spa Menu

Ayurvedic Face Rejuvenation

Experience how this unique combination a gentle balancing touch, use of marmas (vital energy points), stimulating scalp massage, together with the use of aromatic oils can deeply calm, refresh and re-energize both your face and your whole being.

Products and Equipment Needed:

Skin type questionnaire

Massage table or esthetics couch

Top and bottom sheet

Blanket or duvet

Gown or wrap

Head and Neck pillow or equivalent

Cool Eyes Pack or similar and cotton eye pads

Tummy Warmer or equivalent

Natural makeup remover

Wash cloth

Bowl of warm water

Choice of vata, pitta or kapha face massage oils

Nutmeg lotion-optional

Products for facial as needed

Before your client gets changed into their gown or wrap ask them to take a minute to fill out a client intake form and a client Ayurvedic Skin Care Assessment Form if that has not been handled by a receptionist. Briefly describe the treatment and ask if they have any questions or concerns. Give clear instructions on which clothes to leave on and which to take off and where to put both clothes and valuables. It is useful to have a small bowl for jewelry that can be kept close at hand so the client feels more secure. Get into the habit of checking the bowl before your client leaves. It is not uncommon for both client and therapist to feel a little "spacey" after a treatment and a quick check can avoid the inconvenience of favorite gems getting left behind.

Take the time to read through the forms and discuss anything that concerns you with the client. It is annoying to spend time filling in forms and then find they are not used or checked. The forms should help you gain insight into your client's situation and help them feel that you have a level of professional concern. Take a moment to briefly explain about different skin types and ask your client to select a face oil that smells good to them. (For details check the strip test in the assessment chapter.) Trust their nose. It is most important that the client enjoys the smell of the treatment products.

Where to Make Contact and Why

This type of treatment requires a centered focus and open receptivity. It should feel like an inspiring conversation, a full and meaningful interaction. It is interesting to note that one word used in Tibetan for massage, *nye,* means interaction. Once this rapport is established, wherever you make contact with your client change will occur. Not only will your touch affect that particular area, but there will also be a response throughout your client's entire body. This is commonly recognized in reflexology where points on the feet, hands, or ears are massaged to help the cleansing and re-energizing of organs, joints, or limbs. It is also recognized in shiatsu (massage that utilizes acupuncture points), and functions similarly to marmas in some cases, though in the case of marmas the response occurs more in the electromagnetic energy field of the body. In polarity therapy, this reflexive response may be in the thought forms unbound from their fixation to the physical body. The Ayurvedic Facial Rejuvenation Sequence employs all of these techniques and uses aromatic oils that are designed to balance the doshas on the physical, mental and emotional levels.

In this modern world our heads tend to feel busier than the rest of our bodies. Our thoughts and emotions tend to constrict the muscles of the face, head, neck, and shoulders, giving us that tired, pinched, and generally stressed look. Sometimes we are more aware of one area than another; maybe pain around our eyes, jaw, chest, back of the neck, or one shoulder. These pains are the way our bodies have of communicating messages to us. Releasing underlying tension not only helps the pain in these areas, but may also release memories, emotional traumas, and/or visual images. Releasing neck tension, for example, allows energy to flow more freely between the head and the heart, hence facilitates better connection between our thoughts and emotions, our habits and behavior patterns. The shoulders are often tight due to unexpressed or repressed feelings. We even talk about "putting your shoulder to the wheel" to mean working hard, or "having the weight of the world on our shoulders". When this tension is released, communication flows more naturally with more confidence and less anxiety and the face blossoms into its own beauty and perfection.

By working on the head, neck, and shoulders, changes can be facilitated on many levels. With such potential it is very important to work with concentrated care and gentleness. Keep in touch with your client throughout the session and help them to keep in touch with themselves. If anything of a serious nature comes up, such as strong emotions or difficult memories, be supportive and kind but do not get into a counseling role. It is better in everyway to suggest further professional help if something very overwhelming surfaces.

Starting the Treatment Session

A great treatment takes work and a giving attitude. In order to do your best work, make a habit of taking a few moments for yourself before starting the treatment to charge your own body and settle the atmosphere. Consider the treatment time as space for both yourself and your client to divorce yourselves from the mundane world to experience the magic of touch for an hour or so. You may choose to sit quietly and take a few deep breaths imaging that as you breathe in, all negative thoughts and feelings are draining out of your body into the floor beneath you whilst your body fills with light and positive energy. It is very powerful to wish that your work not only benefits your client but everyone and ultimately the whole environment. As it is your hands that will be in closest contact with your client, take a few moments to gather energy there. Tarthang Tulku, Rinpoche's books on Kum Nye, give an excellent exercise for this purpose.

1. Begin by sitting or standing comfortably with your back straight, breathing gently through your nose and mouth. If you are standing, allow your knees to be slightly bent and allow your back to feel soft.
2. Put a little warm oil on your hands.
3. Bend your arms at the elbows and hold your hands open, with palms up, at the level of your heart. Allow the tension to drop out of your shoulders. Cup your hands as if holding glowing balls of light in them. Sense the energy in your fingers, then let it pass into your hands like a flame licking and spreading.
4. From your hands let the energy pass into your arms, up through the elbows, shoulders, and into your heart.
5. Allow yourself to feel deeply nourished by these sensations.
6. Now slowly bring your hands together and rapidly rub the back of your left hand with the palm of your right. Reverse hands and continue to rub vigorously.
7. Next rub your palms together in a rapid motion until they definitely feel hot.

8. Once again hold your hands open, palms up at the level of your heart, cupping them a little as before.
9. Take a minute to sense your own body and thoughts.

You are now ready to begin the treatment.

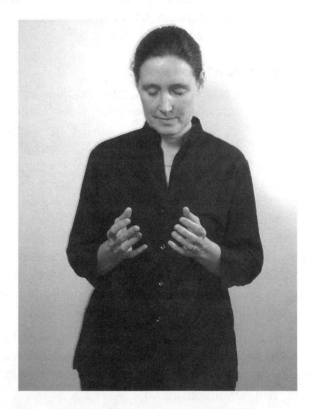

Another preparatory exercise is to stand quietly and rest your right hand over the *svadhisthana* chakra, just below your navel, and your left hand over your forehead, the area for *ajna* chakra. Breathe in a quiet and relaxed manner. This exercise will strengthen your aura, which will benefit your client and keep you strong and protected during the treatment.

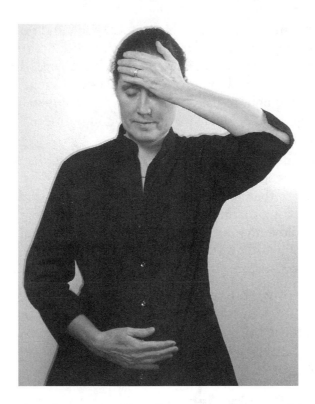

This only takes three minutes of treatment time and it makes a big difference in terms of setting a relaxed tone with a sense of having time for nurturing. It is also sets a good example for your client, showing them that work does not have to be a stress-producing activity. In order to get the desired results from the exercise, you can also practice it when you don't have clients as it will improve your proficiency. If you are shy or feel your client may be upset by it do it in between clients as time allows during the day.

People's different constitutional types will generally prefer or benefit from different styles of treatment. Check with the Ayurvedic Skin Assessment Form and go with what you understand about Ayurvedic body-mind types when you are customizing your treatment.

VATA—dominant clients enjoy subtle, energetic work; light touch, warmth, and gentleness. When talking to them, be soft, supportive, and use feeling tones and music. (A sample dialogue for VATA types using imagery: "Allow yourself to float back and enjoy the warmth and aroma of the oil as it caresses your face and melts away your tensions, taking you to a quiet, creative space within.")

PITTA—dominant clients enjoy direct, firm, cool, and refreshing touch. They also enjoy logical explanations of the work and use color visual images easily. (A sample dialogue for PITTA types using imagery: "Lie back. Notice each point where your body touches the table. Allow a cool blue light to pass through you, relieving your tensions and transporting you to a place free from competition, filled with soft colors and luxurious sensations.")

KAPHA—dominant clients benefit most from firm, deeply stimulating touch. They need to be motivated to keep in touch with the massage process rather than sleep. Any insights you share with them will go deep and be long lasting. (A sample dialogue for KAPHA types using imagery: "Allow my touch to gradually penetrate deep into your tissues bringing with it a sense of light, fresh, tingling, dancing energy to awaken and inspire your deepest thoughts and sensations.")

Allow your intuition to guide the rhythm and pressure of the treatment. Stay focused and relaxed. When you concentrate your face will often start to tense in a scowl. The forehead wrinkles and the jaw tightens. Remind yourself to smile every ten minutes or so to help break the tension habit.

PHASE ONE: Calming Technique

1. Standing behind your client, cradle the back of their head in your cupped hands. Close their ear holes with your thumbs and place your finger tips along the occipital ridge of the skull at the back of the head. Feel the weight of their head in your hands. The more relaxed the client is, the heavier their head will feel in your hands. Note that if you relax your own arms, you will assist them in letting go more easily. Let tension fall from your own shoulders.
   Ask your client
   - to try to let go. Avoid the words "just relax".
   - to allow their head to be heavy in your hands—if you feel a change in the weight let the client know they are doing exactly what you asked and thank them.
   - to allow you to do the moving—so many clients do what the they think is helpful to you and miss the chance the let go completely.

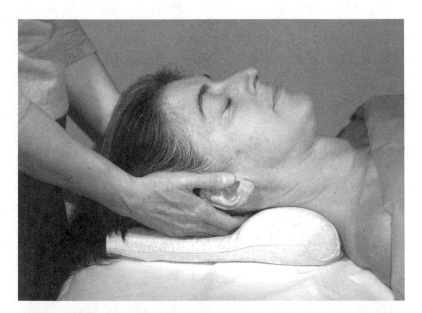

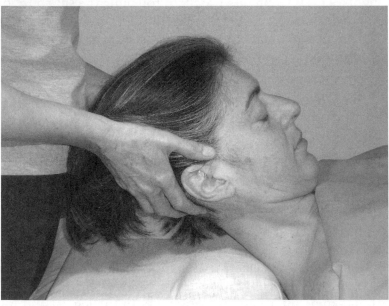

Bring your client's chin forward to their chest, stretching the back of the neck, holding their head in this position to the count of three just as you might hold a yoga posture. If there is slight pain or stiffness, rock the head from side to side very gently and subtly. Never push through uncomfortable pain. Then take your time to lower the head back onto the table. Allow the head to rest on the table for a moment and take a breath yourself. Repeat this process two more times, raising and then gently lowering the head. This begins to build a trusting rapport. (Sometimes during the treatment, the neck tightens again. You will notice this by the chin pointing more in the air than being in the preferred slightly tucked position. If you see this, re-adjust the head using this gentle stretch technique again.)

This movement establishes a non-invasive contact with the client, building rapport and mutual confidence. Releasing neck tension initiates a "relaxation" response through the whole body by opening up the flow of energy in the spine.

2. Keep the head cradled in your hands, moving only your thumbs so they are in front of the ears. Then allow your fingertips to meet and rest at the temples. Breathe in as your client breathes out and out as your client breathes in. Try breathing in and out deeply through your nose only. Center yourself by breathing down into your belly to a point two to three inches below your navel. Send out positive thoughts. This is technique is called "touching the subconscious". It creates a deeper contact with the client and is a way of harmonizing your energies. You may use verbal suggestion at this point, as well. Use any of these short prompts.

   • Let your breathing nourish and relax you.
   • Enjoy the feeling of deep rest and letting go.
   • Let the breath bring renewal to your body and a greater sense of calm and clarity to your mind.
   • Allow your breath to sustain and nurture you. Feel how your senses are coming alive, giving all of your life a magical spicy flavor.

Remember: the more present and relaxed you are, the easier it is for your client to relax. If at any point you feel that you have lost your focus or contact, return to this breathing pattern.

This hold balances the electromagnetic energies in the right and left side of the brain. This is energizing as it increases the brain's ability to deal with incoming information, bringing both the logical and intuitive responses together which really helps alleviate mental stress.

3. Change your hand position so that the left hand is cradling the back of the head and the right hand wraps over the forehead. Use the same alternate breathing as in STEP TWO for about 90–120 seconds.

   This hold balances the electromagnetic energies of the front and the back of the brain. This can help bring forward deeply buried memories to the conscious mind and then comfortably release them.

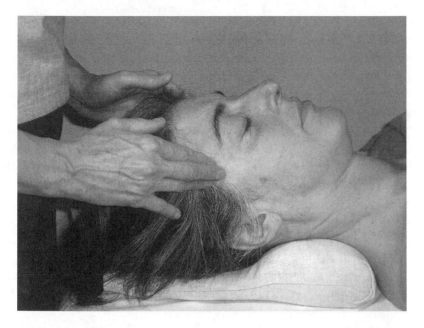

Steps 2 and 3 help to create an alert, balanced state of calm and receptivity.

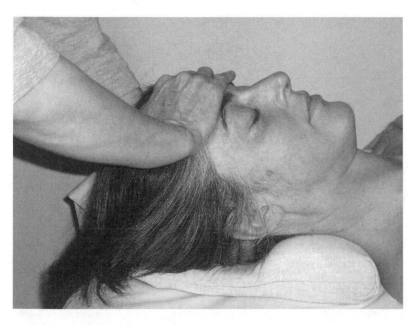

4. Rest the heels of your hands midway between the neck and the tips of the shoulders. Lean forward, keeping your elbows straight, using the weight of your body to push the client's shoulders down towards

their toes. (This is less tiring than using only the strength of your arm muscles.) Release the shoulders and ask the client to take a deep breath in with you. Make a good amount of noise doing this so your client can feel comfortable to really take a deep breath. Ask them to let the breath out and as they do, press on the shoulders again. Repeat once or twice more making three deep breaths in all.

After holding a stretched posture, the muscles of the shoulders naturally relax, balancing the position of the shoulder girdle. As the shoulders relax the pelvic girdle responds by adjusting slightly as well. When the two girdles release their tension, energy can flow more freely between them throughout the torso. Breathing will become deeper and easier. Sometimes the client will sigh or take a very long, deep breath that will be visible. This type of breath is a good sign of deep release.

Ask the client if they would like an eye pillow and explain how it is restful for the eyes and helps the body rest more deeply. Always mention it can be taken off any time.

My experience indicates that clients who have more pitta are the most claustrophobic to the point of not liking their eyes covered, but that these are the very clients that would benefit most from the cooling effect of the eye pillow.

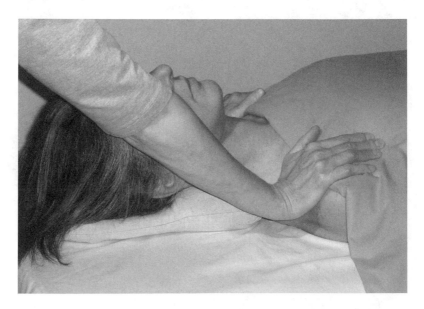

5. Move to the right side of the client but keep your hands in contact with the client as you move. Stand on their right side level with their

knees. Rest your left hand on the large thigh muscle on the front of the right leg and hold the right knee cap between your finger tips and the heel of your hand. Rotate the kneecap five times counter-clockwise and five times clockwise. Counterclockwise movements are more stimulating and clockwise movements are more calming. So first we stimulate, then calm the energy. Remaining on the client's right side, reach over to the left leg and repeat the same movement on the left knee.

Generally speaking, keeping both hands in contact with the client is more balancing and reassuring. Try to do this for each move, even when only one hand is active.

This movement releases hidden tensions that tend to accumulate around the knees. Those that stand a lot at work or carry extra weight tend to have more knee joint tension. Work very gently if the client has had knee problems as these clients seem extra nervous about touch, and never push down through the knee. All movement should be in the horizontal plane. A bolster or pillow under the knees can be very helpful in easing tension in the lower back.

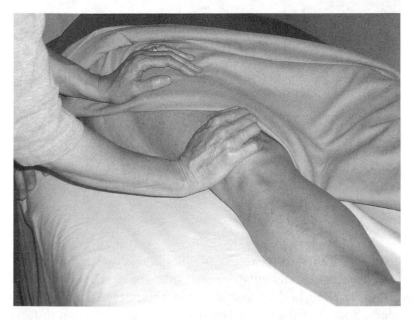

6. Move to the end of the table and stand so that the corner of the table near your client's right foot is pointing at you. Lift their right leg, supporting it with your left hand over the Achilles tendon. Don't allow the heel to rub on the sheet when you move it. Take hold of

the top of the foot and rotate the ankle three times counterclockwise and then three times clockwise. Move slowly enough to feel you are moving the ankle through as full of a rotation as possible. Beware of the pitta in any client that wants to do the moving for you. This is a sign of a need for control. Just say something like, "you don't have to work so hard here, try and let me do the moving". Cover the foot if you have a chilly client, then do the same movement for the left foot, standing at the corner near the left foot. Remember, the client's right foot will be on your left if you stand at the foot of the table. Standing at the corner gives you more room to move and work. Raise the sheet to expose both knees.

Extra vata tends to collect around the joints, so taking the client through these basic stretches of neck, shoulders, knees, and ankles helps settle them down by taking away the fidgits.

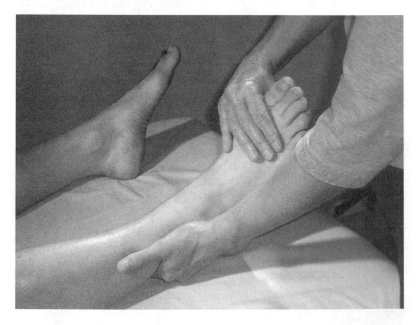

7. Allow your hands to move down the client's lower leg as you move to their feet and stand at the end of the table so that you are looking straight up their body. Make a "V" shape between your thumb and fingers. Slide your hands up the lower legs over the calf muscle until they are just below the knees. You will feel a soft hollow just before the knee joint on the inner side of the knee. Allow your thumbs to rest in these hollows.

This hold helps balanced energy to gradually flow from the head, neck, and shoulders down to the legs. The point to the inside of the knees helps build strength and stamina. It is particularly useful for those who have been under long term stress and before long journeys.

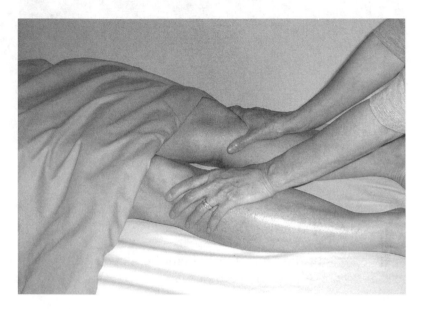

8. Move your hands down towards the ankles. Rest the thumbs at the point midway between where the bottom of the foot would touch the ground and the bone which protrudes on the inner side of the ankle. In polarity therapy these points are the negative pole points of the body as the head is the positive pole. Apply gentle pressure and notice if you feel a pulse. If you, do hold until you feel the pulse in each ankle pulse together. This is energy balancing.

   Touching first the head or positive pole and working down to the ankles or the negative pole while focusing on the breath moves and balances the body's electromagnetic flow, harmonizing and relaxing the body.

9. Move back to the client's right side at the level of the chest. Rest your left hand over the forehead and the right hand on the belly, three to four finger-widths below the navel. Rub the belly slowly in a clockwise direction five times. Then rock the belly by moving your right hand across and back, up and down along the whole abdomen. The belly is the neutral pole of the body.

   If the client is particularly stressed or anxious, apply a tummy warmer to the lower abdomen. (Note contra indications mentioned in equipment section.)

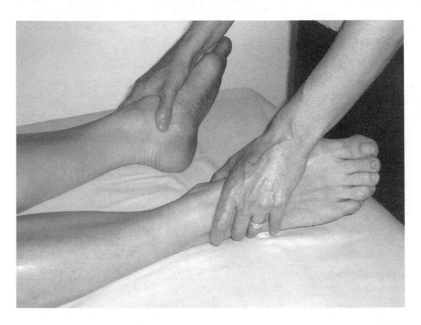

Much anxiety and tension is held in the muscles of the abdomen and diaphragm. Gentle movements ease out the stress and feel very nurturing.

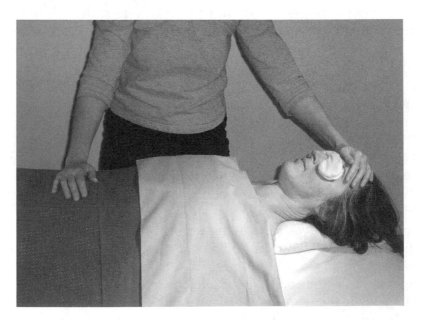

10. Still at the client's right side, move to the waist level. Facing their torso, hold your hands about six inches above their belly, (this is the

distance the average person's aura extends out from their body) palms down, left hand slightly below right hand. Starting at the navel level, make small clockwise circles over their body with your hands, spiraling outward over their torso. Then bring the left hand over the chest, up over the head and touch the table above the head then bring the right hand down over the hips, legs and feet and touch the table below the feet. Imagine you are creating an imaginary capsule that encircles your client six inches from their body surface. You can imagine this capsule being a protective shield filled on the inside with healing light.

Creating this type of protected space, the client feels safer to experience the sensations and emotions that arise.

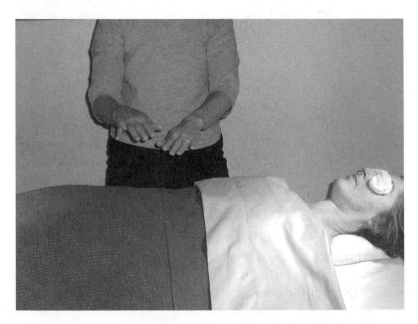

11. Standing behind the head of the client again, rest your thumbs on the middle of their forehead, a point midway between and slightly above the eyebrows. Rest your palms around both sides of the head. Hold for a short time, breathing down into your belly.

This brings focus back to the face and head which is where the greater part of the massage takes place. It also helps you to still and focus your own energy once again.

Although STEPS ONE through TEN are preliminary to the main portion of the Ayurvedic Face Rejuvenation Sequence, it is best if you have time to work through them thoroughly. If, however, you do not have time, at least spend a few minutes holding and focusing your attention on your client's head, knees, ankles, forehead, then belly, keeping your focus and mentally creating a positive environment. This sequence is great to use before any treatment as a relatively quick way to help the client feel comfortable with you and in your space.

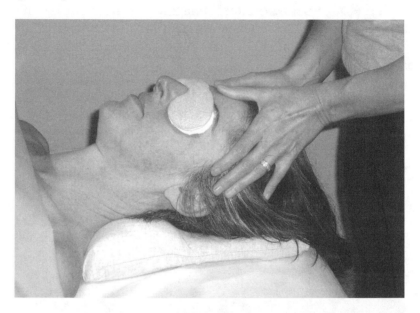

PHASE TWO: Touch to the Head

1. Point 1 is at the crown of the head on the midline. To find it easily and accurately, ask the client to put their right hand over their forehead with the heel of the hand at the top of their nose with fingers pointing up over the head. Then, with their left hand, measure three finger widths back from the tip of the middle finger of their right hand. This is the crown point or MURDHI marma. You can also find this point if you draw or imaginary line over the middle of the top of the head and another line from the tip to tip of each ear. Put your thumb where these imaginary lines cross.

   All marma points should be touched with great care, rubbing in gentle, small, clockwise circles, gradually increasing, then gradually releasing pressure spiraling in and spiraling out.

   Massage this crown point for 30–60 seconds, about the time it takes to do 35 clockwise circles. Remember this point and use it as a measuring reference for the other points.

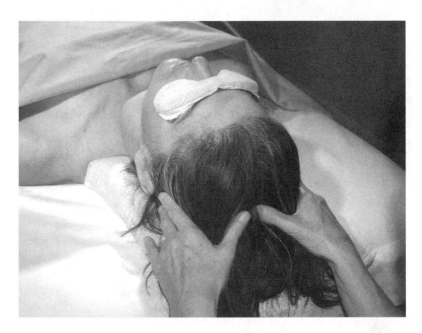

2. Point Two is three finger widths in front of the crown point, still on the midline. (Remember to use the client's hand as a reference, not your own; or, make appropriate allowances if you just "eyeball" it.) This point is called BRAHMA RANDRA and is found resting over the anterior fontanel. Sometimes you will feel a slight ridge or depression where the skull bones come together. Rarely, the bones do not meet at this fontanel point. However, if they do not, do not use pressure, only gentle circular movements brushing the surface of the scalp.

   Massage as in STEP ONE in small circles for 30–60 seconds.

3. Point THREE is four finger widths behind the crown point. It is called SHIVA RANDRA and is over the posterior fontanel. As with the anterior fontanel mentioned in STEP TWO, you may feel a dip or ridge where the bones of the skull come together.

   Massage as in STEP ONE. Sit if you want to use your thumb again. If you want to remain standing you will find it more comfortable on your wrist to use your middle finger.

   These three points on the midline of the head are key to taking the client to a deep level of relaxation. Even—or especially—the more talkative client should be encouraged to be quiet for these three points. One diplomatic way to achieve this is to simply ask, "Can we be silent together while I touch a few points on your head? It will help you relax more easily."

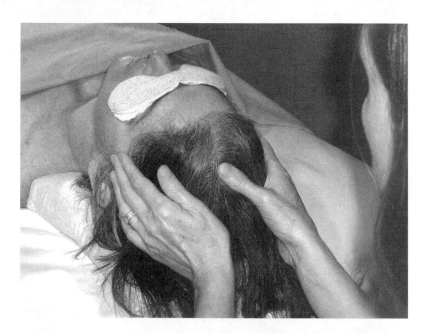

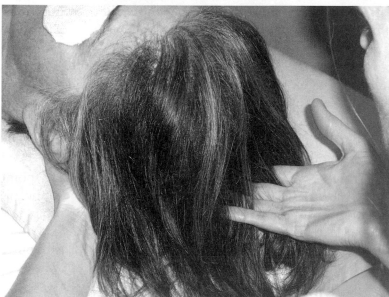

4. Turn the client's head to the left, cradling it with your left hand. With
   the index and middle finger of your right hand find the bony bump
   behind the right ear lobe. This point is called KARNA marma.

   Massage this point in gentle clockwise circular movements. Then,
   progress with a firmer touch using all the finger tips of your right

hand along the occipital ridge of the skull working toward the back of the neck. When you get to the base of the skull at the midline, use your left hand to work up the back of the left side of the occipital ridge to the bump behind the left ear. Circle clockwise around the left KARNA marma, then do the reverse of what you have just done working your way back to behind the right ear. Repeat this back and forth process 2 more times. As you repeat this process, you will pass over two other marmas called MANYA marmas. Give these points special attention by massaging them in five gentle clockwise circles. All circles will be five times from here on.

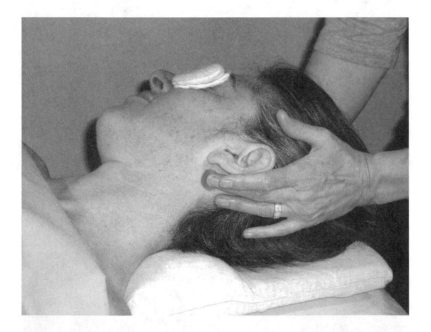

5. Keep the head turned to the left, cradling it in your left hand. Use all of the fingers of your right hand to stimulate the right side of the scalp in "zigzag" movements, from the back of the skull over the head to the hair line. Apply sufficient pressure so that skin is moved back and forth on the skull bones. Be sensitive to the individual. Thin people usually need less pressure and do better with slower, gentler, circular motions. Heavier people with thick scalps get more from firmer zigzags.

Work over the whole of the right side three times. Then turn the head to the right and repeat the process on the left side of the scalp. (Working with your left or non-dominant hand takes a little practice. However, it is very difficult to cross over and work with the right or dominant hand again on the left side.) Always support the side of the head you are not working on so the client does not have to brace their neck to hold it in position for you.

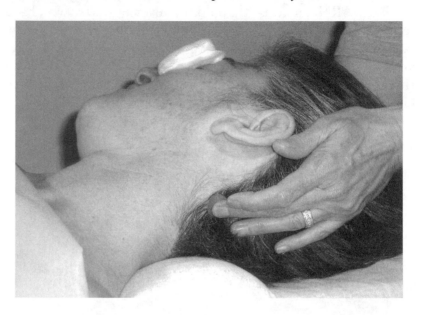

Cradle the head so the neck is straight and the face in the mid position with both hands to once again calm and ground the energy.

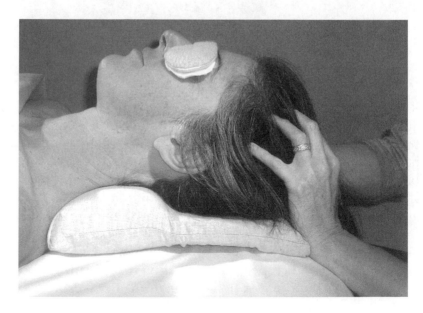

PHASE THREE: Touch to the Neck and Upper Chest

1. Raise the head slightly with your left hand and pinch down the spine from the base of the skull to the top of the shoulders using your right hand. Repeat twice.

    At this point, moisten your fingertips with warm massage oil. Warm oil is more soothing and relaxing and penetrates the skin better than cool oil. It also deepens the effect of the massage by nourishing the muscle tissue and lubricating the layers of connective tissue. Use sufficient oil from now on to allow your fingers to easily flow over the skin. You can use nutmeg lotion as additional help to ease tension.

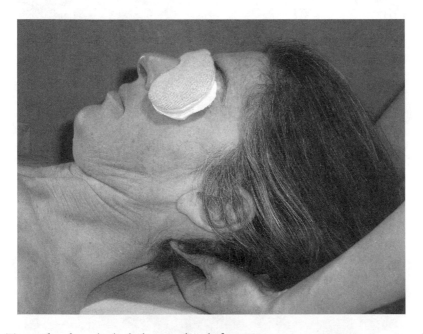

2. Turn the head slightly to the left again, supporting it in your left hand. Find the bony point behind the earlobe again and make five gentle circles around this point. Then use the flats of your middle three fingers to stroke down the large flat muscle that is attached to the skull at this point and wraps around the side of the neck, connecting to the collarbone near the windpipe. This is the sterno-mastoid muscle. Use your thumb to find the point where the muscle attaches to the collarbone and press three times down towards the feet. Repeat this twice more on the right, then turn the head and do the same movement three times on the left.

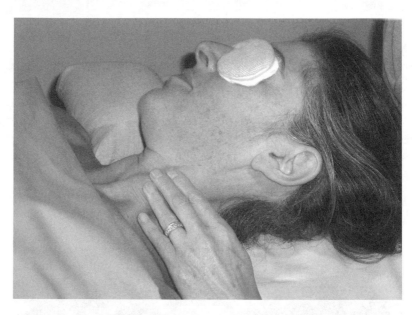

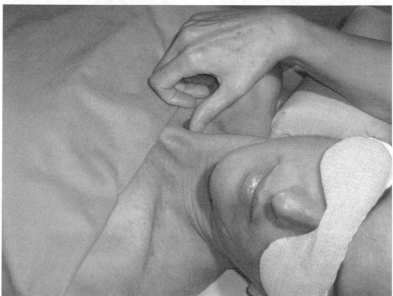

3. Stand to your client's side so you are looking at them face to face. Apply a small amount of oil to your palms and fingers. With the head back in the central position, tilt the chin slightly upward and stroke down alternate sides of the windpipe from underneath the chin down to the collar bone. Repeat stroking on the right then left until you have completed ten strokes in all, five on each side.

This loosens and tones the muscles on the front of the neck and stimulates the thyroid gland, which generates a flow of fresh energy throughout the body.

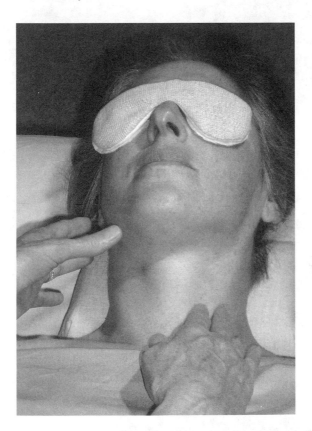

4. Stand at the head of the table again and stroke from the underside of the tip of the chin down the midline of the neck, pause in the middle of the neck (SVARA marma) and make five gentle clockwise circles, then continue on down the midline and let your thumb find the point on the top of and slightly behind the breast bone.

Hook your thumb behind the notch at the top of the breast bone (sternum), in the natural hollow that is there. This point is called the KATHANADI marma. Gently press and release three times, pressing down towards the toes. This point is a cough reflex point, so don't be surprised if some clients need to clear their throat at this time.

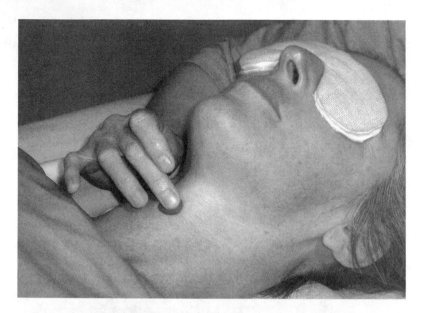

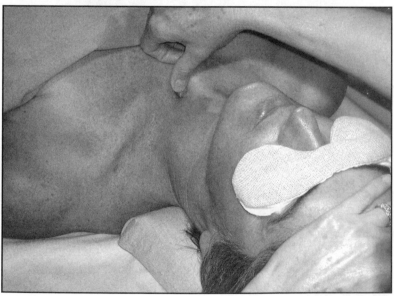

5. Make your hand into a fist with your thumb on the outside of your fingers. Use the tips of your thumbs to feel for the point on the top surface of the collar bone where it joins the sternum. Feel into the angle made by the neck (sterno-clavicular) muscle and the top of the collar bone (clavicle). These are the ARSHAK marmas. Use your thumbs to press down towards the toes, then press and release alternately with right then left thumbs as you work your way out to

the tips of the shoulders. Hold your fingers in a fist to support the thumb so it doesn't wobble.

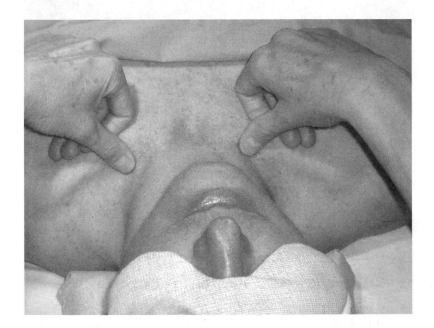

Work your way along the top of the collar bone, pressing and releasing with your thumbs to the tips of the shoulders. Apply slight pressure to the tops of the shoulders, releasing quickly. Repeat once or twice starting at the medial end of the collar bone and moving out to the tips of the shoulders.

With a loose wrist, tap from the top to the bottom of the sternum three times. This stimulates the KATHANADI marma, helping to build immunity. Then stroke gently over the top of the chest. Cover the shoulders with the sheet.

Rest both of your hands on the tops of the shoulders. Relax. Focus your breathing deep into your belly. At this point, let your client know that you are now going to start to work on their face. Remove the eye pillow if you have used it asking that the client keep their eyes closed. Even with eyes closed, shield them from the light to help with adjustment in sensation.

When working directly on the face, use cold-pressed, preservative-free vegetable oil or combinations of oils. Top quality essential oils may be added for their aromatherapy effects (check the list of suppliers at the back of the book). Be sure to dilute essential oils as even the best quality ones can burn and cause long-lasting irritation.

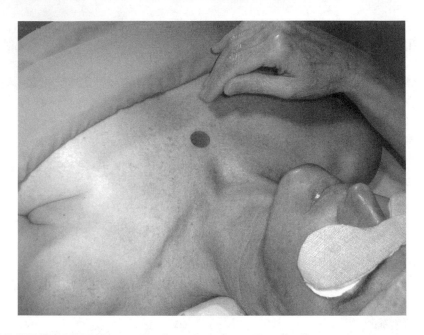

PHASE FOUR: Face Rejuvenation Technique

The smooth strokes release subtle tensions underneath the skin. The marma points work on the deeper tissues of the face corresponding to organs of the body. They awaken the processes that heal and renew tissues and they restore the flow of subtle energy that brings a healthy glow to the complexion.

1. Drop 5–10 drops of the face oil into the palm of your hand. Press your palms together and then coat your fingers with oil. Avoid rubbing your hands together as this is sufficient to create enough heat to diffuse the essential oils out of the product too quickly. Hold your hands over the client's face so they can first smell the oil above them, then touch it to their cheeks, chin and forehead. Take a moment, then use gentle strokes that start on the midline and move up to the sides of the face to get a fine, even application of oil. If your hands or the client's face absorbs the oil quickly, take a drop or two more of oil in the palms of both hands as a "store" where you can touch your finger tips to provide enough lubrication for your stokes to move smoothly without pulling on the skin.

2. Using the tips of the second, third, and fourth fingers of your right hand stroke underneath the chin from the left to the right side. Use a little pressure to feel into the soft tissue between the jawbones. Use your left hand to stroke in the opposite direction. Repeat right

then left until you have done ten strokes in all. Rest two fingers of each hand at the tip of the chin.

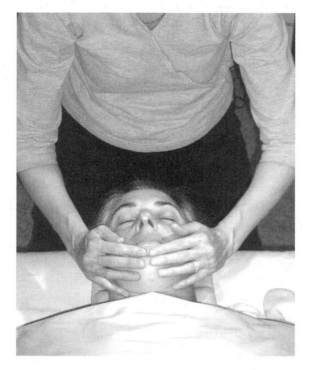

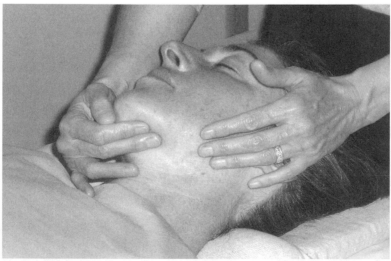

The rejuvenation technique works a lot on the jaw to release the tension that gets trapped there. The jaw muscles are the strongest muscles in the male body, beaten only by the uterus muscle of the female body, so their ability for holding on is tremendous. Once the tension is eased circulation improves, emotions are released, clients are better able to express themselves and the whole face opens and looks more alive.

3. Stroke from the tip of the chin following the jaw line. Let one finger of each hand rest below the jaw bone and one above so you are stroking the underside of the jaw and on top of the jaw bone as you first follow the angle of the jaw, then move up in front of the ears and eventually find the hollow of the temple. Pause at the temple SHANKAR marma and take a breath or two. Put a smile on your face and feel a deepening sense of connection with your client. Use your finger tips to move in five gentle circles about the size of a quarter. Traditionally both little circles should be clockwise so your right hand is moving as if you were beckoning towards yourself, and the left hand is moving the opposite way as if you were making a courtly bow. If these movements are slow and the therapist can re-lax into it, clients that are more vata and kapha dominant are very soothed by this movement. Consistently I find that the more pitta dominant clients feel uneasy and do better if your fingers are mov-ing together both "beckoning".

Repeat twice more.

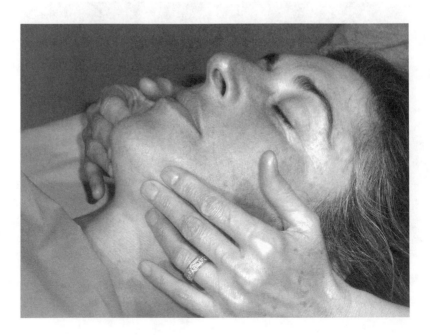

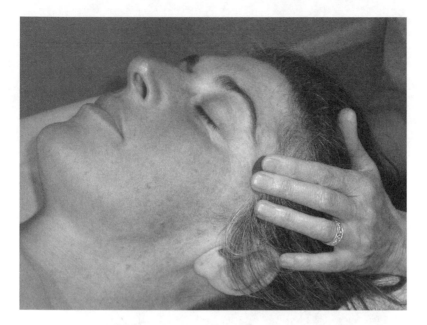

4. Let your fingers slide down the cheeks and let one finger tip from each hand rest in the middle of the chin. You can also break contact and move directly to this point. This is not classic European face massage and it is allowed. If you do choose to break contact, focus your mind on the point to which you are going to move your hands, and the energetic will be there for your client.

   Press and release three times at this mid chin point, HANU marma, keeping your fingers on the surface of the skin.

   Stroke out to just below the corners of the mouth and make five clockwise circles in the area where fine lines develop or are visible if you turn down the corners of your mouth in a frown.

   Stroke up and out into the middle of the cheeks and feel for the front surface of the muscle that opens and closes the mouth. If you are not sure, ask your client to open their mouth wide and then close it. The muscle will move forward under your fingers. Press and release three times on the front surface of this muscle, pressing towards the back of the teeth. Press fairly firmly as it takes a little pressure to ease the tension locked into the muscle. Stroke up to the temples and repeat the five circles there as in step three.

   Repeat twice more.

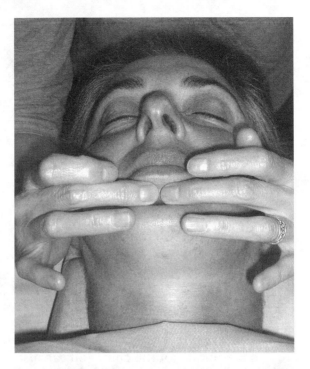

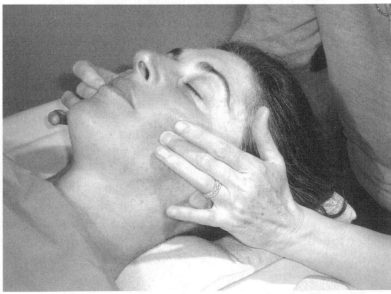

5. Place the index fingers one on top of the other at the point in the middle of the upper lip, USTA marma. Press and release three times. Stroke out to just above the corners of the mouth and make five gentle circles in the area where fine lines form. Continue by

stroking out to the points in the middle of the cheeks. Press and release three times as before. This time, as the movement started above the mouth, the stroke goes up over and behind the ears. Rub thoroughly behind the ears where the ears join the head, then find KARNA marma again and make five gentle clockwise circles there.

Repeat twice more.

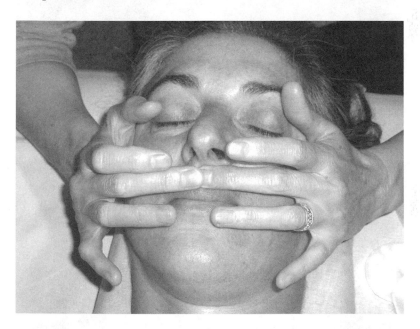

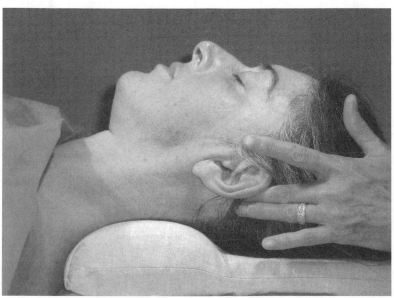

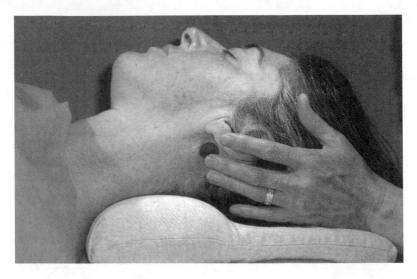

6. Cover the left side of the head with your left hand. Place your right index finger in the hollow where the flare of the right nostril joins the face, NASA marma. Press and release three times, then stroke under the cheek bone up and over the ear as in step five.

   Repeat twice more on the right side, then switch hands and do three strokes on the left side.

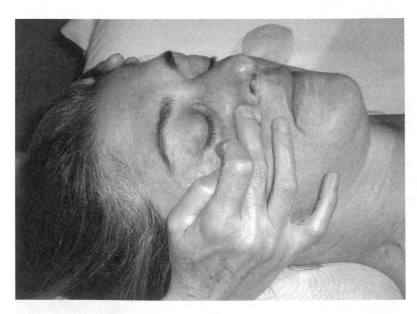

7. Working with both hands together, touch the tips of index fingers to the points on either side of the nose and half way up, GANDU

marma. If you press these points on yourself and talk, you will sound nasal. Gently rub in five clockwise circles. Take the stroke out over the cheek bones and again over the ears ending again at the KAR-NA marma where you do five clockwise circles.

Repeat twice more.

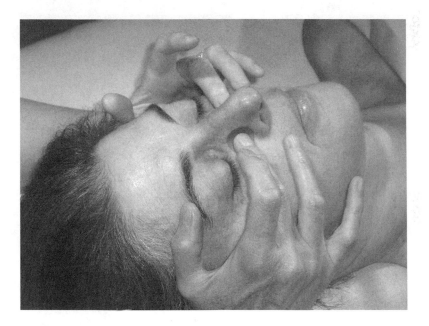

8. Now quietly tell your client that you are going to be touching them gently underneath their right eye. Say it even if the client is dozing. Rest your left hand on the left side of the head then let your fingers "walk" over the cheek until your thumb touches the top surface of the lower bony orbit of the eye just below the tear duct. Use the tip of your thumb to gently press on the top edge of the bones that you find under the eye. Lift your thumb completely and move a fraction to the right, away from the inner corner of the eye, and press gently again. Press and release in this manner working from the inner corner to the outer corner of the eye three times. Be sure to lift before you press again so there is no drag on the tender skin here.

   After the third time, use your index finger to find APANGA marma the point in the outer corner of the eye just on the inner surface of the bony eye socket. Some clients have a lot of space between the eyeball and the socket, and some have very little. Do not press deep into the socket or toward the eyeball itself. Place your index finger at the corner of the eye. Point in toward the middle of the head, then press gently away from the eye and jiggle your finger up and down. Jiggle for a slow count to ten.

Repeat for the left eye. Always work around each eye separately. It is easier to feel tensions that way, and also easier for our bodies to release tension.

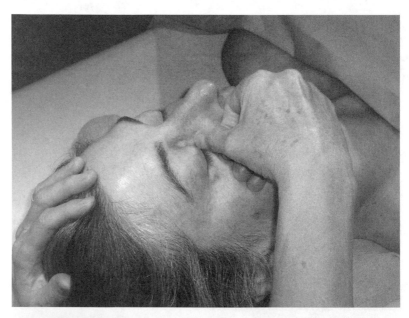

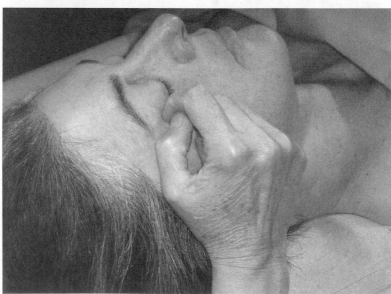

9. Using two fingers of each hand, stroke from the tip of the nose up along the sides of the nose to either side of the bridge. Let the tips of your right index and middle fingers rest just below the inner end of the eyebrow. Take your left hand and let it rest over the left side of the head. With your right hand, find the little bumps on the upper bony orbit of the eye that are closer to the bridge of the nose. Gently rub here, then the press and release in tiny steps along the upper bony orbit of the eye to the outer corner of the eye. Again, do not press deep into the eye socket or toward the eye. Press toward the top of the head releasing completely in between steps so as not to pull on the skin.

Repeat for the left eye, starting at the tip of the nose again.

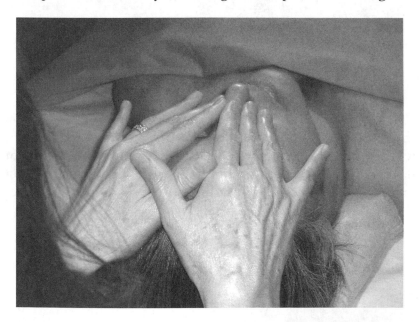

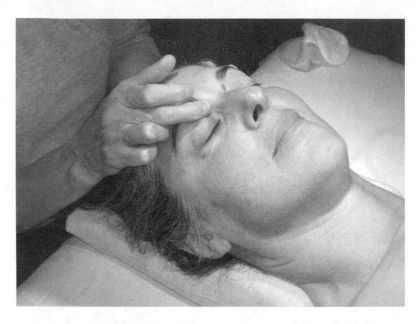

10. Pinch both eyebrows from the inner to the outer ends fairly firmly three times. It is interesting to know that we tend to store tension where we think we cannot be seen from front view: the back of our neck, our backs, under the chin, the scalp hidden by hair, and even under our eyebrows. Touch reminds the body to let go of the tension and is essential for stress relief.

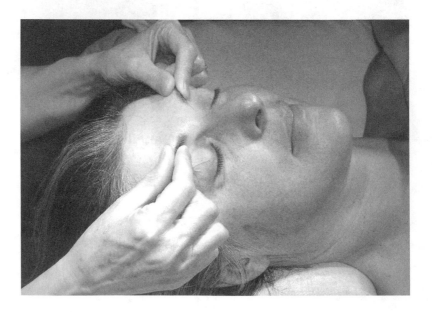

11. Stroke from the tip of the nose as in step nine. This time the left hand moves to the top of the head and rests over the crown while the middle finger of the right hand moves to the center of the forehead, AJNA marma. Draw a clockwise spiral that starts small and gradually moves out to fill the forehead. Return to the middle of the forehead and make two more spirals. Take your time as this is the last slower move of the sequence.

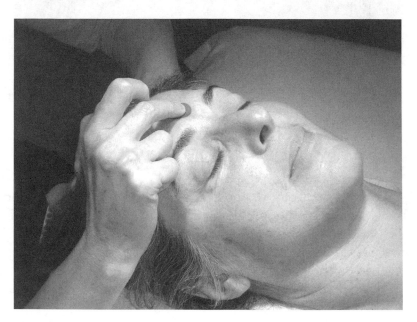

PHASE FIVE: Closing Movements

These movements are designed to gently and effectively bring the client back from the deep state they have been in so they feel rested, completely fresh and clear and ready to move into the rest of their day.

1. Transition from the spirals to gentle zigzag patterns back and forth over the forehead. Gradually let the movements get a little quicker and a little firmer.

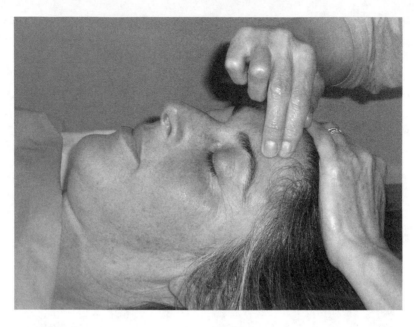

2. Stroke from the tip of the nose again, and this time both hands go all the way up to the middle of the front hairline. Use your finger tips to work in vigorous little circles following the hair line behind the ears and eventually to the very back of the neck.

   Move up the back of the head on either side of the midline with the same circular movements upward and outward. Continue over the top of the head to the front hairline.

   Go around the hairline twice more.

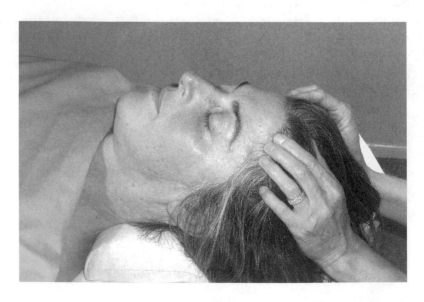

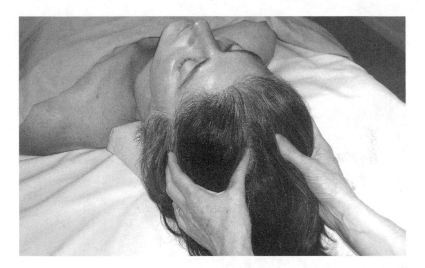

3. Cradle the head so that it is slightly turned to the left. Have your left hand underneath the head so it is well supported. Take hold of the right ear so that the index finger is behind and the thumb is in front rubbing and smoothing first the outer edge, the next ridge then right next to the ear hole. Fold the ear forward, stretching the muscles behind the ear. Cup your hand over the ear and turn your client's head so it is resting on your right hand.

Repeat these movements for the left ear. Move the head back to the middle position and rest for a moment with your hands over the ears.

Stimulating the ears awakens all parts of the body reflexively but is especially effective for getting energy to the kidneys. When the kidneys are energized, you have ease getting up and getting a move on. Clients should not feel sluggish after this treatment but calm, clear, and refreshed.

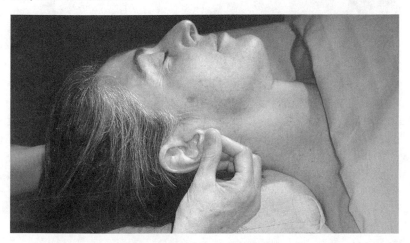

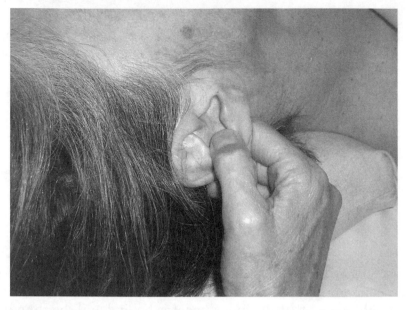

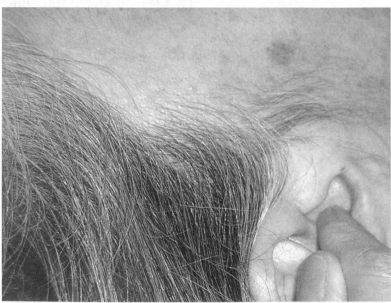

4. Close the ears with your middle fingers and very lightly rest your thumbs over the closed eyelids. Take time to mentally extend the wish that what you have done will be useful in someway. Take your hands away as if they were the petals of a flower gently opening to reveal the perfect newborn center.

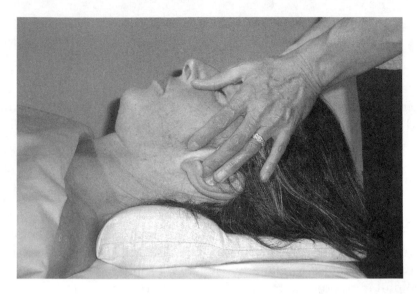

Touch your client's shoulder and let them know you are finished. Let them know the time so those with busy schedules will not worry and allow them to rest for five minutes. You can sit, leave the room, or quietly clean up but do not let the client get up without your help.

If the client has shared any concerns or you have discovered particular areas of tension you might show them marmas that may help if touched gently and regularly at home. A face chart showing the marmas is a helpful reminder.

■ *Helpful Marmas on the Face, Head, Neck, and Chest*

I call these points magical marmas because they are so helpful and make such a difference so easily and comfortably. We are lucky now that more is being published about this wonderful system so we can better understand the depth and subtlety of this work. In these texts you will find clinical information about the treatment of medical problems and detailed descriptions of how marmas work energetically to help balance the doshas. This is a profound study and best done under the guidance of an experienced teacher. My goal here is different. I simply want to help you find these points accurately, be able to describe these points to your client without using clinical terms, and share with you general uses that might be of interest to your clients. I am not suggesting they should be used to diagnose or treat any particular problem, just that they maybe helpful in some ways to ease discomfort. You might find that names vary slightly text to text. I have tried to use the names used by my teachers and those most commonly published. The names themselves very often translate into very ordinary terms such as ear point or chin point, and sometimes relate to deeper functions such as father of the sensory system. I am sure the names have power but the love and confidence in which we touch is more important. If touched gently and with respect, magic will happen.

Side Face   Skull

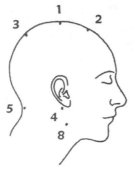
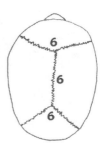

Whole Face

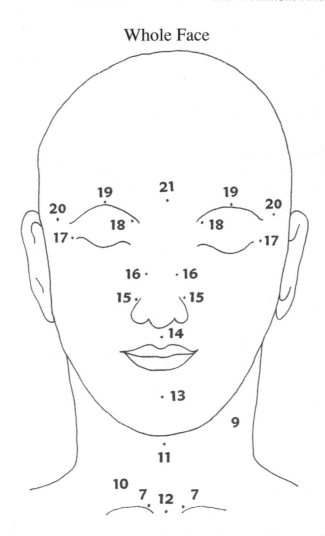

(1) MURDHI (ADHIPATI)

Put the heel of your hand on the bridge of your nose. Wrap your palm over your forehead and your fingers over the top of your head. With your other hand measure three finger widths back from your middle finger on the midline.

- Helps relax the whole body, easing back and neck tension.
- Helps bring tranquility, clarity, and joy to the mind.
- Encourages restful sleep.

(2) BRAHMA RANDRA
This is located on the midline, eight finger-widths above the eyebrows.
- Helps relieve insomnia and irregular sleep.
- Helps regulate body weight.
- Helps balance hormonal functions.

(3) SHIVA RANDRA
Put the heel of your hand on your front hairline. Wrap your hand over the top of your head and feel the point at the tip of your middle finger.
- May help normalize blood pressure.
- May help improve memory.
- Might help with ringing in the ears. Use with karna marma and a few drops of warm sesame oil nightly.

(4) KARNA (KARNA MULA or VIDHURA)
This marma is located behind and slightly below the mastoid process (round bone) behind the ear lobe.
- Helps to relax the muscles of the face and jaw.
- May help with pain, ringing or congestion in the ear.
- Helps relieve fear and anxiety.

(5) KRIKATIKA
Find these on either side of the spine just where it goes up to meet the skull.
- Helps to relax the whole body, easing tension in the neck and upper back.
- Helps relieve pain in the back of the head.
- Might assist in improvement of hearing.

(6) SIMANTA
These are all the joints between the skull bones.
- Helps to ease tension that hides in the scalp.
- Helps you feel nourished and satisfied.
- Helps improve the quality of rest and relaxation.

(7) ARSHAK
Turn your head to the left. Let your finger run down the outside of the large neck muscle that comes forward as you turn your head. Press down

toward your feet at the point in the L angle made by this neck muscle and the top of your collarbone. Find the collarbone by moving your shoulder up and down.

- The point on the right may be tender after drinking, eating fatty foods or being angry. Gentle touch supports liver function and helps remedy these habits.
- The point on the left gets tender when you have eaten lots of sweets or have overextended yourself for others and feel like you are running on empty. Gentle touch supports spleen energy that helps restore energy reserves and moderate mood swings.
- Helps stimulate lymphatic drainage helping to clear the complexion and balance swelling

Minor marmas are found either side of the wind pipe. Stroking down alternate sides of the neck from the face toward the chest eases congestion and fluid accumulation, helps balance the thyroid and can help the voice.

(8) MANYA
Find this one on the side of the neck, four finger-widths below the ear lobes.

- Gently stroke over this area to help improve circulation to the face, stimulate lymph drainage and help ease a sore throat or upper chest congestion.

(9) SIRA MATRIKA
This is on either side of the windpipe on the upper half of the neck.

- Gently brush with your oiled fingertips to improve circulation and improve the voice.

(10) NILA
This one is on either side of the windpipe on the lower half of the neck.

- Gently brush with oiled fingertips to improve the voice and ease a sore throat.

(11) SVARA (KATHA)
This can be found in the middle of the front of the neck, around the Adam's apple. Do not press, just gently rub around.

- Helps in the regulation of the mood swings.
- Helps us to speak up for ourselves and voice our opinions, worries, or inner feelings.

(12) KATHANADI (JATRU)
This is in the hollow on top of and slightly behind the breast bone.
- Very helpful in the relief of sore throats and loss of voice.
- May help with chesty cough and congestion.
- Helps circulation to the face.

(13) HANU
This marma is located in the middle of the chin.
- Helps improve circulation to the face, which will help clear the complexion and normalize skin tones.
- Helps to make a better connection between our head and our heart—what we think and what we feel inside.
- Helps relive jaw tension.
- May help with the health of the prostate or cervix.

(14) USHTA
Find this marma in the middle of the upper lip.
- Helps you feel relaxed but more alert and have better concentration, so it is a wonderful study aid.
- Helps overcome dizziness.

(15) NASA (PHANA)
These marmas are where the flare of the nostrils join the face.
- Helps the right and left side of the brain work better together so we will be clearer about and less stressed by our problems.
- May help improve breathing.

(16) GANDU
These are located halfway up the nose on either side.
- Helps moisten and brighten the eyes.
- Helps drain extra moisture and congestion around the eyes.
- May help with eye strain or eye pain.

(17) APANGA
These are found in the outer corner of each eye slightly inside the eye socket. Never press on the eyeball.
- Can be very helpful to sooth tired, inflamed, or stressed eyes.
- Can help resolve congestion, puffiness, or discoloration around the eye.
- Can help with recovery from minor eye surgery.

(18) BHRUH
Look for these below the inner ends of the eyebrows on the upper bony orbit of the eye. Feel for tiny bumps of bone end that contrast with smooth bone above the eye. These points are often tender.
- Again, can be helpful in the relief of eye strain.
- Can help relieve burning sensation in the eye.
- Can help with migraine pain especially if associated with acid indigestion.

(19) AVARTA
These can be found in the middle of the eyebrow.
- Helps with feeling more centered and alert.

(20) SHANKHA (SHANKHAR)
Find these in the hollow of both temples.
- Can help you to tune into yourself.
- May be helpful with memory.
- Very soothing, calming, and emotionally nourishing.

(21) STHAPANI (AJNA)
This marma is located in the middle of the forehead, approximately ½ inch above the eyebrows. This point is sometimes called the "third eye".
- Helps relax and energetically balance the body, mind, and emotions.
- Yogis focus to bring harmony, order, and sound judgment to the mind and body.
- Touch here can help with peace of mind, build inner confidence and stability, and awaken our own perfect wisdom.

Regarding Ayurvedic Facials

The moment we say facial, there is an immediate expectation of a more product-oriented treatment. The Ayurvedic Face Rejuvenation sequence can easily be included in part or full within any facial and of course is a perfect fit in an Ayurvedic Facial. The focus of this book is not beauty in the usual sense or skin care in particular but as the question about Ayurvedic facials does comes up we feel we want to give some suggestions.

One of our Diamond Way Ayurveda trainers, Jon Alan Vice, does a considerable number of facials at his spa and has made extensive use of our techniques. In terms of product there is plenty to choose from. We use simple oil blends and a product Jon developed as a gentle herbal cleanser/exfoliatior made with flour, milk powder, and essential oils. If you have the knowledge to create such products yourself or already work with a particular line of these products that is available, they can be used as well.

Ayurvedic Facial Procedure:
1. Pre-cleanse with an oil on damp cotton pads .
2. Cleanse with a cream made with the flour/milk blend.
3. Allow to dry for a brief time.
4. Gommage—roll off.
5. Rinse residue off and cleanse with warm wet cotton pads.
6. Put warm compresses on the whole face while you do a hand and arm massage.
7. Massage face using stokes and marmas from the Ayurvedic face rejuvenation sequence.
8. Apply a simple mask.
9. Remove mask.
10. Mist.
11. Add a touch of oil on a damp face as moisturizer.

The selection of the oil, the timing of each step, and the quality of touch and temperature should be customized to match the client's skin type. See appendix for details on oil selection. Customized touch is discussed in the section entitled "What makes a treatment Ayurvedic". In brief, the guidelines are as follows:

Vata—more oil, warmer temperatures, lighter touch

Pitta—less oil, cooler temperatures, precise touch

Kapha—less oil, warmer temperatures, firmer but comfortable touch.

■*Himalayan Mountain Abhyanga*

This is a full body massage with warm oil that is designed to bring the subtle energies of the body into balance through the use of customized essential oil blends and touch techniques. It is both deeply revitalizing and relaxing while at the same time being gently cleansing and detoxifying.

The term "abhyanga" literally means "loving hands". If we were in India, went to an Ayurvedic clinic or practitioner, and were told that we were going to receive abhyanga, a standard term used for oil massage, this meaning would be immediately implied. It is important for us to know this as it should inform the attitude we take when offering this service.

Traditionally abhyanga is offered in a variety of ways and is usually followed by keeping the body warm in some way for 10 to 20 minutes. In the treatment offered here, this accomplished by keeping the client covered after the completion of the massage for a period of 5 minutes to allow the oils to penetrate deeper, followed by an additional 5 minutes from the time an ubtan powder is sprinkled on the body to eliminate the excess oils that are deep in the pores. This last 5 minutes, when the ubtan is left on the body, is a critical and necessary part of abhyanga. It guarantees that the oils that have been worked into the body and thus contain concentrated lactic acid and toxins is removed from the pores in a way that a shower alone cannot do. The result is that much of the stiffness and tiredness that many people complain about on the day after a through massage is completely eliminated. In fact, after this treatment, beyond feeling deeply revitalized and relaxed, the client will feel clear, alert, and light.

There are many styles of abhyanga. Rest assured, if you look at other texts, you will find different ways of offering this service. This has to do with how doctors in different regions of India would interpret the texts and offer what they thought was most beneficial. Do not get caught up in any parochial idea as to which one is better. They are all beneficial and wonderful to give and receive.

However, one point is critical. This is an *oil* massage. We emphasize this because in offering pancha karma under the guidance of various Ayurvedic physicians and hearing the stories of other massage therapists and clients who have gone to India for treatments, it seems that what matters most is getting the oil on the body. Whereas we in the west may think of the oil as just creating enough slip to get from point A to point B, the quality of the oil and what it mobilizes in the body to detoxify and rejuvenate is what matters. You are literally feeding the body oil through the pores. Consequently, *what you chose as an oil is critical*. Beyond the obvious mechanical results that can come from easing someone's pain by working on their muscles and tissues using baby oil or lotions, we see no other benefits. If done too frequently, we would say that such poor quality or inappropriate oils and lotions can create more toxicity than they help to release.

Thus while your strokes and style will probably be what gives you rave reviews with your client initially, in Ayurvedic terms when it comes to Abhyanga, they are almost of secondary importance. The bottom line is *use good quality oils*. Check where they come from, whether they are organic, how they smell, if they have fixatives or preservatives, etc. If you do not have access to oils for the different body-mind types or the daily condition of your client, at least use the best quality oils you can find.

This being said, there are a number of ways one can receive abhyanga. The most common include:

- Self-massage with warmed oil appropriate to your dosha followed by soaking in a warm bath. After a relaxing soak mix the ubtan powder into a thin paste with pure water, milk, or herbal tea and apply all over the body and the face like a lotion. Gently massage over the body again as the paste starts to dry. Rinse off with a warm, then a cool shower. This is a great suggestion to offer your clients for home care and to bring the experience they have had with you into their home routine. A self-abhyanga series will be shown following the spa protocol.

- Full body massage by one, two, or more massage therapists, which can then be followed by steam in a steam room or steam tent, that is herbal (herbs of choice include ginger, eucalyptus, and bay) or with essential oils appropriate for dosha balance. A herbal linen wrap, sauna, or   bath may also be used to warm the body. As before, the treatment ends with the application of ubtan (either as a paste or warmed dry powder) and a shower.

In the protocol offered here, the abhyanga is offered by one therapist. Two-person abhyanga can be a very luxurious treatment, but it can also create some difficulties. For one thing, it requires that two therapists are in the room, which can be costly and create staffing dilemmas. Secondly, the two people offering the abhyanga have to be well trained to work in tandem; their touch and speed has to be well coordinated. If one person has a light touch and the other a heavier touch, the effect can feel quite unbalancing. Lastly, bi-lateral symmetrical strokes on both side of the body at the same time, while feeling luxurious and delightful *if* the therapists are really in harmony, is actually physically weakening for the client as it causes a Vata-like reaction in the central nervous system; they get overloaded with too much stimulation. Thus, if one wants the client to have the benefits as described earlier, a two-person abhyanga is not recommended.

As above and given daily, this ritual is part of PURVA KARMA as a preparation for the deeper cleansing procedures of PANCHA KARMA. Here abhyanga is given daily until the hair and bowel movements become oily. This is the outward sign that the linings of the digestive organs are well lubricated and protected.

Suggested Menu Description

Himalayan Mountain Abhyanga

Abhyanga means "loving hands". In the ancient tradition of Ayurveda, this is the name given to a full body massage by one or more therapists. Our treatment calls for one therapist working on one part of the body at time using warmed aromatic oils to nourish the skin and mobilize deeper tissues. During the massage, marmas (secret energy points) are used to freshen and revitalize the body. Finally, warmed ubtan (herbal powder) is sprinkled over the whole body to polish the skin leaving you feel light, energized and relaxed.

Equipment, Products and Materials
General Requirements
Massage table and head cradle

2 sheets and face cradle cover

1 blanket

Gown and/or wrap and slippers

Oil and ubtan warming equipment (hot towel cabi, warmer, or a crock-pot work well)

Shaker for ubtan powder

1 or 2 oil application bottles

Dosha-appropriate body oil

Dosha-appropriate face oil

Pomegranate Oil or Shatavari Ghee (if breast massage is offered)

Brush for face mask

Small Bowl

¼ cup of pure water, milk, or herbal tea

Shower access or warm towels to get ubtan and excess oil off

Refreshment (Suggestions: Lemon and/or honey for tea, and fresh fruit)

Additional Specialized Equipment May Include

Head and neck pillow

Tummy warmer

Cool eye pillow

Ubtan rose or sandalwood

Herbal hair powder (optional)

Music that is up-beat and keeps you as a therapist moving along. If it is too dreamy, you'll probably find that the treatment takes longer and longer.

Table set-up

Top and bottom sheet

Blanket for extra warmth

Head cradle and cover

The Treatment:
PHASE ONE—Choosing the Right Product

Use the diagnostic procedure indicated earlier for the three points on the back while the client is still dressed to determine the appropriate Ayurvedic dosha blend for your client. Warm the oils, ubtan and tummy warmer while the client is changing. This will also help you in knowing what style of touch, type of music, lighting, etc. will work best for your client.

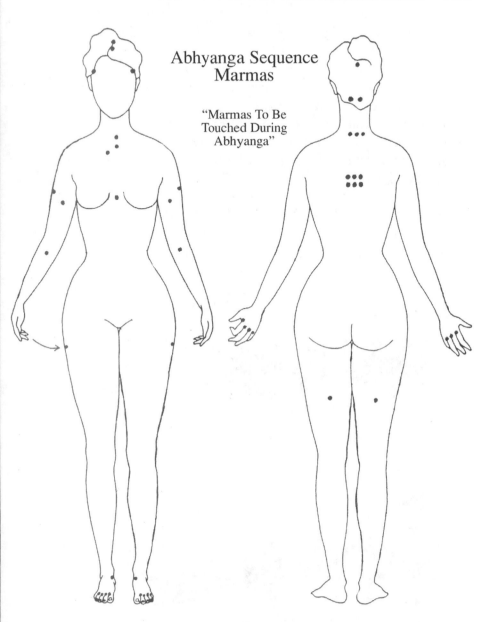

Abhyanga Sequence
Marmas

"Marmas To Be
Touched During
Abhyanga"

PHASE TWO—Work on the Head (Client On Their Back)

When your client has settled on the table, tell them the following:

"The massage I am about to give you is very deeply nurturing. It is both relaxing and dynamic and you may experience it at different levels. I'll start the massage on your head and gradually work on your neck, shoulders, face, chest, abdomen, arms, legs, and finally your back. I shall focus on your joints and muscles with massage strokes as well as touch subtle energy points on

various parts of your body. Together we have selected an oil that will bring your
subtle energies into balance.

After a short rest, I shall rub a warm, dry, herbal exfoliant over your entire
body and a cool paste to leave your skin soft and fresh. You'll then have time
for a warm shower and a refreshment.

Feel free to ask me to concentrate on certain areas or to comment at any
point. Are there any questions to start with? (pause) Let's begin . . ."

Do a centering/mindfulness process to prepare yourself to touch your
client. Then begin.

Head, Neck, Scalp and Shoulders, Face

1. Having the head turned so that the client's face is to the left and your
   left hand is cradled around the client's left ear, start the rotational
   digital kneading on the right side of the base of the skull and move to
   the forehead, using circular strokes. Do this three times on the right,
   then turn the head to the right and do the same on the left side.

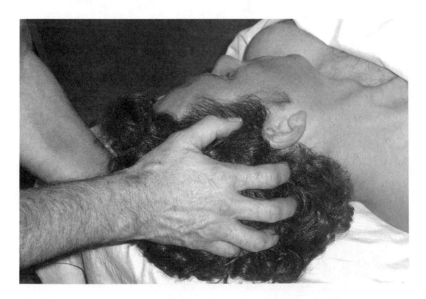

2. Hacking-style percussion is next (remember to keep your fingers
   slightly separate to ensure that the soft impact you make will have a
   powerful effect). Contra-indications to this procedure are if a person has a headache or if they have a plate in their skull.

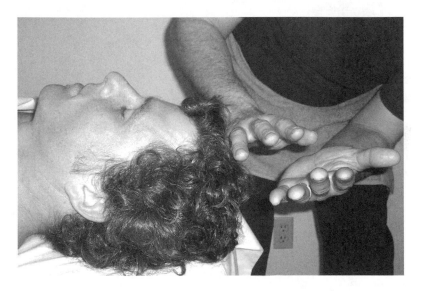

3. Reach through the scalp and gently pull the hair. Have the client breath in and as they breathe out, pull on the hair. Do this 3 times. (For men with short or no hair, place your palms on their scalp and draw the skin upward.)

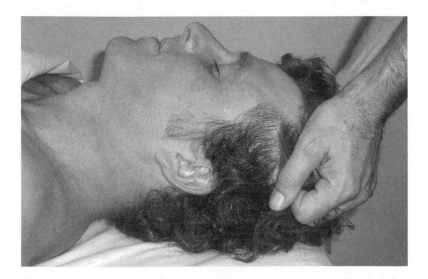

4. Next, massage the three primary head marmas—murdhi, brahma, and shiva—7 circular motions on each, 3 times in sequence.

              1 Murdhi

              2 Brahma

              3 Shiva

Side Face

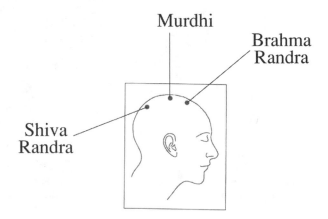

5. Roll the pinna of ears (both together), from top to bottom 3 times.

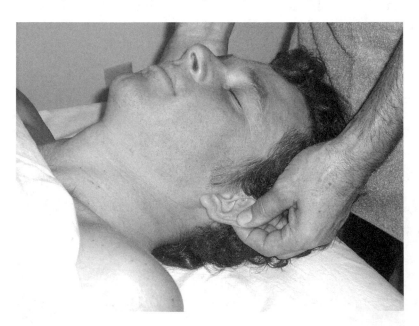

6. Next, massage the Karna marma points in 7 clockwise rotations, 3 times.

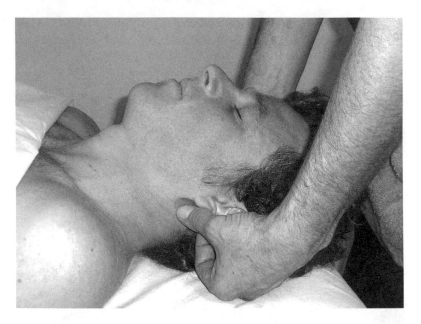

7. Turn the head to the left as in step "1" and apply friction downwards along the right side of the neck and shoulder 3 times.

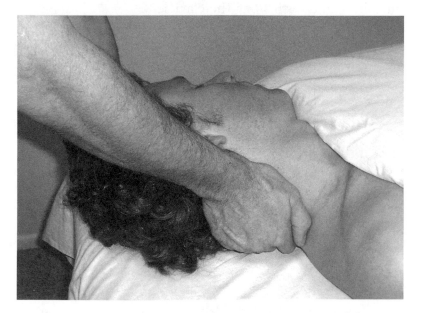

8. Knead the right side of the neck, starting at the base of the skull and working down over the shoulder. Repeat twice for a total of three times.

9. Using your hand in a fist, knead along the right side of the brachial plexus and along the back of the shoulder.

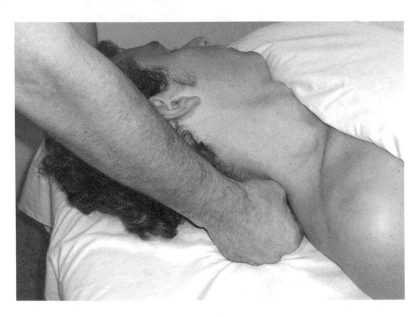

10. Chuck back and forth along the clavicle

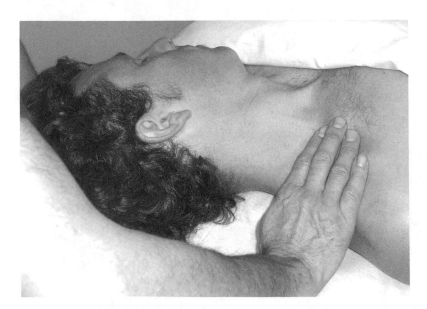

11. Apply thorough friction over the shoulder joint, using the fingers to build up heat and drive the oil deeper.

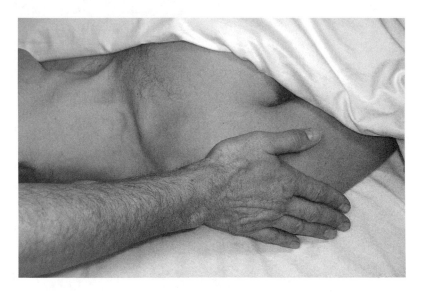

12. Then apply friction from the side of the neck down over the shoulder. Do this a total of three times.

13. Cross stretch—with your left hand on the base of the skull and your right hand on the top of the shoulder, have the person breathe in and as they breathe out, stretch. Do this three times.

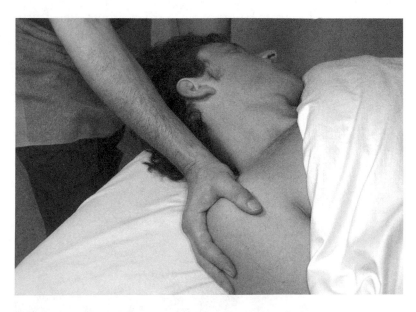

14. Press into the *ansa* marma in the hollow of the acromium process. Do seven rotations three times (helps release tension in shoulder and arm).

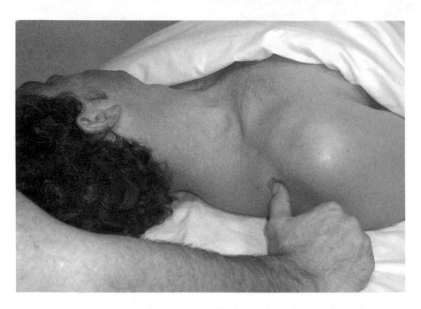

15. (Repeat '7' through '14' on left side)

16. Massage the client's face using a dosha-appropriate face oil:

    a) Three strokes from the mid-line out starting on the chin and moving towards jaw joint. On the last time, do seven clockwise rotations on the TMJ.

    b) Three strokes from below the mouth moving towards jaw joint. On the last time, do seven clockwise rotations on the TMJ .

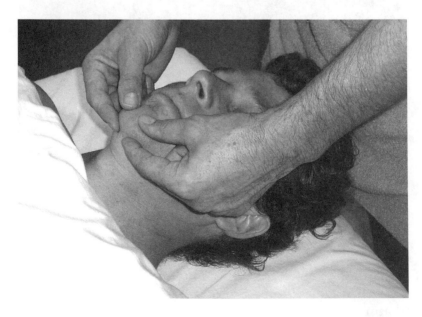

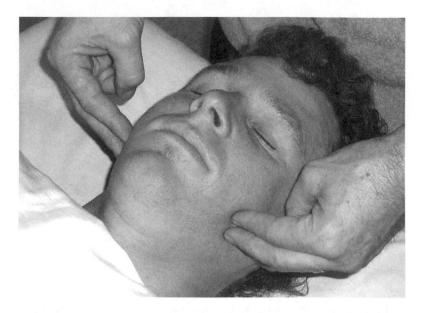

c) Three strokes from above the top lip to the TMJ. As before, do seven rotationson the last stroke.

d) Three thumb strokes along the nose and along the crease to the sides of the mouth.

e) Three strokes from under the eyes to the cheeks, ending with seven clockwise rotations on the TMJ after the last stroke.

f) Smooth out the forehead with your palms. Do this seven times.

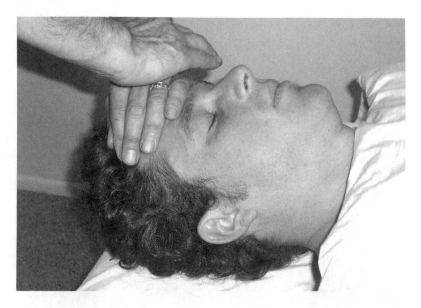

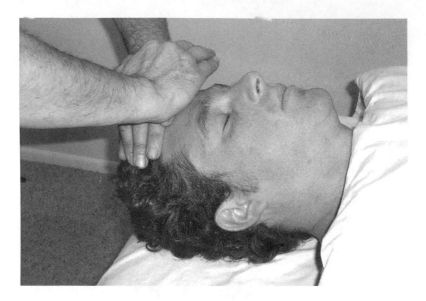

g) Do seven clockwise rotations on the Shankar marma—at the temple 3 times, then hold—thinking good thoughts. (You want to imagine a place that represents a state of being that supports each client. You could send them a good wish, a prayer, or use the following ideas for relaxing places for each. For the VATA client, think of a place that is warm, cozy, and secure. For the PITTA client, think of a green open space where there is a fresh breeze. For the KAPHA client, think of a sunny, exotic place with beautiful birds and interesting things to see.)

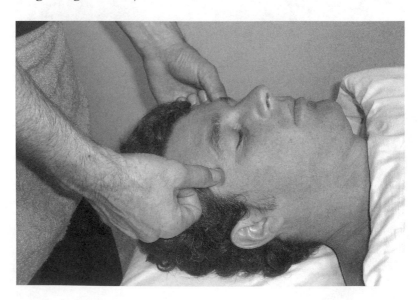

h) Apply circular friction on the cervical vertebrae, starting at the 7th and finishing at base of skull with mild traction. Repeat twice more for a total of three times.

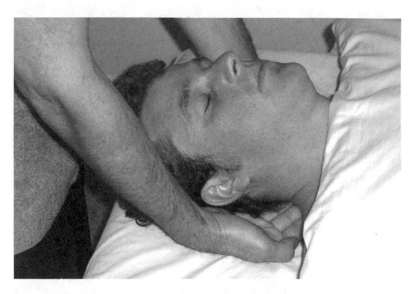

(Or, as an option, raise the head toward the chest as the client breathes out, then turn the head to the right for a deep breath in and out, then the same on the left side.)

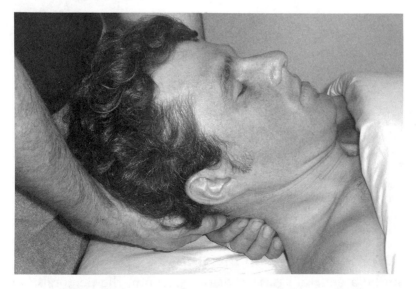

17. At the end of the head, neck, and shoulder massage, hold the 2 *krikatika* marmas (either side of the spine where it enters the skull)

until there is a sense of balance (weight, pulsation, temperature, imaged color).

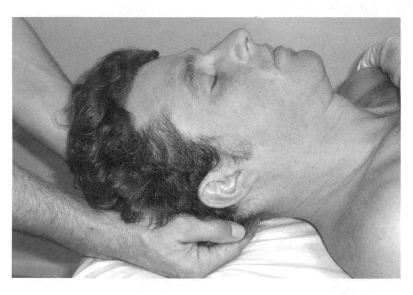

18. Place the Head and Neck Pillow under the bottom sheet for head support.

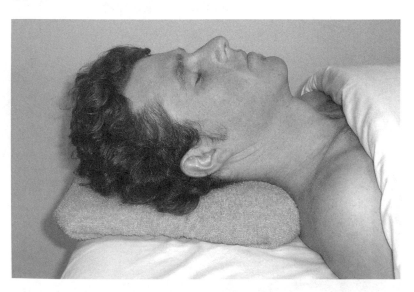

PHASE THREE—Work on the Chest

This can be a general massage of the sternum, the pectorals, and the sternum *or* it can be the Ayurvedic Breast Massage Protocol. Ask the client at this time which they would prefer.

For your female clients, to find out whether or not you will need to keep the chest and breast area partially draped at this time, say to them something like, *"I am now going to massage your chest area. Would you feel comfortable if I worked on you undraped or would you prefer to be partially covered?"*

1. The general chest massage

a) Standing to the client's side, stroke down the right, then left, side of the neck to the clavicle, on either side of the sternal notch. This is going from KARNA to ARSHAK marmas. As you come to the arshak marma, press on this point with clockwise circular motions seven times. Go from karna to arshak in this manner 3 times.

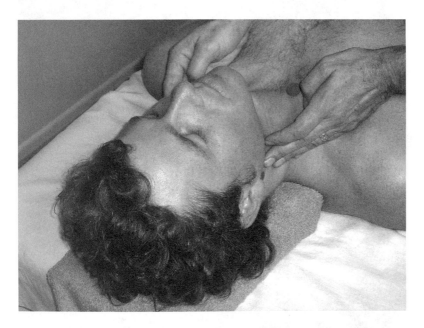

b) With your four fingers on both clavicles, press down from the upper edge of the clavicle, towards the feet. Work from the center out to the edge of the shoulders in an alternating fashion.

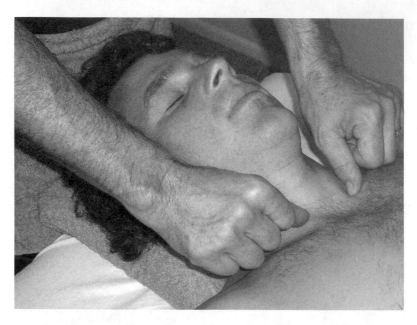

c) Pinch the upper and lower sides of the clavicle in a similar fashion as in 'b'.

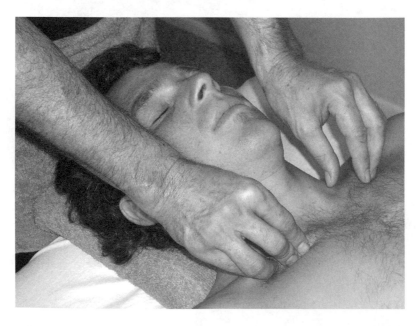

d) Do strokes from the sternum along the upper pectorals.

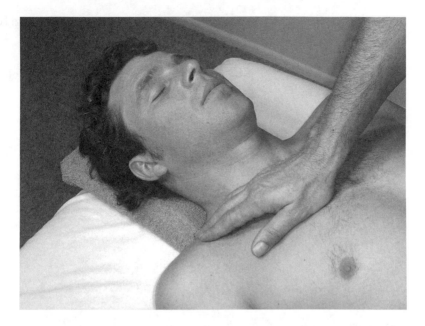

e) From the sternal notch to the xyphoid process do clockwise circular motions along the articulations of the sternum.

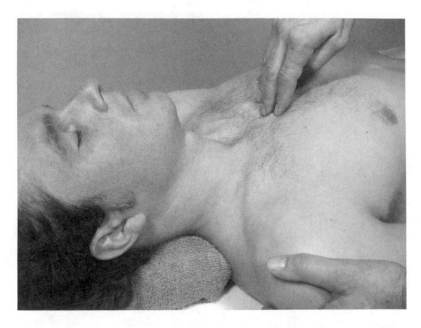

f) Starting on the client's right side, apply digital friction from the sides of the body along the ribs towards the sternum. Follow this with a pulling motion from the side of the body towards the midline. Pull from the sides of the ribs towards the sternum. Be sure to also go over the pectorals towards the sternum as well.

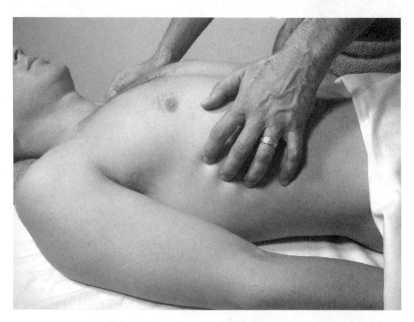

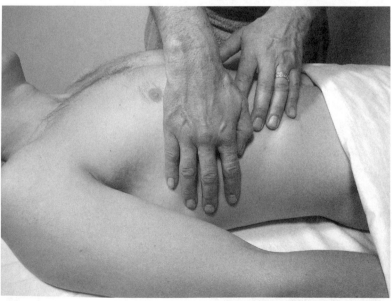

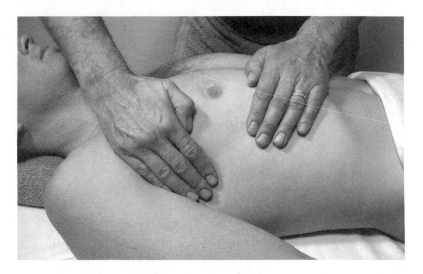

e) Perform 7 clockwise rotational circles on the upper HRI-DAYAM marma, approximately 3 fingerwidths below the sternal notch as the sternum begins to climb. Do this 3 times.

f) Touch the APASTHAMBHA marma (on right side only), which is approx. 4cm or 1.5 inches down the sternum from the up-per HRIDAYAM point and to the right in the intercostals space in the upper and inner quadrant of the breast area. Do 7 clockwise rotations, 3 times.

g) Do 7 clockwise rotations on the mid-point of the sternum (HRIDAYAM--an anxiety reducing marma).

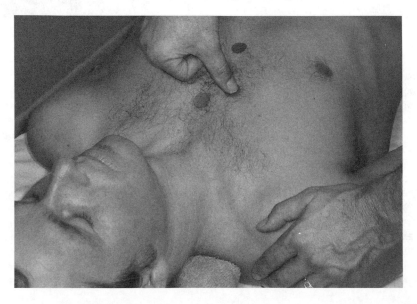

h) Keeping the right thumb or three fingers on HRIDAYAM marma, place your left hand on the forehead. Feel a sense of balance, take the hand off the forehead, then off the center of the chest.

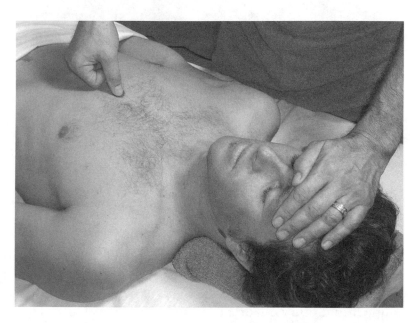

If the client consents to a breast massage, use the following protocol.

Ayurvedic Breast Massage Protocol

Using Shatavari Ghee or Pomegranate Oil
The Technique—Ayurvedic Breast Massage

Ayurvedic massage for women has always included extensive work on the breast area. This is done not only as a means to beautify the breast, encourage a delightful shape, and for greater comfort, but also for deeper therapeutic reasons. Ayurveda, like a number of oriental healing traditions, teaches that massage over and around breast tissue improves or helps maintain health in all parts of female reproductive tissue as well as assisting with hormonal balancing.

Like many Ayurvedic massage techniques, this breast-touching technique relies on a combination of modalities; the use of herbal oil, stimulation of marma points, and gentle strokes. The traditional oils most beneficial for the breasts are either Pomegranate Oil or Shatavari Ghee. Most women we have worked with prefer the Pomegranate Oil with its thick, slightly stimulating warmth and light sensuous aroma of amber—an Indian essential oil blend traditionally used on breast tissue. Along with the marma points, the massage strokes one uses are applied as strongly as one would pet a cat and are intended to activate the lymphatic system. Together, the points and strokes on the breast tissue itself help mobilize toxins, fats, and the collection of excess subtle energies and hormones which are then carried away via the lymph system, allowing for increased blood flow with fresh nutrients to revitalize the breast tissue. Strokes around the breasts, on the neck and above, below, and to the sides of the breasts further support this action. My own experience (corroborated by friends and clients) tells me that this technique helps my breasts feel more comfortable, look more beautiful, and gives me a calm confidence and a feeling of liking myself as a woman. Before you begin, tell the client exactly where and how they are going to be touched.

Because this can be a highly emotionally charged area to work on, it is important that your client is able to see you and that you keep both hands on the body so that they feel re-assured and in control.

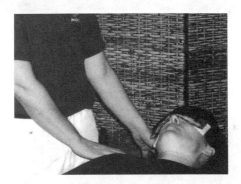

1. Turn the client's head slightly to the left and place the right hand over the region behind the right earlobe. Touch the marma called KARNA just behind the ear lobe, moving in little clockwise circles five times. Then stroke down the right side of the neck to the point (ARSHAK) on the top surface of the right collar bone where it joins the breast bone, applying light rotational pressure to this ending point. Repeat four more times. Now turn the head to the right and repeat the same procedure on the left side using the left hand.

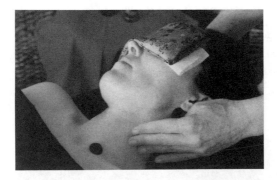

2. Turn the client's head slightly to the left, and use the right thumb to press down toward the client's toes, working along the top surface of the right collar bone from the breast bone out to the tip of the right shoulder. Repeat twice more, then turn the head to the right and repeat the same touch technique on the left side. If your client is pregnant, apply this technique using very gentle touch especially at the shoulder tips.

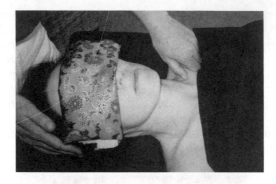

3. *Again working on first the right side then the left use the flat of your thumb to apply clockwise rotational pressure in the hollow space behind the collar bone, starting again from the breast bone and moving up along the tops of the shoulders. This helps the body relax and combats fatigue. The looser we keep our shoulders the less likely we are to pick up any "problems' physically or mentally.*

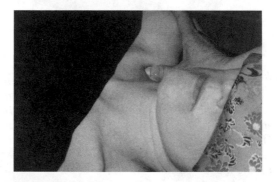

4. *Starting under the right arm, press gently into the deep hollow of the armpit and apply clockwise rotational pressure into the APALAPA marma. For greater client comfort support the arm at the elbow. Do this 3, 5, or 7 times. Repeat on the left side. This point activates the lymphatic system in the upper torso and releases tension around the shoulders and arms.*

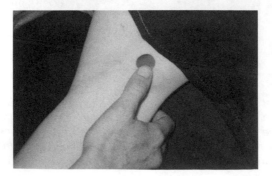

In our photos we have undraped the client so you can see the points more clearly. Normally, you can touch each of these points over the sheets.

5. *Touch the point four fingerwidths below the top of the breast bone, approximately 1.5 inches below the sternal angle. Press and release this point (upper HRIDAYAM marma) in a gentle, pumping action 3, 5, or 7 times using your index or middle finger. This point allows us to more joyfully connect with our body and the world around us.*

6. *In the same way you touched HRIDAYAM in step 5, find the point that is approximately one and a half inches below and to the right of HRIDAYAM. This point, known as APASTAMBHA marma, balances energy in the lungs and helps the body let go of grief and sadness, emotions which are often stronger in clients that have issues concerning breast tissue.*

7. *Locate a point that is midway on the sternum, roughly at the level of the nipples. Apply gentle clockwise rotational pressure to this marma, also known as HRIDAYAM, and then proceed down the remainder of the sternum with circular massage strokes. This helps to alleviate depression.*

The picture shows the third of these three points being touched.

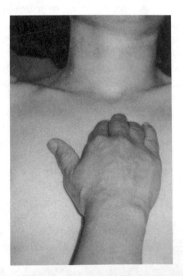

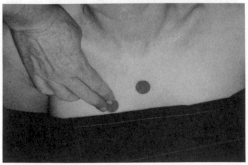

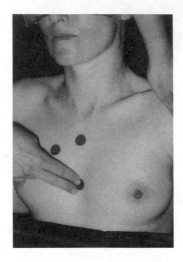

8. Using ½ teaspoon of Pomegranate Oil or Shatavari Ghee per breast use your right hand to apply the oil on the right then the left breast.

9. Stroke over the topside of the breast with flat of your hand, moving from the breast bone towards the armpit, using the pressure you would use to pet a cat. Repeat four more strokes. Next stroke similarly this time under the breast, as before ending the stroke in the deepest part of the armpit. Again five strokes total. Be sure to touch every part of the breast. Pay particular attention to the outer upper quadrant of each breast as this is the most common area for problems to arise. ***Remember to end each stroke at the armpit.*** *Stroke five times over, then five times under the breast. Repeat on the left side using your left hand. Arrange the sheets to expose one breast at a time. Stand at the corner of the table and support the arm at the elbow to avoid discomfort in the shoulder.*

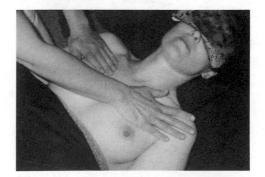

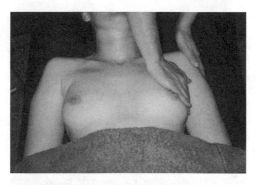

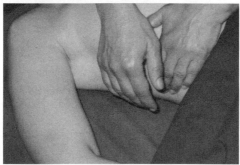

10. *Do twenty-one strokes in a figure eight pattern over the breast tissue itself follow-ing the pattern of the infinity symbol—this is done by starting in the middle of the chest, moving up and over the right breast, down and around and under the right breast, then up and over the left breast, down and around and under the left breast coming back to the middle of the chest. Keep your own shoulders relaxed and project positive thoughts towards your client. The movement should cover the outer portion of the breast and the tissues just slightly above, below, and to the sides of each breast. Allow the movement to get gradually smaller, working towards the nipples so the whole surface of the breast is touched. Massage to the area directly below the breasts stimulates blood circulation. Massage to the portion of the breasts below the nipple increases sensuousness and a sense of self-confidence. All in all, this step helps maintain a pleasant shape to the breasts.*

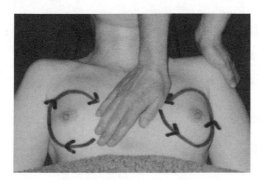

11. *Pull the nipples, using gentle pressure between the thumb and index fingers. Nipple stimulation excites the finest capillaries and lymph tissue in this area of the breasts. If you don't feel comfortable with this step tell the client this is something they should do for themselves at home.*
12. *Repeat the massage of APALAPA marmas as in step 4 to work gently into the deepest part of the armpit.*

TO CLOSE—Rest your left hand on the top of the client's head and the fingertips of the right hand in the middle of the chest. Let your hands and mind rest there for a minute to end the treatment.

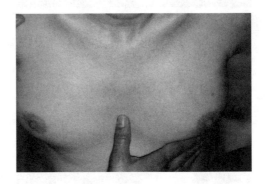

Cover the breast area and shoulders with a towel.

PHASE FOUR—Work on the Abdomen

The abdominal massage is often an area not addressed in conventional massage. Here is a simple protocol that is a standard part of this abhyanga, but can also be done on its own. It is not possible to offer Ayurvedic massage that does not have some work done on the abdomen. The benefits are that circulation is increased into the large intestine, hence encouraging toxins in the blood to accumulate for elimination. Furthermore, the colon is the seat of Vata. Thus excess Vata in the body is attracted to the colon more easily and creates a deeper sense of balance and calm in the client.

CONTRAINDICATIONS: Some people will just not feel comfortable receiving an abdominal massage. Once you have explained the benefits, most people will be willing to go along with it. In fact, from that point on, they will probably always want you to do it. At the same time, if they do not want one, one can alternatively place a Tummy

Warmer or hot water bottle on the abdomen to ensure that a rich supply of blood is moving to the abdomen for the purpose of detoxification.

Other contraindications may be if they have a heavy menses, are pregnant, or have some medical condition where moving the abdominal organs and muscles would cause discomfort. Then again, ask. Some women feel that abdominal work helps their menses. A modified version of what is offered here can feel wonderful for someone who is pregnant. Even medical conditions may be benefited when this treatment is done. *Tune in and trust yourself.*

To perform this abdominal massage, **have your client bend their knees** so as to soften the tummy and allow for deeper benefits. If they need additional support, you may put a bolster underneath their knees.

1. Place warm oil in your palms, gently pour into client's navel, and spread the oil in an outward, clockwise circular motion from there.
2. Rolling, using the heels of the palms and the fingers, pushing from the right side of the abdomen with your palms and pulling back towards yourself on the left side of the abdomen with your fingertips.

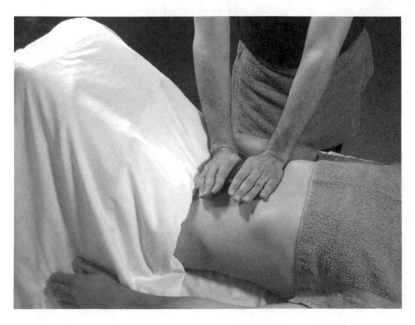

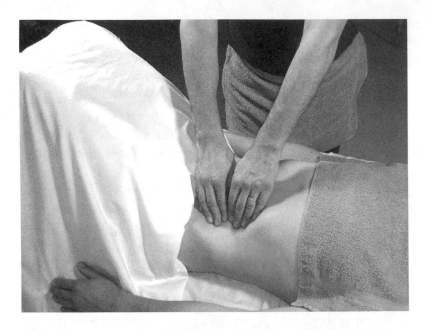

3. Circular kneading in clockwise strokes around navel region.

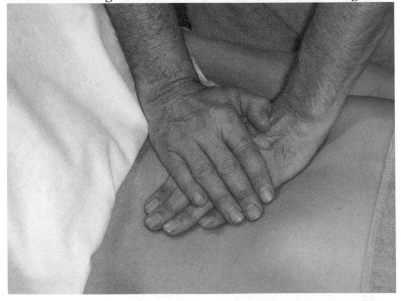

4. Circular strokes with the palms and fingertips, which go deeper and deeper, done in a clockwise motion around the abdomen. This is the main stroke to be done continuously. Do this for a minimum of 3 minutes. This may seem monotonous, but it is very soothing to Vata and takes the client very deep.

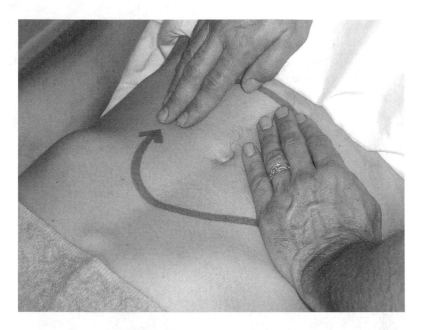

5. Repeat rolling as in "2".
6. Place your thumb at a point about 3 fingerwidths below the navel. Have the client breathe in and when you tell them to breathe out sink your thumb into this point until you meet resistance and do seven clockwise rotations. As they breathe in, lift off the pressure and as they breathe out, go in again. Do this a total of three times.

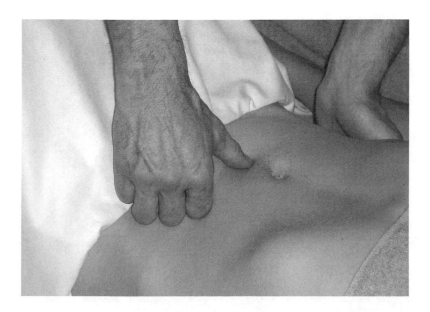

7. Finish with a polarity hold where left hand is under the lower back and the right hand is just below the navel. Hold for a sense of balance. Remove the hand underneath the back and place this hand on top of the right hand (still resting on the abdomen). Then, lift both hands from the abdomen.

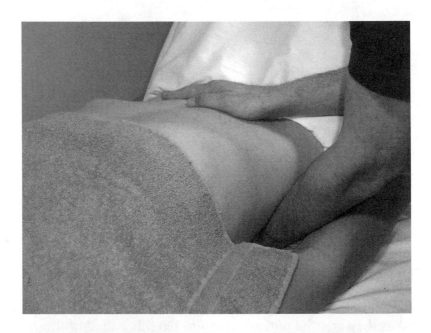

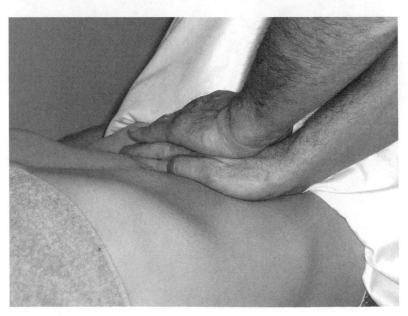

8. Cover abdomen. Ask the client if they would like a *tummy warmer*. If they do, apply the *tummy warmer*.

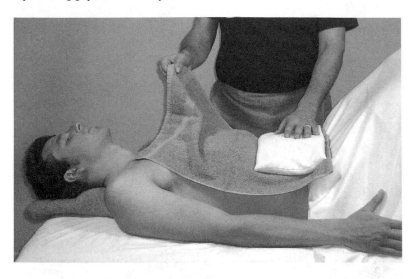

Client may lower their legs if they wish.

PHASE FIVE—Work on the Arms

1. Starting with the right arm first, spread oil over the arm, starting at the shoulder and spread and coat down to the fingertips.
2. Use friction strokes on the front and then the back of the arm working from the wrist to the armpit or over the shoulder. Stroke 3 times on the front, then 3 on the back.
3. Digital kneading of fingers, starting with thumb—do each finger thoroughly 1 time.

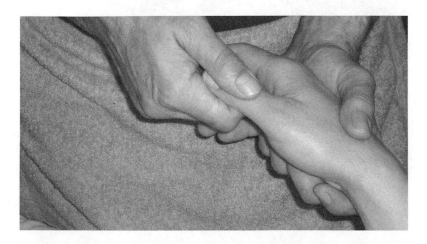

4. Marmas in webs of fingers, starting between thumb and index finger, 7 rotations each, 3 times in sequence.

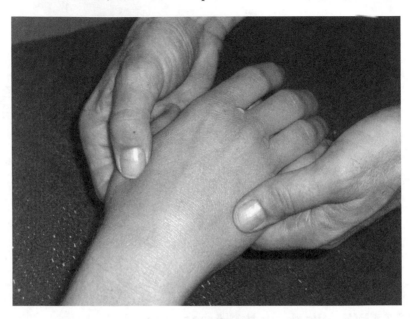

5. Spread the fingers and massage the palm.

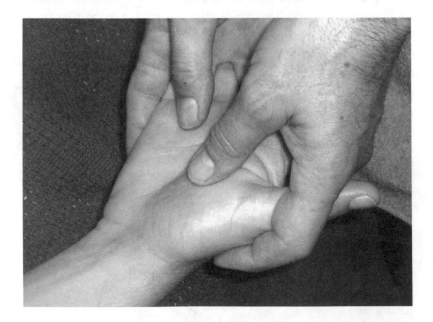

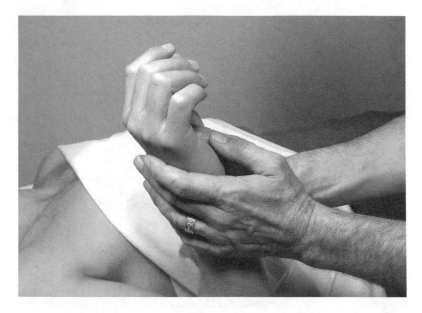

6. Use an 'Indian rope burn' style of friction over the wrist to drive the oil in. Then, press with 7 rotations, three times, the Vata marma in the 'anatomical snuff box.' This marma is excellent for headaches as well as jetlag and stress from travel.

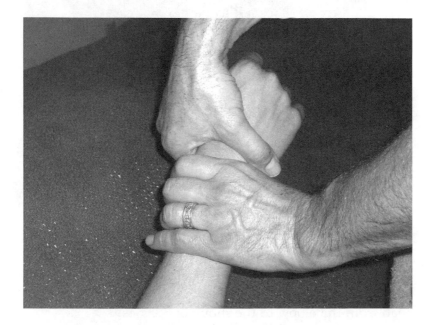

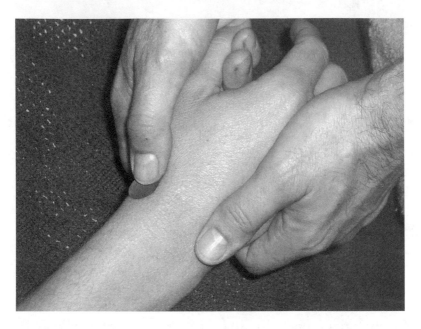

7. Knead from the wrist to the elbow 3 times. Drive the oil into the entire elbow joint.

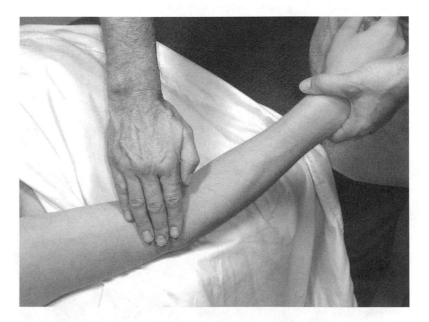

8. Knead from the elbow to the shoulder 3 times.
9. Apply friction up the arm 3 times.

10. Light meridian stroking, down the front of the arm from the shoulder to the palm and up the arm from the back of the hand to the shoulder 7 times.
    (Refer to Meridian Stroking Diagram found at the beginning of this chapter on page . . .)

11. 3 marma points in sequence, center of anterior forearm or INDRA-BASTI (for improving digestive fire and blood quality), middle of bicep or URVI (for improving water metabolism, plasma health, and healthy tissue growth), then base of deltoid (for lung health), 7 rotations, 3 times.

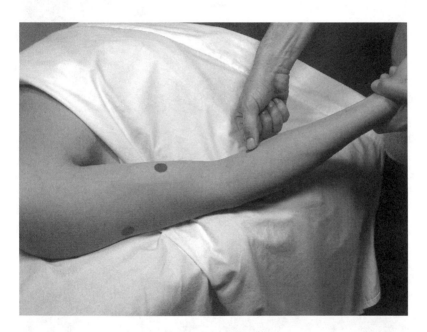

12. Armpit Marma—This is the deepest marma point in the body. It is excellent for activating the movement of lymph. It is also a vital point in helping to clear the breast tissue in the Ayurvedic Breast Massage. With fingers resting on the shoulder, have your thumb drop into the armpit (to make this even more comfortable, you can place a cotton pad on the tip of your thumb and then press this into the armpit). Ask the client to breathe in and as they breathe out drop your wrist and allow your thumb to go deep into the armpit. Do 7 clockwise rotations. As they breathe in lift the thumb pressure and as they breathe out, repeat. Do this three times.

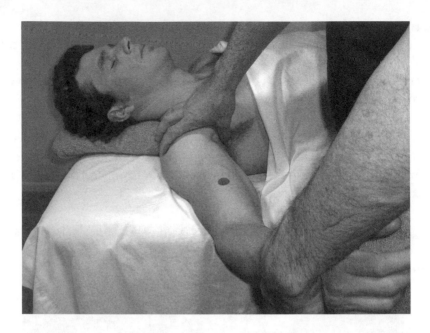

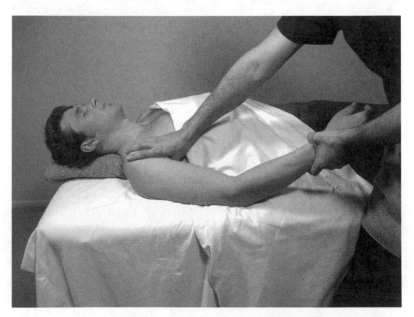

PHASE SIX—Work on Front of the Legs

1. While applying oil, use friction strokes with the flat of your hand up the front of the leg, right side first. Repeat strokes 3 times.
2. On the right foot, digitally knead the toes thoroughly, starting with the big toe. Do this only once.

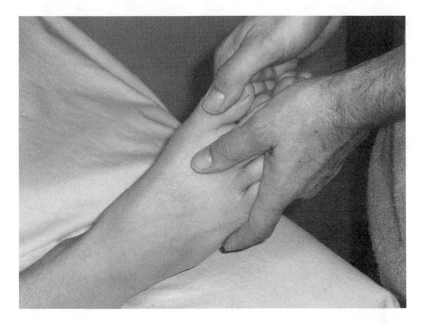

3. Massage the marmas in the webs between the toes. Do 7 rotations 3 times.

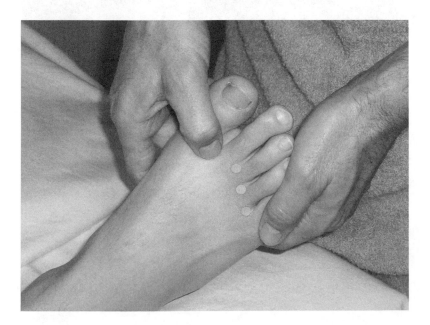

4. Generally knead and stretch the entire foot. Reach your fingers between the toes to spread them.

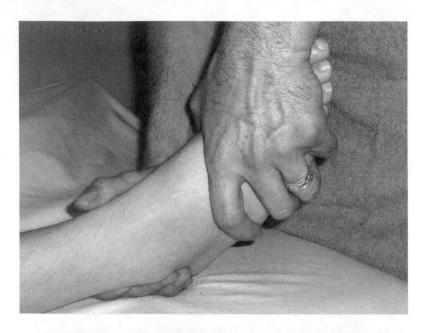

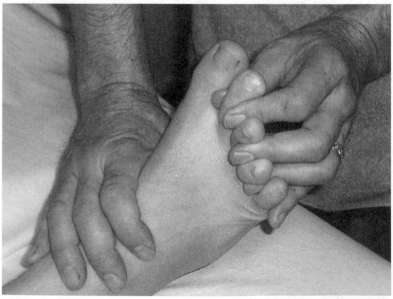

5. 'Indian rope burn' style friction around the ankle to drive in the oil.

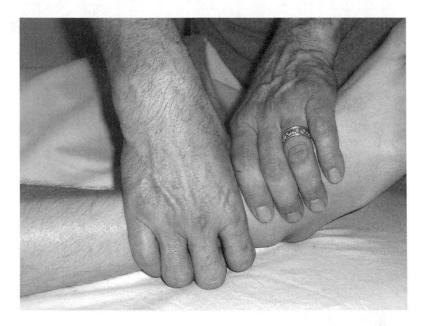

6. Knuckle or palm-knead from the ankle to the knee 3 times.

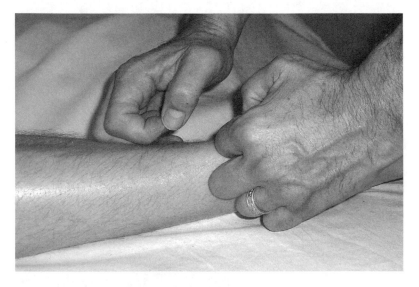

7. Apply circular friction around the entire knee joint.

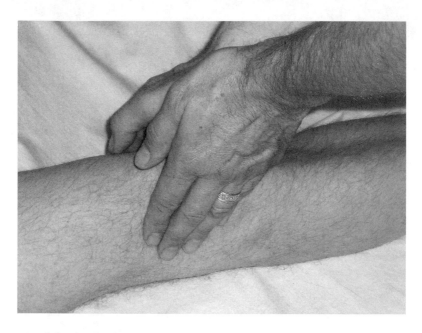

8. Knead from the knee to just below the groin 3 times.

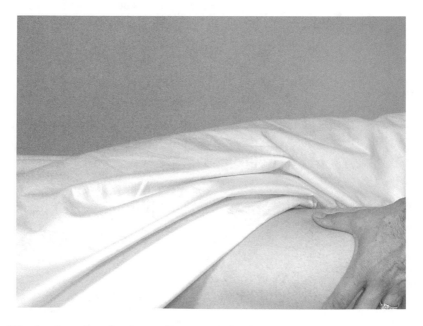

9. Clockwise circular kneading into the hip joint 21 times.

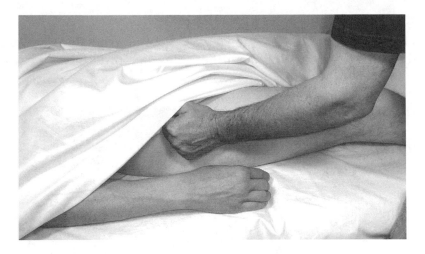

10. Apply friction from the foot up the entire leg 3 times.

11. Meridian stroking lightly up the inside of the leg and down the outside 7 times.
    (Refer to Meridian Stroking Diagram found at the beginning of this chapter on page . . .)

12. Locate the vata marma point on outside of the upper leg by having your client bring their arm down to their side. Where their middle finger touches their thigh is where this marma is located. (Excellent for leg health in general, and for easing colon congestion.) Have the person breathe in and as they breathe out, apply clockwise rotational pressure 7 times. Repeat 3 times.

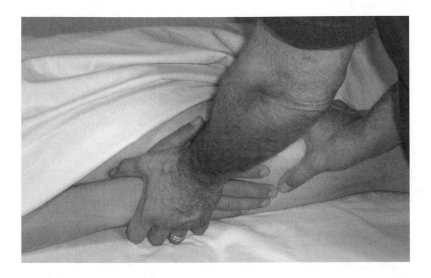

13. REPEAT '2' through '12' ON LEFT SIDE

14. Hold the marma that is midway between the medial malleolus and the edge of the heel on both feet. The therapist comes away only after there is a sense of balance.

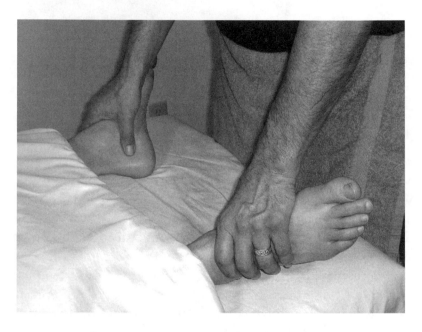

*Remove the tummy warmer and the head and neck pillow
and have the client turn over onto their stomach.*

At this point, your client may need to relieve their bladder and may also want something to drink. If they want a drink, offer them a small sip of room temperature water, just enough to relieve thirst.

PHASE SEVEN—Work on the Back of the Legs

1. Apply warm oil from the buttocks down toward the heel, right leg first.
2. Use friction strokes to work oil into the back of the legs from ankle to buttock. Repeat 3 times.
3. Stretch and loosen the foot, then apply compression to the heels, followed by press and release techniques.

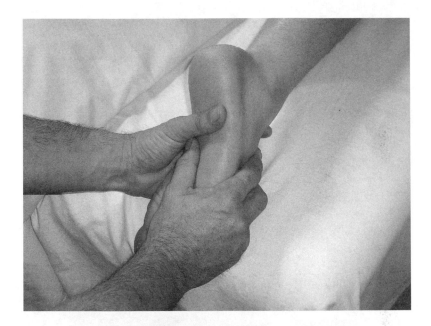

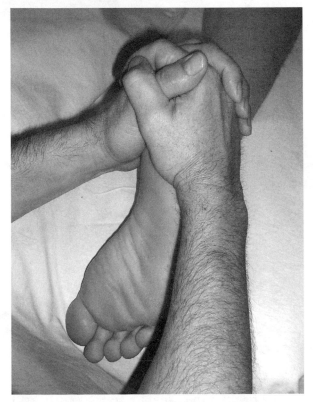

4. Apply friction all along the back of the ankle joint.

5. Knead from the ankle up to the back of the knee 3 times.

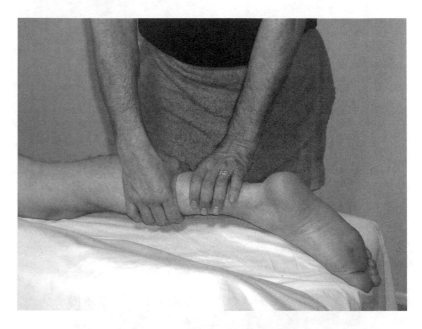

6. Knead thoroughly around the back of the knee.

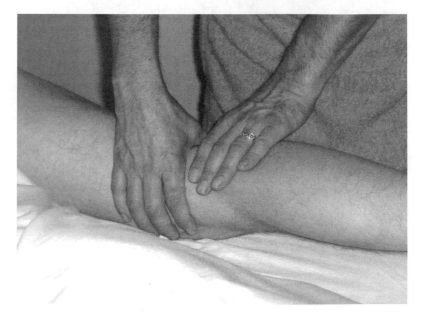

7. Knead from the back of the knee up to the buttocks 3 times.

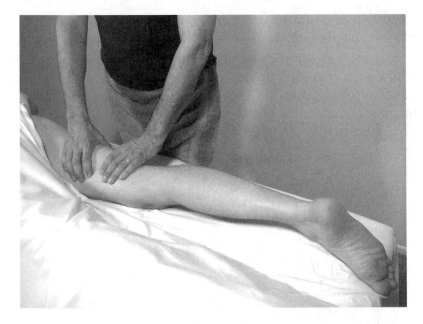

8. Do clockwise circular kneading of the gluteal muscles of the buttocks deeply 21 times.

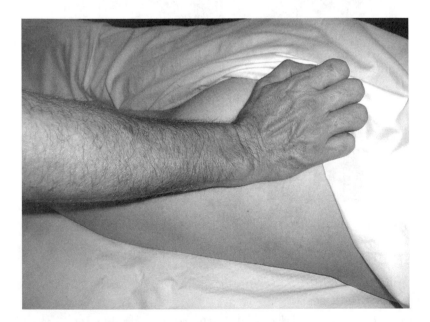

9. Repeat friction as done earlier in '2'.
10. Light meridian stroking from the buttocks down to the heels, then to the toes 7 times.

(Refer to Meridian Stroking Diagram found at the beginning of this chapter on page . . .)

11. Locate the vata marma point in middle of the back upper leg on the hamstrings, midway between the crease of the back of the knee and the base of the buttocks. Have the client breathe in and as they breathe out press deep into this point with 7 clockwise rotational movements. As they breathe in, lift up and then repeat. Do this 3 times.

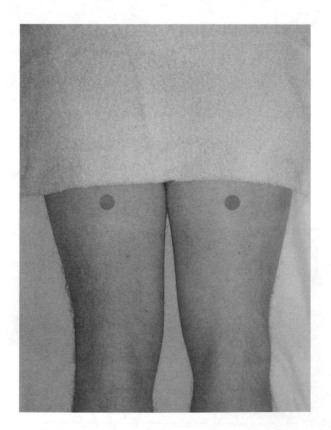

12. REPEAT '2' through '11' ON LEFT LEG.

PHASE EIGHT—Work on the Back

1. Apply warm oil from the shoulders down towards and over the buttocks.
2. Start at the base of the back with friction strokes using the flat of the hand to work up the back. Repeat 7 times, starting on right, then left side of back.

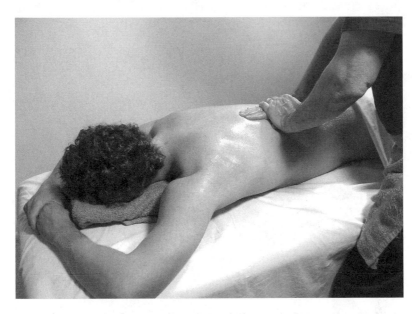

3. Hacking up and down along spine (ask client first if they have any problem areas/discs on the spine—skip over these areas).

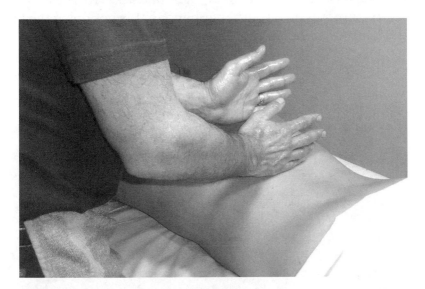

4. Center, right, then left marmas of the spine at C7 (for Vata), T5 (for *prana*, the vital force within the breath and the subtle aspect of Vata), and T6 (for the heart), using 7 rotational pressure movements on each point. Do this 3 times, from C7 down. The points to the right and left of the spinous process (middle point) are about ¾ inch away (traditionally, the length of the first articulation of the client's index finger).

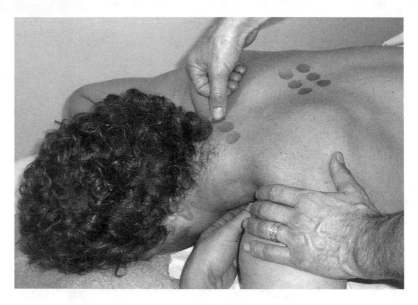

5. Knead in circles up and away from the spine, moving towards the top of the shoulders. Work all around the scapula. Repeat 3 times.

6. Knead down along the side of the right buttocks (REMEMBER: for polarity purposes, rest your other hand that is not doing the kneading on your client's opposite shoulder).

7. Start on the side of the right buttock and draw from lateral to medial towards the spine, moving up to and over the shoulder. Do this several times.

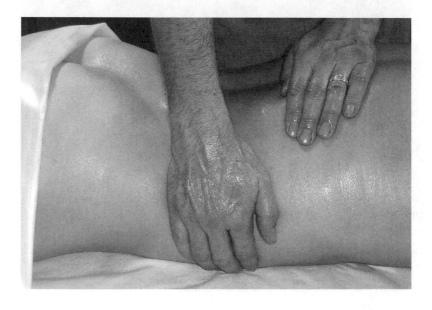

8. Repeat last three steps ('5' through '7') on left side.
9. Apply friction up both sides of spine 3 times.
10. Meridian stroking down spine 7 times.
    (Refer to Meridian Stroking Diagram found at the beginning of this chapter on page . . .)
11. Rest one hand on the back of the base of the skull and the other on the top of the sacrum and hold until there is a sense of balance. (A special visualization you can do here is to imagine that there is a column of deep sapphire blue light between your two hands along your client's spine. In meditation, sometimes it is visualized that the deep blue column of the central spiritual channel runs anterior to the spine. Here, just try to see a deep blue column and if there are any areas of lightness or discoloration in that deep blue column. Imagine that deep blue healing light is coming through your hands and into the body. See in your mind's eye that you are filling in the color so that the entire color of the column is radiantly blue. When you have accomplished this, go on with the instructions as indicated next.) Take your left hand off the back of the client's head first and rest it on top of the right hand. Then breathe in and remove both hands together.

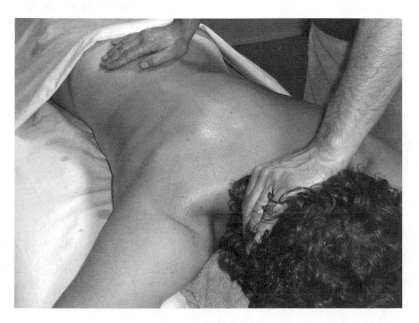

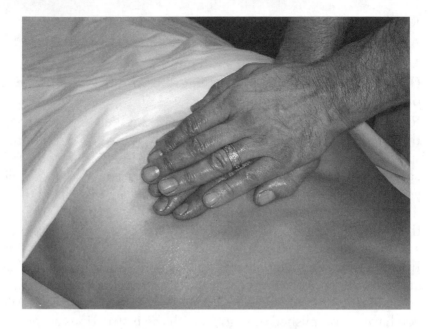

Cover the client thoroughly to keep them warm.
You may also place a tummy warmer on the small of their back
to provide additional heat and allow them to rest for 5 minutes.

This may also be a time that you give a form of hydrotherapy such as sauna (Kapha) or steam room or cabinet for Vata or Pitta. If you have a client with more Pitta symptoms, give them a cool towel or cloth to wrap or cover their head with. Once they have done this for 10 minutes, return them to the table and have them rest covered for an additional 5 minutes.

(NOTE: This will increase your treatment time to 1.75 hours)

PHASE NINE—Apply Ubtan

If a tummy warmer was on the back, remove it now.

1. Uncover the back and apply warmed ubtan to the whole back surface in the following order: Back, back of right leg, back of left leg, (Have the person turn over), front of right leg, front of left leg, abdomen, chest, right arm, then left arm. **Throughout, make sure that your client feels appropriately draped** and at the end make sure the body is completely covered again.

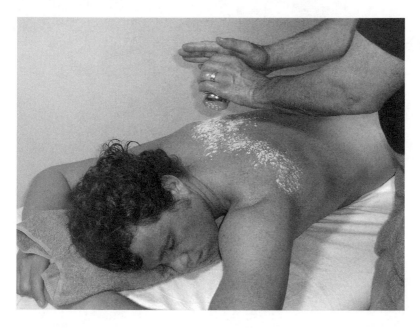

2. Mix a little of the ubtan with milk, cool herb tea, or cool water. (NOTE: Tell your client that the mixture that you are about to apply will feel a bit cool.) Apply to the face with your fingertips, using the same stroke order as that used for the face massage portion. (If the client is Vata based on your initial diagnostic assessment, you may want to use warm to hot water, tea or milk.)

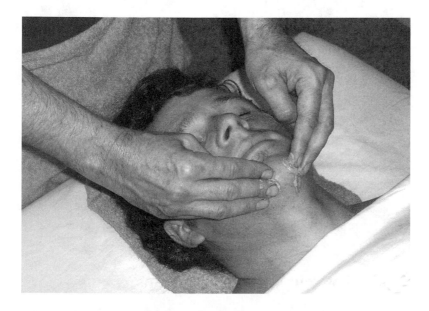

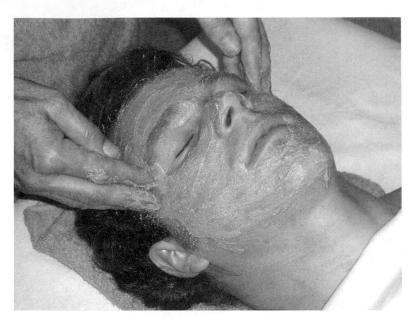

3. Place finger tips either side of the spine where it goes into the skull (*krikatika* marma). Hold until there is a sense of balance, then come away.

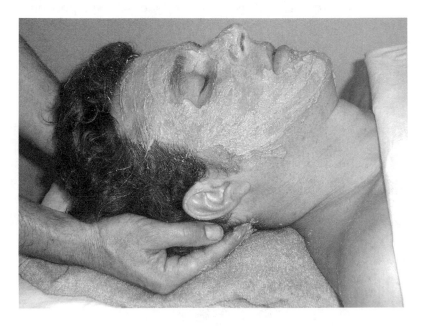

Allow your client to rest for five minutes.

PHASE TEN—Hair Care/Shower/Refreshment

If you do not have a shower available, you can use warm towels, either dry or moist, to remove the ubtan and extra oils from the client's body. Encourage them to go home and shower within a few hours.

If you have a shower available, be sure that the shower area has adequate natural soap and shampoos. There are even excellent Ayurvedic herbal hair washes available. In any event, guide your client to a shower.

When they are dressed, offer them refreshment consisting of a dosha appropriate herbal tea, lemon and little fresh fruit. For other ideas, see the "Recipe" section of the book.

■ *Tibetan Shirodhara Sequence*

Shirodhara is probably the most sought after Ayurvedic treatment in the spa and beauty industry. Specifically, it is the pouring of a fine stream of oil onto the forehead or the crown of the head for a period of time. In short sessions, it facilitates the release of serotonin and can lead a client into deep relaxation, and for some, psycho-spiritual experiences. For that reason, Tibetans call it psycho-spiritual massage. Within the context of Ayurvedic medicine, Shirodhara done for long periods of time and with great frequency can have profound effects on the Vata dosha, specifically in treating any number of neurological and psychological conditions.

What follows is a specific treatment ritual that we see have excellent results for the spa environment. Each phase of the ritual is a treatment unto itself. They can be used together as suggested, used separately, or combined with other treatments. **The shirodhara itself, which is the last phase in this particular treatment ritual we suggest should be the last or final phase or treatment offered if a series of treatments is offered. And nothing else should be done when the oil is pouring onto the head.**

This sequence involves bringing together four Tibetan massage protocols in a seamless rhythm that will lead your client into a very peaceful and profoundly deep state of relaxed awareness.

The sequence starts with a simple touch test on three points near the back of the neck to discover which dosha, or body energy, is most in need of balance at the time of treatment. One of three delightful essential oil massage blends is then selected and the treatment begins.

Phase One is the Tibetan Psychological Stress Series as taught by Dr. Lobsang Rapgay. This a gentle anointing of twelve marma, or vital energy, points with essential oils to begin the process of deeply calming the mind and feeling more present on both the mental and physical level. **This Tibetan marma sequence is an excellent beginning for almost any treatment you are offering. It helps to calm any distraction or agitation in the mind of your client, making it much easier to go deeper and be more effective with whatever treatment comes next. As a result, you will get better results with less effort.**

Phase Two is an abdominal massage. Warm scented oil is poured into the navel and then gently and rhythmically massaged into the belly to physically nurture and calm the body.

Phase Three is the Tibetan Eye Rejuvenation Sequence, a spa version of what was taught to us, again, by Dr. Lobsang Rapgay. A "cool eyes" eye pillow coaxes the eyes to rest and relax as the feet are massaged with anise lotion and the hands are massaged with essential oils. The feet are then cleaned with rose powder and warmed on hot clay stones.

This is a wonderful treatment just by itself. Spas in the US offer this as a thirty to forty-five minute service at lunch time for secretaries and others who spend a lot of time in front of computer screens. Although the emphasis of the treatment is on the feet, the drawing of the winds of Vata downwards away from the face whilesimultaneously stimulating the eye reflexes of the feet relaxes the face and helps to re-hydrate the eyes. It is a very safe treatment to offer and is sometimes an excellent substitute for Netra Basti. It can also be taught to clients so they can do it at home. This will be evident when you see how simple a protocol it can be.

Finally, in Phase Four, a continuous fine stream of warm sesame oil is poured over the

middle of the forehead for ten to twenty minutes. By stimulating the marma, or vital energy point, on the middle of the forehead with the warm oil stream, a message is released in the brain that allows the body to enjoy the experience of letting go and relaxing on the deepest level. Energies around the spine are freed which helps to calm and clear the mind. This is the Shirodhara. In Tibetan it is called 'psycho-spiritual' massage.

It is a process that demands a mindful attitude on the part of the therapist. If given in a place that feels safe, a 'sacred' space, the client will have an experience that is physically nurturing, mentally calming, and which will help them become more in touch with their inner being.

Treatment Ritual Time: 90 minutes should be booked for this entire ritual.

Suggested Menu Description

Tibetan Shirodhara

This spa ritual brings together four Tibetan massage treatments to create a seamless rhythm that will lead you into a very peaceful and profoundly deep state of relaxed awareness. Special energy points help to release mental tensions, gentle warmth and massage to the abdomen and feet settle the mind and relax the face, all of which lead into an anointing of the forehead with warm sesame oil. This deceptively simple technique of playing a fine stream of warm oil on the middle of the forehead recharges the body, brings clarity to the mind, and offers a quiet space to experience our true selves.

Environmental Considerations

Although the following recommendations could apply to any treatment that you offer, the subtle nature of shirodhara almost demands adherence to these considerations:

- The treatment room must be quiet with as little foot traffic as possible moving past the door.
- As a therapist, you must be able to sit quiet and still while the oil is pouring.
- The room should have independent lighting and sound systems.
- A silent aromatherapy diffuser is a wonderful addition.
- Candles help make a special atmosphere.
- Music that is calming but does not suggest a particular place or scene is best.

Shirodhara is Recommended for Clients to

- promote deep relaxation.
- gently reenergize the body.
- help relieve stress headaches.
- alleviate insomnia.
- improve sleep quality.
- improve mental clarity and decision-making ability.
- help nourish the nervous system.

Shirodhara should not be given to people who . . .

- are under the influence of alcohol or recreational substances.
- suffer from a seizure disorder.
- have open lesions on their skull.
- are receiving cranial-sacral therapy during the same time.
- have an aversion to oil (some Pitta-types will even panic if they are exposed to this amount of oil).

The reason why these considerations are mentioned is because shirodhara is a very subtle, yet powerful treatment. Clients are actually more open to impressions around them. Thus, if they are going into stressful situations or into situations that are challenging to them, they will feel more vulnerable, feel the tensions and stress more dramatically. Thus, even when speaking to the client who has experienced shirodhara, one needs to be conscious of being quiet and un-intrusive. They should also be given time to rest and re-orient themselves before they leave your spa or facility. We have known of people who calmly drove through red lights, because they were so relaxed, they focused just on the pretty red color and not what the color meant!

Equipment, Products, and Materials
General Requirements
2 sheets, 1 blanket

1 plastic drop cloth (18"x 48" approx)

1 box of extra soft face tissue

1 roll of very absorbent paper towel

3 small towels

2 washcloths

Cotton or linen dishtowel

Hot towel cabinet or some way to keep various treatment supplies warm (crockpots can work. Also, food warming trays can be good for this treatment.)

Shaker with large holes such as would be used for peppers or Parmesan cheese

Access to shower or hair washing basin (if hair-washing facilities are not available provide clients with plastic shower caps and turbans, "twisty towels" or a small towel to wrap around their head to return home)

Clipboard and pens

Dates and walnuts if you are going to provide the suggested snack after the treatment

Basic Product Needs
Copper or plastic shirodhara set

1 head and neck pillow

1 tummy warmer

1 'cool eyes' eye pillow

1 set of "Body and Soul" clay stones or La Stone Stones or River/Ocean Rocks or equivalents

Anise Tibetan Lotion

Rose and /or sandalwood ubtan

Music—something without words

Shirodhara information and advice sheet

Dosha-appropriate massage oil

Dosha-appropriate essential oil blend

Refined sesame oil—for general purpose in a spa, this is the most effective for creating the desired results—approximately 750ml. or about 1 quart will provide the length of shirodhara treatment you want

Yoni Treats (using dates ad Tibetan Flower Chulen)—See recipes

Preparation of Oils and Equipment

1. Place the refined sesame oil in a jar and place in hot towel cabinet, in a crock of water, or on a food warmer. Keep some room temperature refined sesame oil available as well—just in case the oil gets too warm to use later on. (**NOTE: Do not use a microwave to keep or get the oil warm. Energetically, this will alter the oil enough to negate its benefits.**)

2. The Body and Sole Clay Stones or alternative can be warmed warm in the same manner as the oil. Place Washcloths crock-pot or hot towel cabinet as well.

3. The Tummy Warmer can be placed in the hot towel cabinet for one hour or can be warmed in a microwave for 4 minutes. This warmer (or a hot water bottle) can be wrapped in a towel or store it in an "igloo" to keep it warm.

4. Start the music quietly before the client comes in the room, and put on the repeat function if there is one.

5. Have the Shirodhara Information and Advice Sheet (provided in the Appendices), a clipboard, and a pen or pencil available.

Starting the Treatment Ritual

As there are recommendations and contra-indications for receiving shirodhara, these should have been discussed with your client prior to their appointment. If you have not done this, take some time to discuss with your client the contraindications for receiving Shirodhara in order to determine whether or not they should actually have this service.

Once these have been discussed and the two of you agree that the service is what will be offered to them, have your client read over and sign the Shirodhara Information and Advice Sheet.

Because of the energetic nature of this treatment, along with telling them which items of clothing need to be removed, encourage them to also remove their wristwatch and jewelry other than wedding bands. It is also advisable that they remove eye make-up as well.

Once they are in your treatment room, have them sit on the table. Determine which dosha-appropriate oil you will be using by performing the **Diagnostic Points Test.** Then briefly explain the sequence of the Tibetan Shirodhara treatment ritual.

PHASE ONE—Dzub Nyin Series for Psychological Stress

Your client should be lying down on their stomach to begin this part of the treatment.

1. On each of the following nine points, do 7 gentle clockwise rotation movements using a small amount of the dosha-appropriate oil. You should generally use your thumbs. However, when pressing on the spinous processes (the middle of the three points), use the three-pronged technique as shown in the Himalayan Mountain Abhyanga ritual.

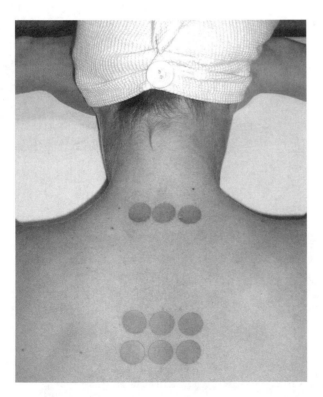

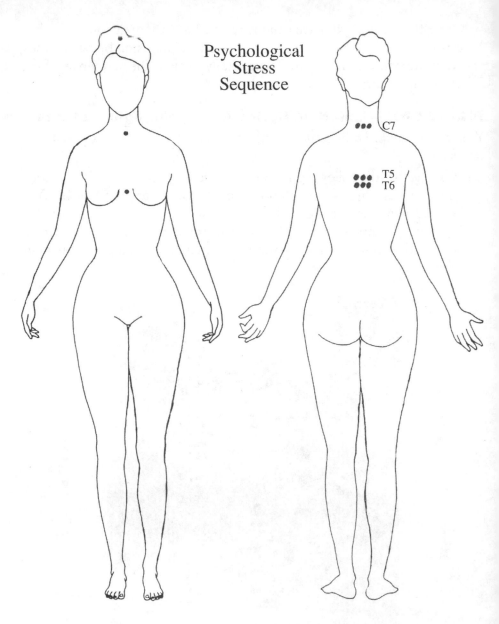

Psychological
Stress
Sequence

C7

T5
T6

a) Cervical 7—center, right, then left (major Vata point)

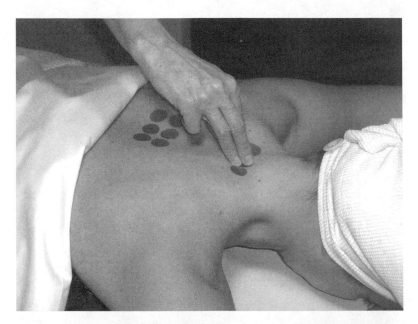

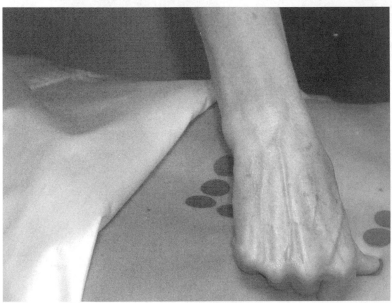

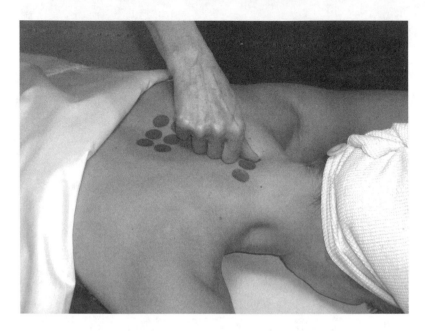

b) Thoracic 5—center, right, then left (subtle Vata—prana or Chi point)

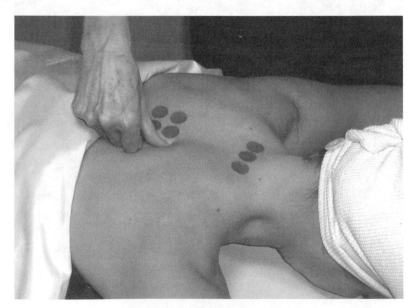

c) Thoracic 6—center, right, then left (heart point)

2. Repeat a–c two more times.

Ask your client to turn over onto their back.

3. Perform 7 gentle clockwise rotation movements to the following
   points, using your thumb.
   a) Jatru—marma point in the sternal notch (PICTURE)
   b) Hridayam—marma at midpoint of sternum

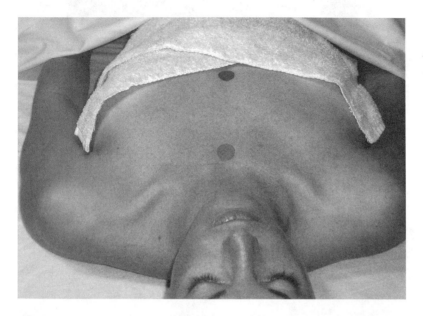

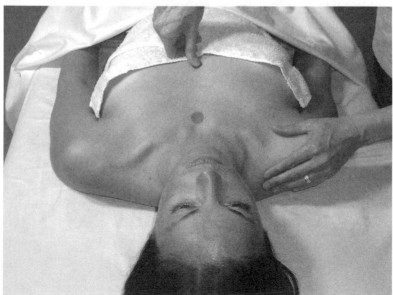

c) Murdhi—central fontanel marma

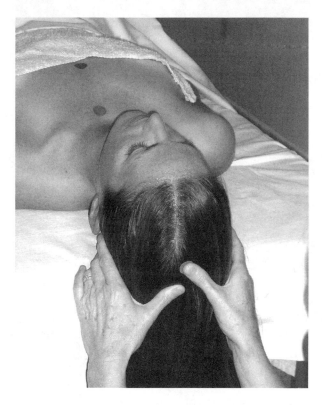

4. Cradle the head with both hands, resting your fingertips on the occipital line with the middle fingers on the *krikatika* marma points that are on either side of the top of the spine.

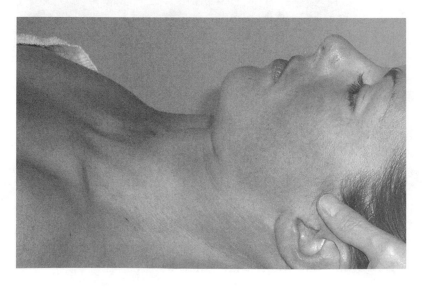

PHASE TWO—Abdominal Massage

This phase helps the digestion, is calming for vata dosha and is both nurturing and grounding. This too may be added to any treatment.

Ask the client to draw up their knees. Use the top sheet to secure the feet.

1. Pour 1 teaspoon of warm, dosha-appropriate Ayurvedic blend in one palm, bring the hands down over the navel, and gently pour the oil into the navel, then spread the oil over the abdomen using a clockwise, circular motion.

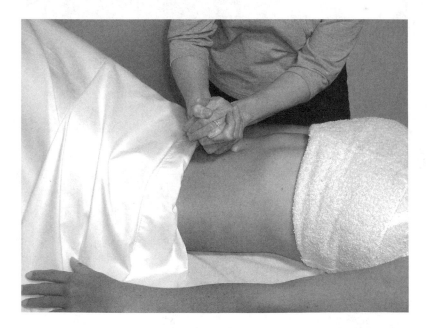

2. Roll the abdomen from side to side, using the heel of the hands on the right side of the abdomen, pressing down, pushing and rolling the abdominal tissues to the left, then drawing the tissues back with your fingers. Watch your client's face to make sure they are both comfortable and secure with your touch. (1 minute)

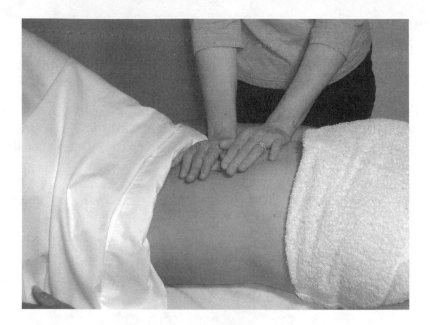

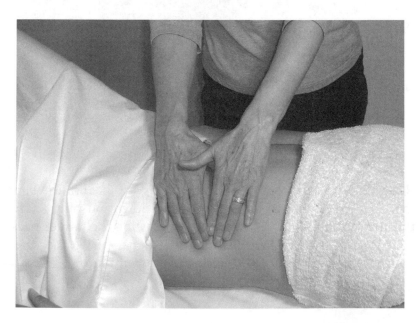

3. With both hands configured as in photo, perform circular kneading around the navel, starting with a downward pressure from the heel of the left hand, the outside of the left hand, the fingertips, the outside of the right hand, then right heel of the hand. Follow ascending, transverse, and then descending colon. (1–2 minutes)

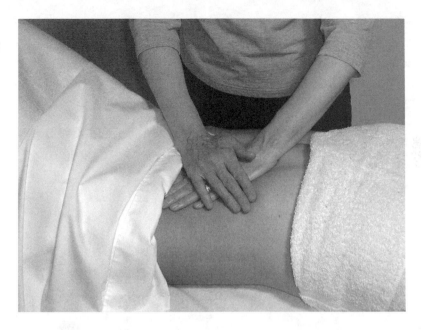

4. Roll the abdomen as in '2'. (1 minute)
5. Deep, slow circular strokes using the flat of the fingers and palms of the hands going up along the ascending, then transverse, and down the descending colon and under the navel. Area covered should be about 3 finger-widths around the navel in all directions. (5 minutes)

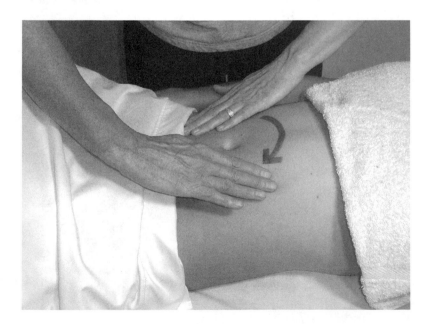

6. Abdominal rolling as in '2'. (1 minute)

7. Apply deep rotational thumb pressure in a clockwise motion to the point approximately 3 finger-widths below the navel. Do this 3 times, having the client breathe out as you press in and as they breathe in, releasing the pressure.

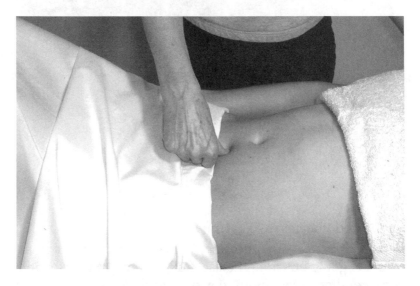

8. Rest your left hand below the navel and slide your right hand under small of the back. Hold this position until there is a sense of balance or a deep pulse felt in the belly region.

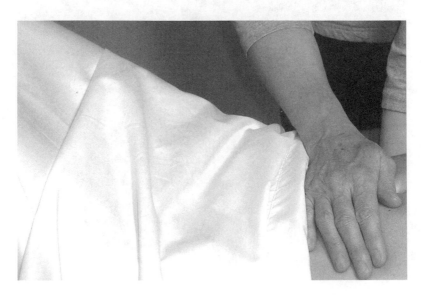

9. Inhale, and draw away the hand from the small of the back first. Inhale again and draw the other hand from away from the abdomen. Step away and allow the client to lower their legs again.

10. Place the Tummy Warmer or hot water bottle on the abdomen, over the sheet, then cover it to hold in the warmth. Encourage your client to tell you whether it is too hot and make it clear it can be taken off at any stage.

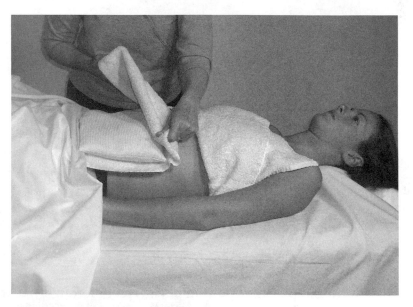

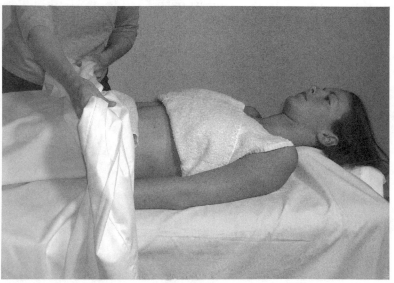

PHASE THREE—Tibetan Eye Rejuvenation Therapy

1. With the client lying on their back, remove or make sure that the client has removed all eye make-up (if you have begun with phases one and two, this has already been done).
2. Having assessed which essential oil is appropriate for their body-mind type, place a dot of this oil at the corners of a folded tissue. Place this tissue directly over the eyes, then apply the cooling eye pack.

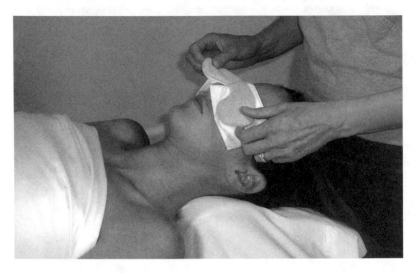

3. With a warm damp cloth wipe your client's feet thoroughly, then pat dry. Position small towels underneath each foot. These will be used to wrap the feet later on.

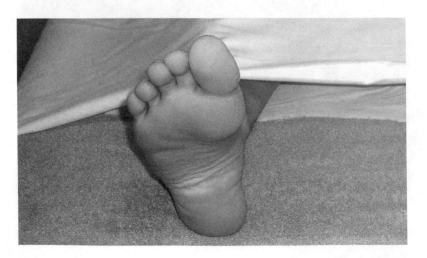

4. Using the Tibetan anise butter lotion or anise lotion, massage each foot for five minutes, starting with the right foot. If you know reflexology, pay particular attention to pituitary, pineal, eye, liver, spleen, colon, bladder, and kidney reflexes. According to oriental tradition, the liver governs the sight in the left eye, and the spleen governs the right. The kidneys govern the actual structure of the eye itself.

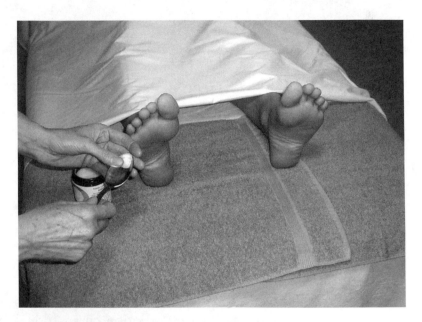

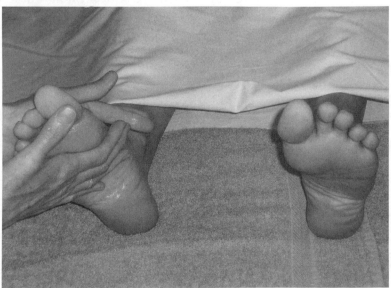

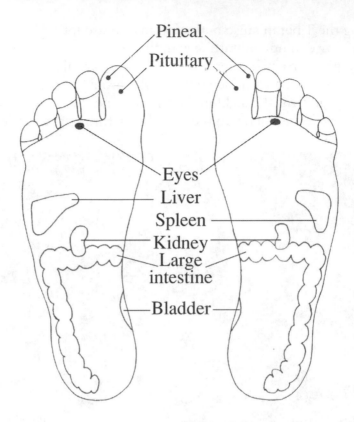

Pineal
Pituitary
Eyes
Liver
Spleen
Kidney
Large
intestine
Bladder

5. After the right foot, cover it and do the left foot in the same manner. Cover the left foot as well and leave the lotion on an additional 5 minutes.

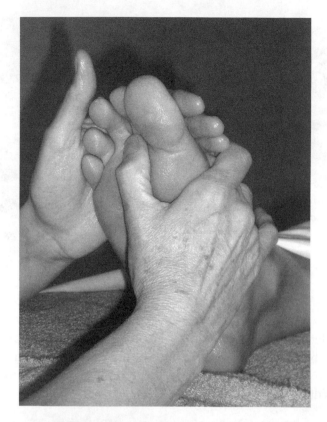

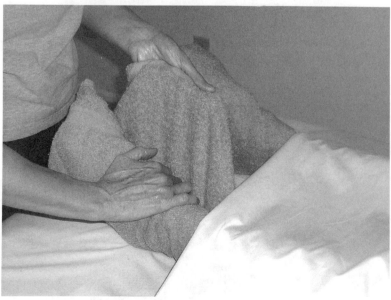

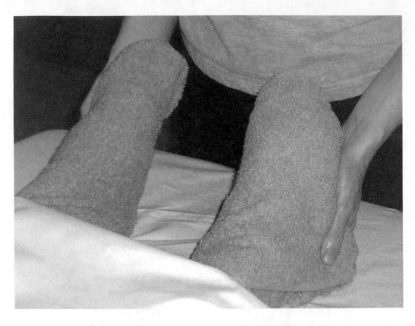

6. While letting the feet soak in the anise lotion, you can perform a general hand massage on the right hand. Use the dosha-appropriate massage oil for this. Do this for approximately 3–5 minutes. The left hand will be done shortly.

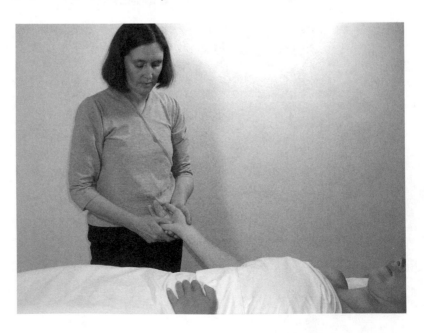

Hand Massage Options

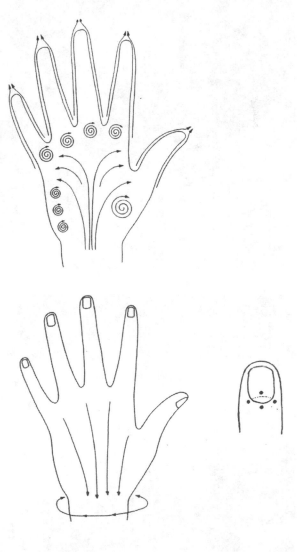

7. Remove the cover on the feet and rub chickpea (besan) flour or ubtan into each foot, starting with the right. Cover, then allow the ubtan to rest on the feet for about five minutes.

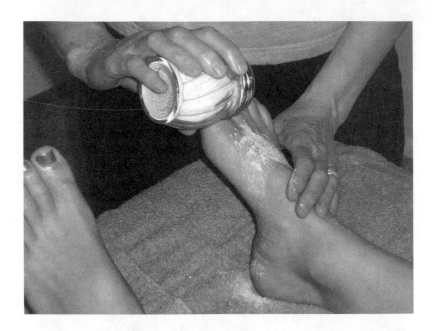

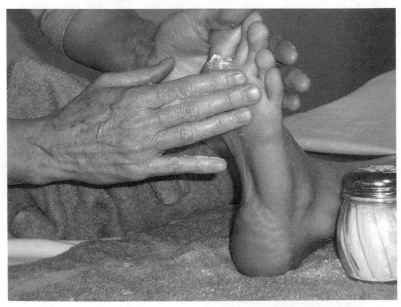

8. While the ubtan is on the feet, massage the left hand.

9. Wipe the powder with a dry cloth and then a warm, moist cloth. Pat the feet dry, right foot first, then left.

10. Place a bolster under the client's knees so that their feet can easily rest on the table. Alternatively, draw their knees up, place their feet

so that they are to the side of the table and the knees touch (so they are knock-kneed) and tuck the sheets and blanket under the legs to keep them in place.

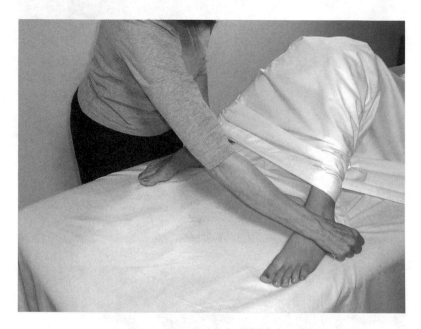

11. Take the warmed 'Body and Sole' stones (or other set of stones) that have been heated up and place them under the ball of the foot, just behind the toes, again doing the right foot first, then the left. If you use the "Body and Sole" stones, the little bumps can be positioned directly under the eye reflexes, found on the under side between the base of the fourth and fifth toes. **Remember to hold these stones in your hands a few moments to check their temperature.** If they feel too hot, place a thin towel or dry washcloth between the feet and the stones. Again, the therapeutic action comes from the earthen quality and consistent deep heat that the stones radiate. Wrap a towel over the feet while the stones are in place. (**Resist the temptation to press down on the feet when you ask the person of the warmth of the stones feels comfortable. The pressure will make the stones feel hotter than they are when their feet are just resting on them.**) The heating benefits of the lotion and the stones reduces Vata which can take the form of stress and tension exhibited in the face. This treatment literally draws this stress and tension away from the eyes and face and out of the body via the feet.

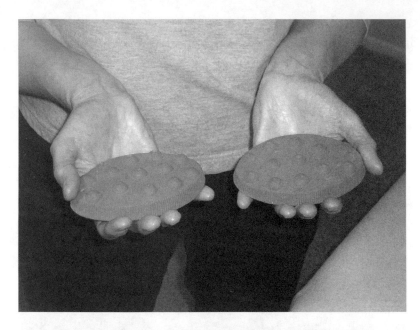

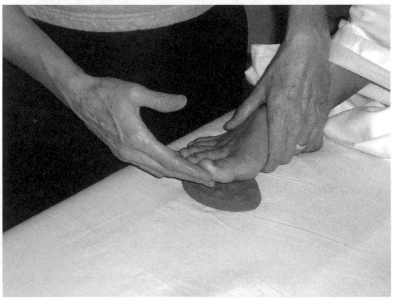

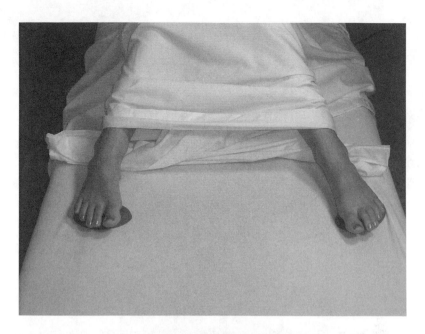

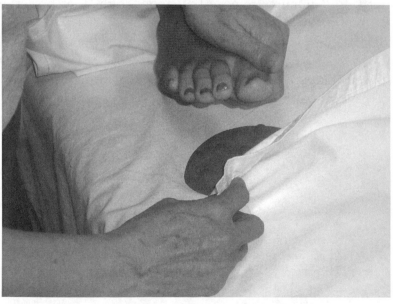

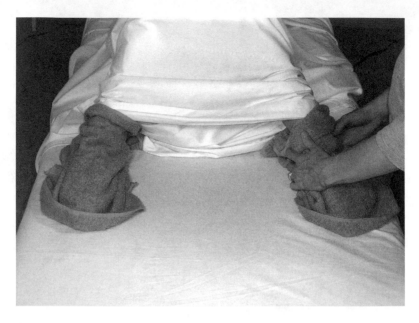

12. After 5 to 7 minutes remove the stones, right foot first, then left foot. Lower the legs down.

13. Hold the marma point that is halfway between the medial malleolus and the edge of the heel on both feet. Notice a sense of balance between the two feet. When you have that sense, breathe in, step away, and re-cover the feet.

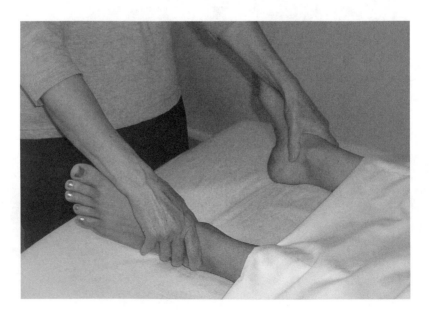

14. (If you are just performing the Tibetan Eye Rejuvenation, at this point remove the eye pad. Hold the tissue down and tell the client to keep their eyes closed while you remove the pack. Then place one hand across the eyes and remove the tissue. Place both of your palms over the eyes. Tell your client to open their eyes in the darkness created by your palms. Have them blink in this darkness for a few moments and then gradually, bring your hands away from the eyes so their vision can adjust slowly.) If you are going on to the shirodhara, keep the eye pack on.

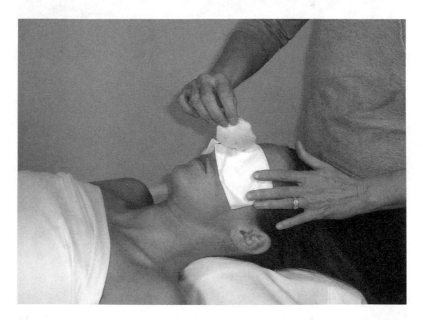

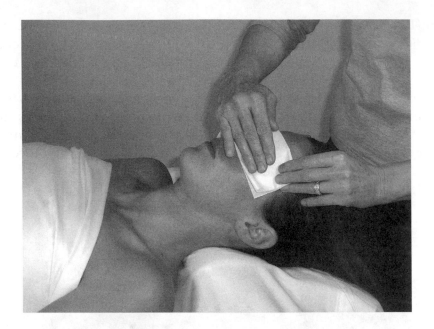

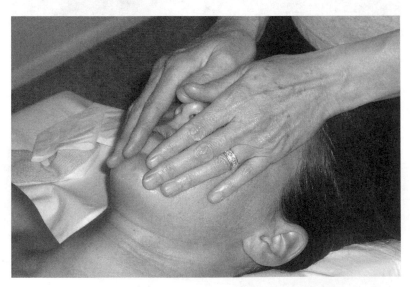

PHASE FOUR—Shirodhara

*If you have been doing the Tibetan eye rejuvenation,
while the stones are on under the feet, spend some time
initially positioning the base of your shirodhara equipment.*

1. Going to the head of the table, ask your client to scoot towards you
   so that you can help them in adjusting the position of their head for
   the pouring of the oil. Make sure there is a gentle slope to their

forehead by allowing their head to hang slightly over the end of the massage table. Use a Head and Neck Pillow or small rolled up towel for extra neck comfort if needed. Position spa plastic sheeting underneath the head so your linens are covered.

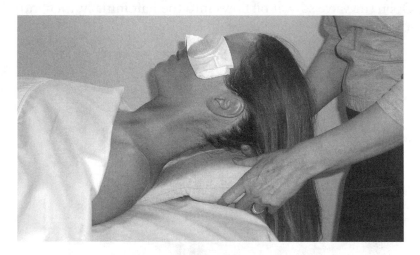

2. Take the warmed Shirodhara pouring vessel and set it into its ring. Position Shirodhara equipment so the spout of the vessel is approximately 3 or 4 inches above the center of the client's forehead. Arrange the catching bowl on the floor, allowing the spa plastic sheeting to drape into the bowl.

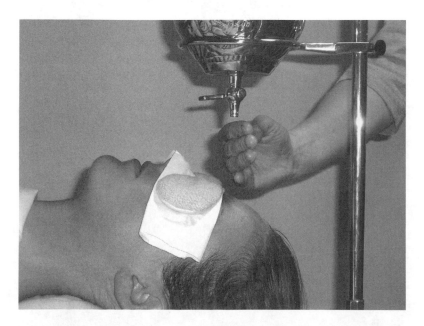

3. Remove the Shirodhara vessel and fill it with the warmed oil and place it back into the ring. **(Remember that when filling the vessel, be sure the stop cock is turned so no oil starts to pour out until you get back to the table and are ready to begin.)**

4. Open the valve so that oil flows into the hair initially, then introduce it to the middle of the forehead.

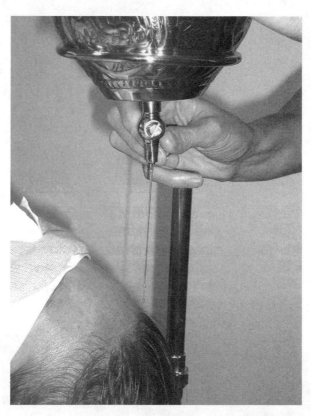

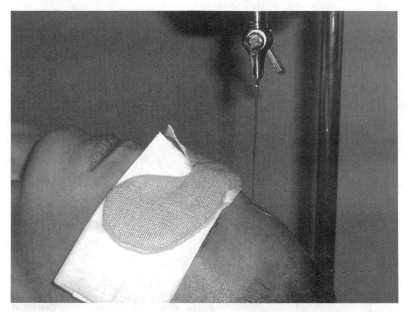

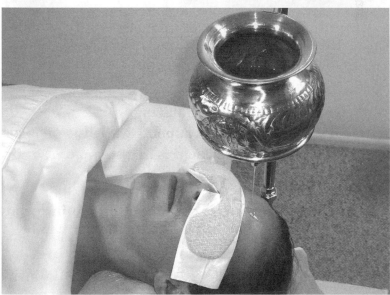

5. Check that the temperature of the oil is comfortable to your client. Pitta clients seem to appreciate slightly cooler oil and/or a moving stream. Vata and Kapha clients tend to appreciate a warmer, wider stream.

6. Watch the stream to ensure that it is staying on the mid region of the forehead. Do the zigzag or figure eight (infinity symbol) pattern if desired. These are especially enjoyed by Pitta types.

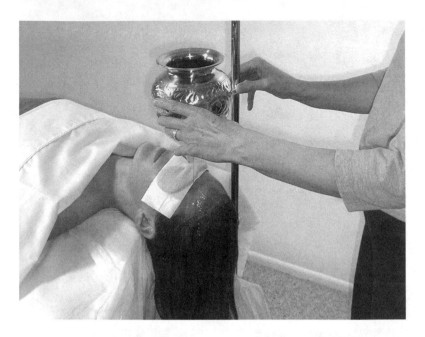

7. Be aware that as the client relaxes the pitch of their forehead can change. They may even begin to make spontaneous head movements as they go deeper and deeper. Thus, we advise:

Never
- **leave the room while the oil is playing.**
- **be tempted to do any other treatments while the oil is playing.**
- **give shirodhara while your client is in a steam tent or or herbal linen wrap.**

If your client becomes upset:
- **Ask if they are all right, but do not get drawn into conversation. Offer to stop the oil but let them know it can be started again at any time.**

8. Be sure that the oil is not allowed to drip at the end. Watch the oil level carefully to ensure that this does not happen. Let the last small amount of oil flow through the hair only.

9. Rest a tissue over the forehead to wipe off the oil. Use a paper towel to wipe oil out of the hair. Remove shirodhara equipment.

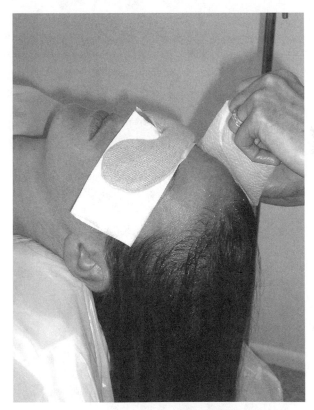

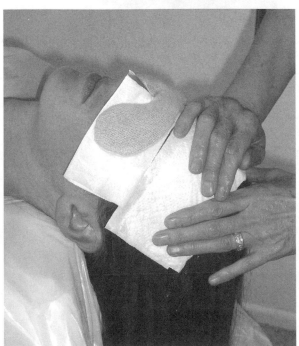

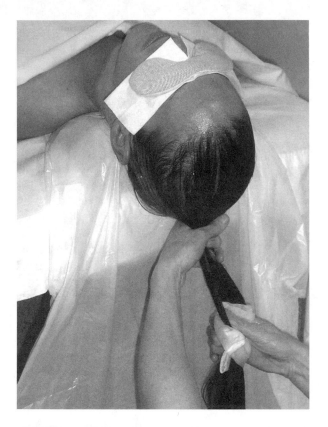

10. Ask the client to move forward or back onto the table so that their head is resting without the neck being tilted back. Hold the polarity point (KRIKATIK Marma) on the occipital crest and get a sense of balance.

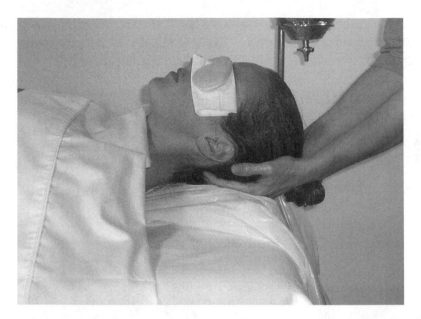

11. Rest your hands over the top of the head with your thumbs resting on the middle of the forehead, the marma where the oil was playing and the SHANKAR marma.

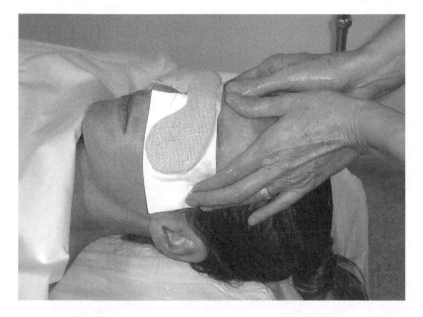

12. At this point you are deeply connected with your client. Silently, think good thoughts. Make a wish that you have done something useful. Breathe in as you take your hands away.

13 Finally, moving clockwise around the table to your client's feet, hold in the middle of each foot (TALHRIDAYAM Marma) with arms crossed. Breathe in again as you take your hands away.

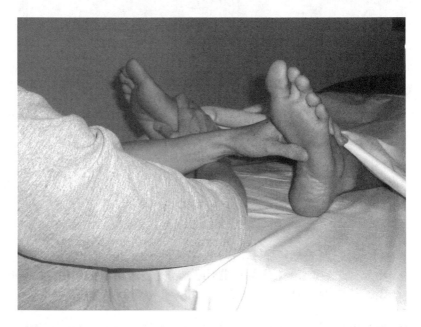

14. Wrap the head in a towel and let the client rest for five minutes. If the eye pad has been on the eyes, tell the client to keep their eyes closed while you remove the pad. Then, place a palm across and over the eyes as you remove the tissue. Cover their eyes with your palms and tell them to blink into the darkness. As their eyes adjust to the light, slowly begin to move your hands away.

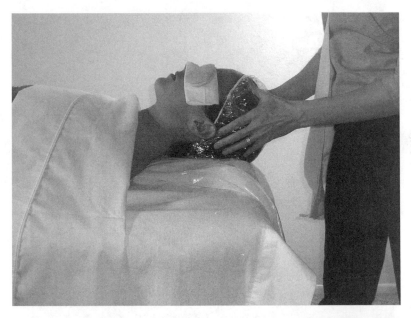

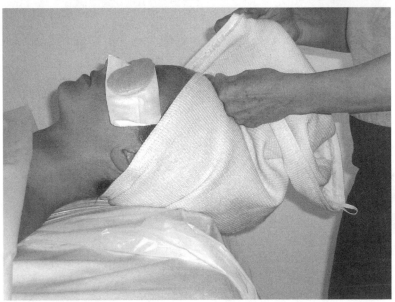

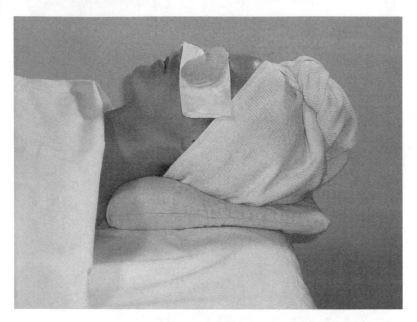

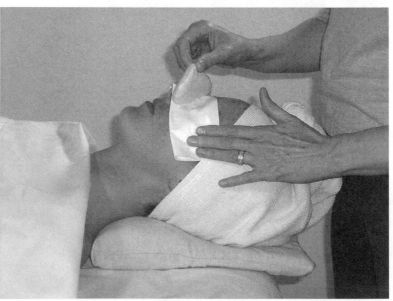

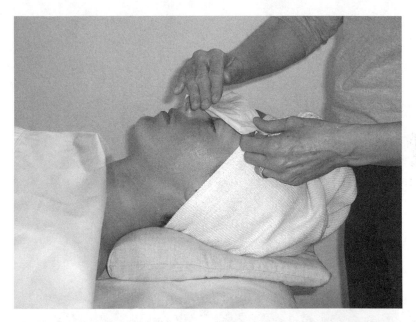

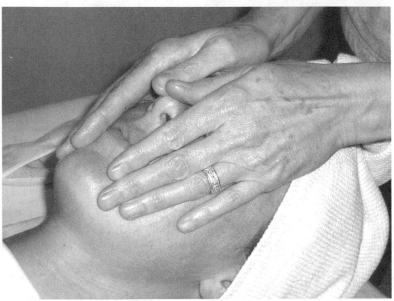

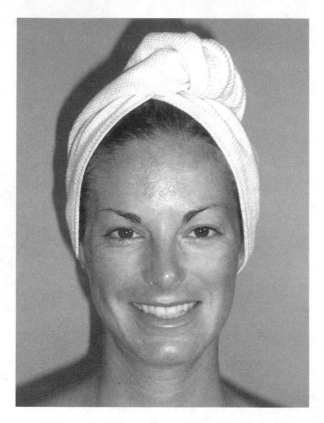

*The only reason to give further work after shirodhara would be to help
a VATA client feel more grounded—hold negative pole of the feet (located
between the medial malleolus and the edge of the heel on both feet).
PITTA clients should stay a while rather than rush off—
give them a short hand massage.
KAPHA clients should be fully alert before they leave—
give a gentle ear massage.*

15. Take the client to the shower or wrap the hair in a shower cap and
turban or towel.

16. Offer tea and a snack.

AGAIN as a reminder: Do not allow anyone to rush out. Remind
them of the recommendations on the shirodhara advice sheet for the
benefit of their own comfort and safety.

■ *Marmas and Mud Magic*

This sequence is, again, a combination of several different rituals all streamed together for a luxurious result. It is also designed to give you, the therapist, an opportunity to talk with your client about stressors in their lifestyle and make some Ayurvedic recommendations that they can work with at home.

The treatment starts off with a warm footbath. Although there are herbal combinations that would work specifically for each body-mind type, in this instance we create a bath salt that uses a tridoshic blend of bay, eucalyptus, and ginger. The effect is very settling. To make the foot-bath a bit more interesting, we suggest putting some whole and half glass beads in the water so the client can stimulate the bottoms of their feet. From the standpoint of an "at home" treatment, having some of these salts available to your client after their appointment is a welcomed treat.

At a point in the foot soak, the feet are taken out and dried. Ghee (clarified butter) or Tibetan Anise Lotion is rubbed over the feet, following which you offer a massage with a very effective Ayurvedic instrument known as a three-metal bowl or *kansa vataki*. These three-metal bowls can be made of copper, silver, and gold, although most are made of copper, zinc, and tin. The effect is tridoshic, balancing to all the doshas, and quite relaxing. When rubbed vigorously over the bottoms of the feet for about ten minutes, the feet can become grey or even black. This has to do with toxins coming out of the body through the feet. Excess Pitta is calmed and heat symptoms are eased. Dr. Smita Naram has told us that she has her clients purchase these bowls for home use. They are easy, beneficial, and fun to use.

Following a short foot massage with the kansa bowl, the feet are soaked again for another few minutes, after which the client is led to a table where they receive the Tibetan "Common Stress" Dzub Nyin sequence. This marma and acupressure point massage is one of the most effective techniques we have seen for dismantling the way in which the mind and body hold onto patterns of stress. This technique, alone, is a great intro-duction to massage for clients who have never experienced the benefits of full-body massage. Also, while this technique is being done with oils in this case, it can be done dry over clothes with very good results, as well.

In the last stages of doing the Common Stress sequence, a fine Ayurvedic mud comprised of pure silt and 12 herbs is applied to the body, from the elbows down to the fingertips, and from the knees down to the tips of the toes. The application of poultices and pastes, known in Ayurveda as *lepas*, is quite common for general health as well as specific medical concerns. In the spa environment, we have not found any product as effective as this proprietary Ayurvedic blend, the source of which you will find in the Resources Guide at the end of the book. Besides its known detoxifying effects, this herbomineral mud allows for a greater intake of prana or subtle vital energy into the body. The client will actually feel as if they are breathing more deeply and feel a greater sense of alertness and vitality.

Suggested Menu Description

Marma and Mud Magic

A warm footbath and foot massage with a special three-metal bowl begins this unique Ayurvedic spa ritual that will help you to unwind and feel a warm glow inside. Following these luxurious and calming steps, certain marmas (vital energy points) are touched from head to toe in a traditional Tibetan sequence with balancing aromatic oils. Finally, your arms and legs are covered in layer of warm Indian clay and herbs that increases the flow of prana (life force) which will help you to feel stronger and more grounded. This wonderful ritual is for anyone wanting the experience of mental rest and more physical energy.

Equipment, Products, and Materials

Chair or pedicure station

Massage table

foot soaking bowl (ideally copper, if available)

10 small towels

2 sheets

Blanket

Kansa Vataki (3-metal) foot massage bowl

Head and neck support pillow or equivalent

Tummy warmer or equivalent

Hot towel cabinet or equivalent

'Cool Eyes' pack or equivalent

Cotton eye pads (for removing eye make-up)

Tridoshic bath salts

Ghee or Anise Tibetan Lotion

Nutmeg Tibetan Lotion

Dosha-appropriate body oil

Auromere's 'Herbomineral' mud

Pitcher of warm water

Small bowl (soup dish size) and a cover for it

Rose Water

Sorig Tibetan Tea (or equivalent Ayurvedic blend)

Sesame Halvah (see recipes)

Coyote Smile Ayurvedic tincture (see Resource Guide)

Preparation:

If you are using a Tummy Warmer, you can either microwave it for four minutes or place it in a plastic bag and put it into the hot towel cabinet.

Dampen and fold 6 small towels and keep them warm in the hot towel cabinet (or equivalent).

Take about 1 cup of the herbomineral mud and add enough warm water to form a slightly runny paste. Cover this bowl and place it in the cabinet to stay warm.

PHASE ONE—Diagnostic:

With your client sitting in the chair or at the pedicure station, perform the Diagnostic Point procedure to determine the appropriate massage oil blend that you will use for the Common Stress Tibetan Dzub Nyin marma sequence.

PHASE TWO—Ayurvedic Bath Salts Foot Soak:

1. Prepare 1.5 Litres (approx. 2 gallons) of comfortably warm water in a footbath with 2 tablespoons of the tridoshic bath salts blend. With the person sitting upright in a chairor pedigree station, place both feet in the water and allow them to soak for 5 minutes.

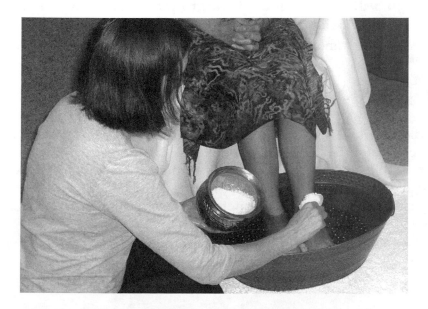

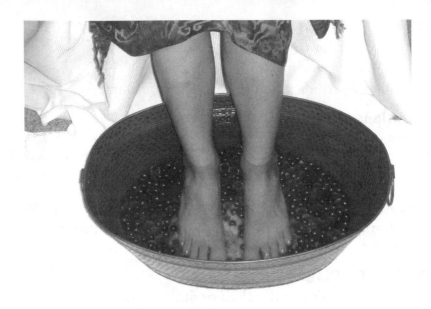

2. Having assessed which of the doshas needs to be brought into balance during the treatment, you can use this time to discuss lifestyle changes to assist this balance. You can talk about the use of the various components of this treatment for home rituals. If you feel more comfortable, perhaps you can share with them about improvements in their diet, various forms of exercise, etc. **Be sure to have printed material available for them following the treatment ritual. Rest assured that after the treatment, they will be in such a different frame of mind that, more than likely, they will forget what you discussed.**

3. After this, remove feet from water and pat them dry. Wrap the left foot in the towel.

PHASE THREE—Three-Metal Bowl Foot Massage:

The Kansa Vataki foot bowl is designed so that you either hold it by its handle (if you have a handled version) or on the edges as it will be the convex side of the bowl that you will use to perform the massage. The edge of this bowl is relatively thin, which means that if you press too hard against the foot, you will feel the metal dig into the creases of your fingers. This will make you instinctively lighten your pressure. The bowl should feel comfortable in your hand.

1. Position yourself so that you are sitting opposite the client or in such a way that you can comfortably massage both feet.

2. Lifting the right foot onto your lap, start coating the entire foot in Ghee or Anise Tibetan Lotion.

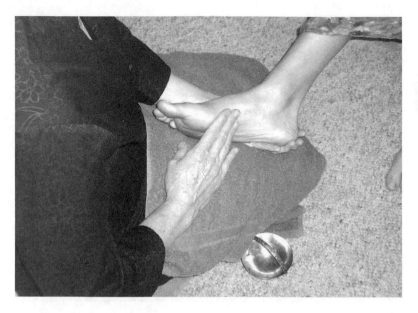

3. For 5 minutes, take the three-metal foot massage bowl and with slow, relatively firm movements, massage the entire right foot:

  a) Rub back and forth along the entire length of the bottom of the foot at least 21 times.

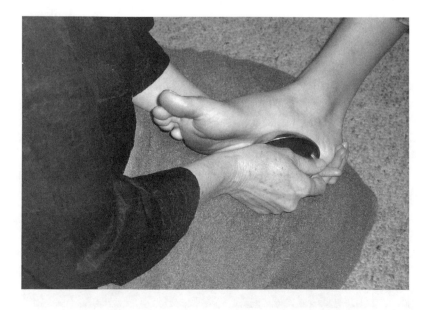

b) Massage the ends of the toes, starting with the big toe; perform 7 clockwise circles on the very tips.

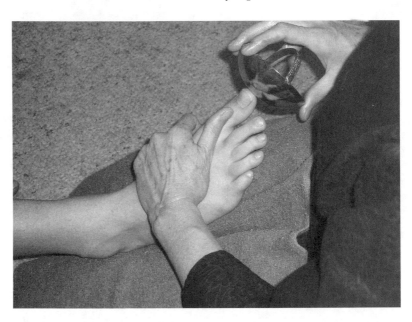

c) Starting at the edge of the big toes, make small clockwise circular strokes along the inner side and arch of the foot, around the back of the heel, and finally up along the enter outer edge of the foot up to the toes. Go around like this 3 times.

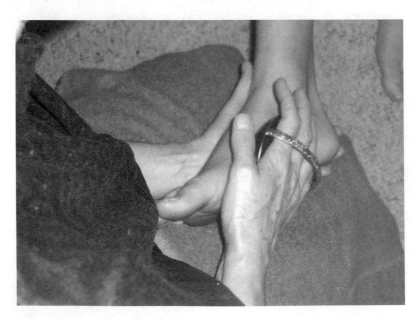

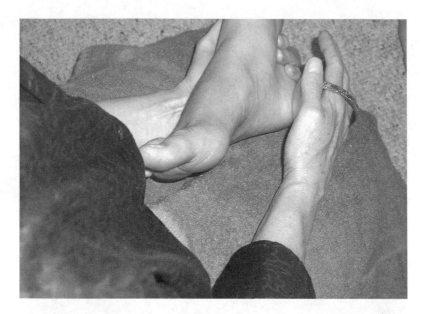

d) Massage the top of foot. As the area is bonier with less dense tissue, use lighter pressure. Go up and over both medial and lateral aspects of the ankle joint. Stroke back and forth along the metatarsal lines.

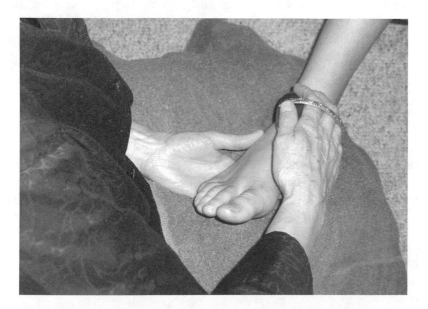

e) Massage the bottom again, this time doing clockwise circular motions, followed by figure eights over the entire bottom, then deep rotations into the arch.

f) Do 3 spins on the tips of the toes, starting with the big toe. The motion is like trying to twist a lid off of a can.

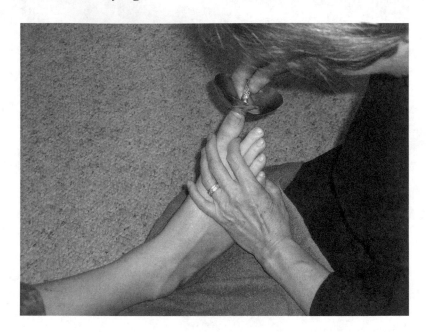

4. Wrap the foot in a warm towel and repeat steps 2 and 3 on the left foot.
5. After completing left foot, unwrap the right foot and return both feet to the footbath for another 5 minutes. (*Top the water off with additional warm water if it has gone tepid.*)
6. Remove the feet and pat them dry.

To help the client become more aware of their body sensations and take them deeper into the ritual, as you direct the client to the massage table, tell them to pay attention to the feel and quality of their feet as a result of the bowl massage. Then, have them lie down on their backs.
Cover them with a sheet and blanket. Ask them if they would like to have a **Tummy Warmer**.

PHASE FOUR: Dzub Nyin Series for Common Stress

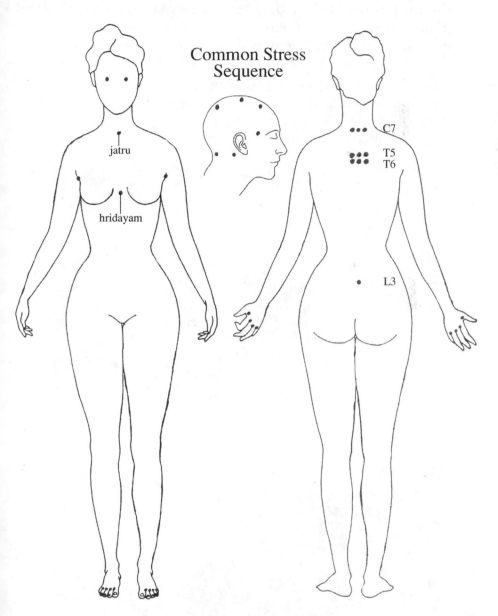

Common Stress
Sequence

jatru

hridayam

C7

T5
T6

L3

Start with the client on their back

1. Turn your client's head slightly to the left. With your left hand cradled around your client's left ear, use the fingertips on your right hand to digitally knead the scalp, from the base of the skull up over the head to the forehead, using clockwise circular motions. Loosen the scalp on the right, then on the left.

2. With your fingers loose, perform hacking tapotment to skull. (**Note: do not perform this if they have a headache or have a steel plate in their skull.** If performed in accordance with the recommendations about the types of strokes for the different body-mind types, this hacking actually feels quite delightful.)

3. Apply 7 gentle clockwise rotation pressure movements to the following points and all subsequent points, using the appropriate Ayurvedic body-mind type massage oil.

    a) Murdhi (central fontanel) marma.

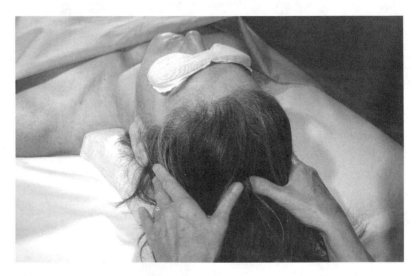

    b) Shankar (temple) marma*.

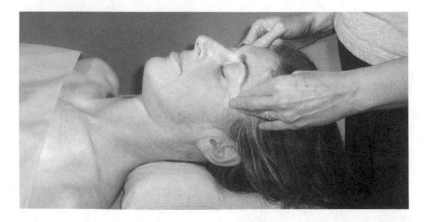

*On third time coming to shankar marma, hold the both sides and be still. This marma helps you to communicate subconsciously with your client. Convey a positive healing message. Then, when you are finished doing that, inhale and move away from these points.

c) Vidhura Marmas behind ears in hollow of mastoid.

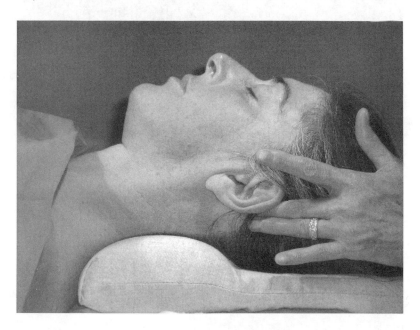

d) Brahma (anterior fontanel) marma.

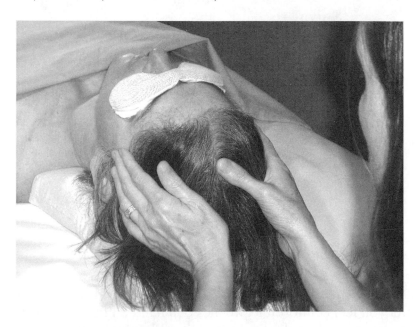

e) Shiva (posterior fontanel) marma.

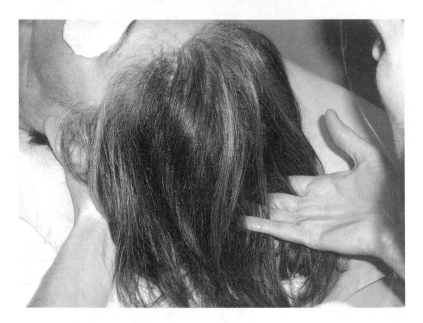

4. Repeat 'a'–'e' two more times.

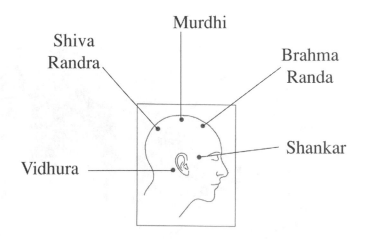

*Remove **Tummy Warmer** if they have one on
and turn the client onto their stomach.*

5. Diagonal stretching of the back. With your hands crossed or however you feel comfortable, anchor one hand on the left buttock and
the other hand on the top of the right shoulder. Keep the hand on
the buttock anchored while the other hand goes down, then back
up the right side of the back– one time down and one time up.

6. Vertical stretch, keeping right hand on sacrum, moving the left hand up the back—do this one time up, then down.

7. Hacking on spine. (NOTE: be sure to note from earlier health questions or now if they have had any spinal injuries. Hack above and below, but not on these areas) Go up and down, from base of spine to the top thoracic vertebrae, three times.

8. If the client reports that their lower back tends to be stiff, take Nutmeg Tibetan Lotion and gently rub it into the back of the neck and lower lumbar and sacral spine.

9. Apply the dosha-appropriate massage oil with 7 gentle clockwise rotation pressure movements to the following points, using thumb pressure to the points approximately ½ inch to the right and left of the spine and the three-pronged approach to the spinous process.

   a) Cervical 7—center, right, then left (major VATA marma point).

   b) Thoracic 5—center, right, then left (subtle Vata—prana or Chi marma point).

   c) Thoracic 6—center, right, then left (heart marma point).

   d) Lumbar 3—center, right, then left (large intestine marma— seat of VATA).

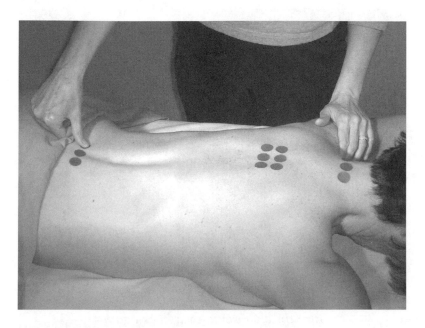

10. Repeat 'a'–'c' two more times.

11. Meridian stroking down back, from shoulders to buttocks, at least 7 times, then cover.

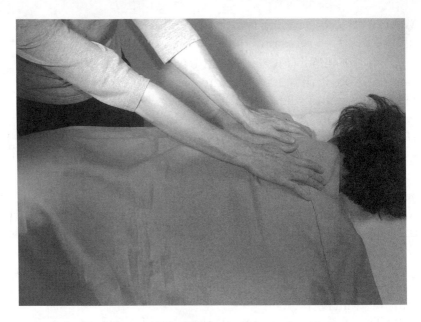

Meridian stroke down the back of the buttocks to the feet, at least seven times, while covered.

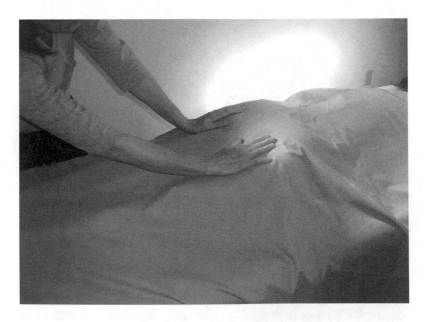

Turn the client onto their back again
Position a Head and Neck *pillow under the client's head.*
Ask them if they would like to have the Tummy Warmer *back on.*
Also, a mini Cool Eyes *pack or equivalent.*

12. Do 7 clockwise rotations on the following points, using your thumbs.
    a) Hridayam—marma that is mid-point of sternum (eases anxiety).
    b) Jatru—in sternal notch (to ease and strengthen upper body).

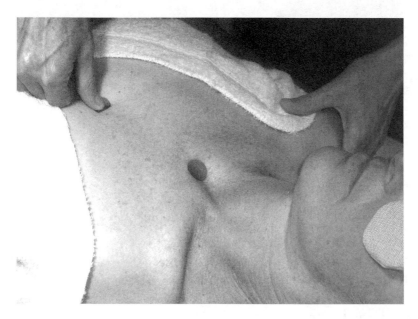

13. Massage the marmas in the webs between right fingers (start between thumb and index).

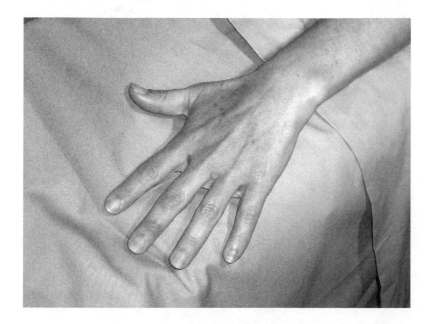

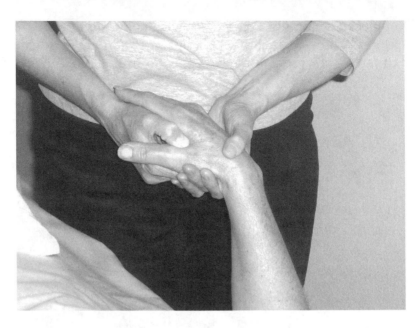

14. Treat the left hand the same as the right (note: remember to move around the client in a clockwise direction).

15. Do the marmas between the right toes, in the webs starting between the big and 2nd toes.

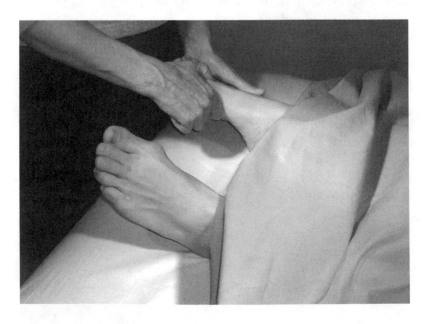

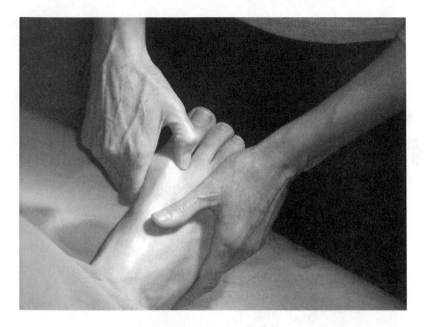

16. Massage the point in the center of the foot (parallel to 5th metatarsal).

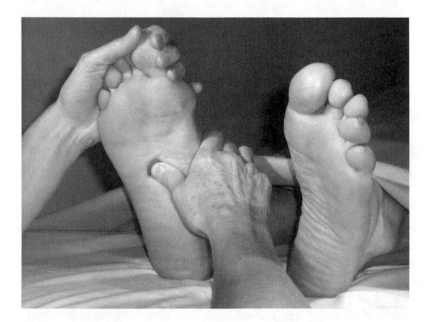

17. Repeat 15 and 16 on the left foot.
18. Repeat this sequence, 12–17 one more time. Then, on third time, add the following for the arms.

19. After doing step 13 on the right hand, do meridian stroking of the entire right arm.

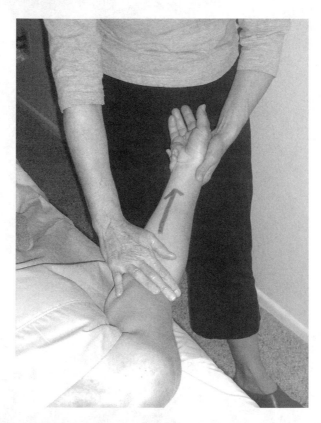

20. Massage the APALAPA Marma in center of the right armpit. This is the deepest marma in body. It activates lymph. As this can be a very sensitive or ticklish area, rest the four fingers of your right hand on the shoulder and the thumb in the crease of the armpit. Stand so that you are holding the client's right wrist with your left hand with their arm extended out to the side. Have the client breathe and as they breathe out, drop your wrist so that the thumb drops into the deepest portion of the pit as you draw the arm to their side. Apply deep clockwise rotational pressure, 7 rotations. As they breathe in, draw the arm out to the side and have your thumb come out of the pit and as they breathe out, repeat. Do this a total of three times. Also: *Before doing this, tell your client that the Lotion you are using will feel a bit* cool).

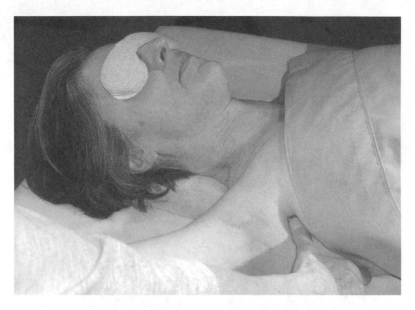

21. Place a small warm, moistened towel under the arm, from the elbow down to the hand. Apply the mud from the fingertips all the way up to the elbows, then wrap the towel around and place the arm under the covers.

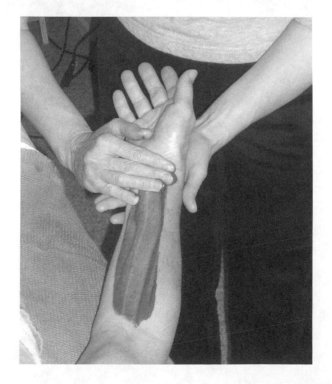

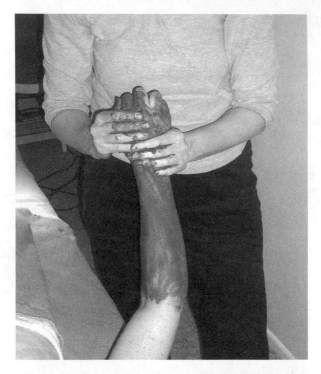

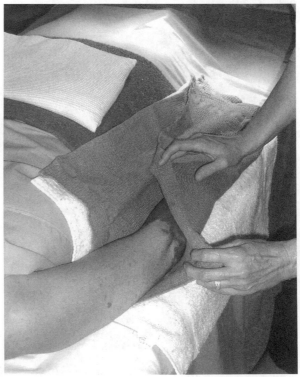

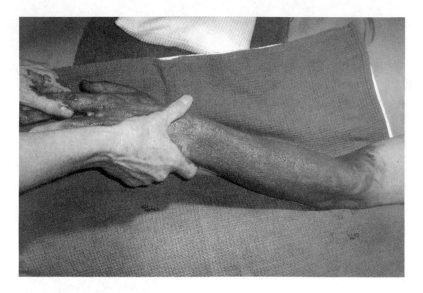

(NOTE: *Before going to the next hand,*
wipe your hands down on a towel as they will be a bit gritty.)

22. Repeat steps 19 through 21 for the left hand and arm, then continue to step 15.
23. After doing the points on the right foot, do meridian stroking, up the inside and down the outside of the full leg. Do this for at least 7 strokes. (PICTURE)
24. Place a moistened towel under the right leg, from the knee down to the foot. Apply mud to the right toes and foot all the way up to and including the knee, and wrap.

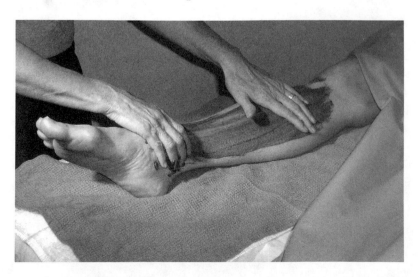

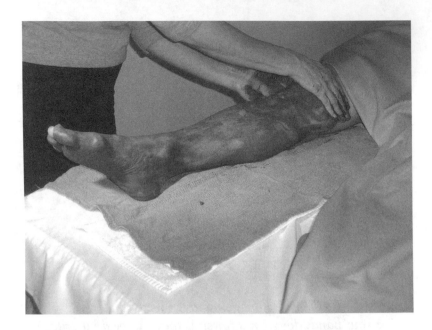

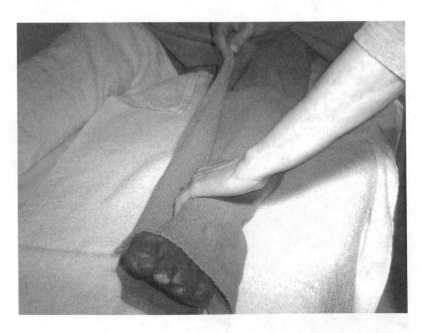

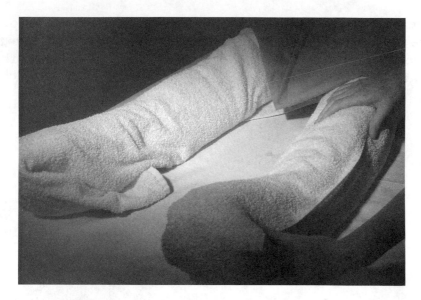

25. Then do the same for the left side, following through steps 23 and 24.

    Wipe or rinse your hands thoroughly and move to the head of the table.

26. (If the person has had an eye pad on, tell them to keep their eyes closed as you remove it.) Then rest your fingers on both eyes with the Tibetan 3-pronged technique. Instructing your client to breathe in, your fingers are just resting there. As you instruct them to exhale, push and rotate gently inward on the closed eyes for 7 clockwise rotations. As they inhale, lift off the pressure, then as they exhale repeat. Do this 3–5 times.

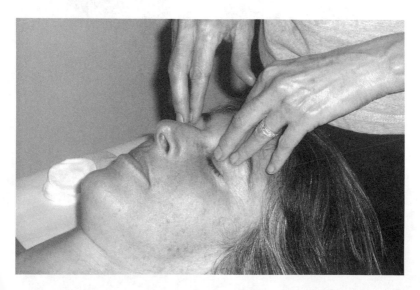

(Alternative: If the person has contacts in that they cannot or have not removed, place your palms over the eyes and allow the person's eyes to rest in darkness, suggesting that they allow their eyes to sink into the sockets as they breath out . . .)

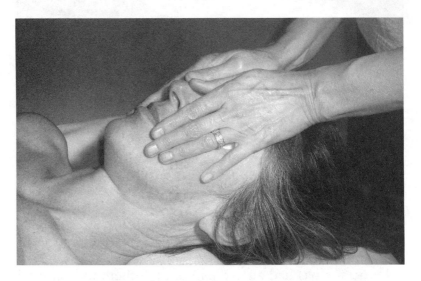

27. Dip two eye pads in the Rose Water and place over both eyes.

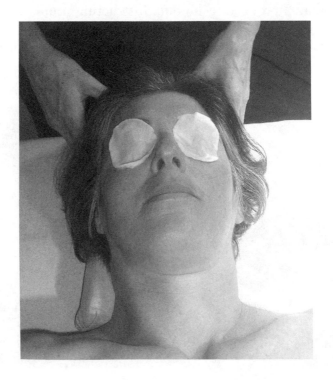

28. Do meridian stroking over the head at least 7 times.

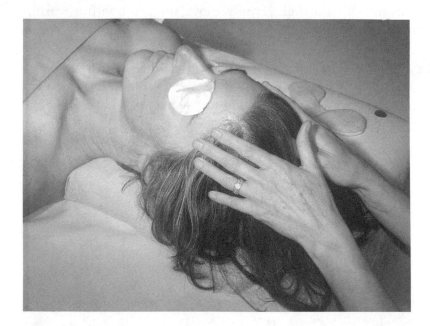

29. Find the KRIKATIKA Marma at the occipital protuberances and hold both of these marmas at once until there is a sense of balance.

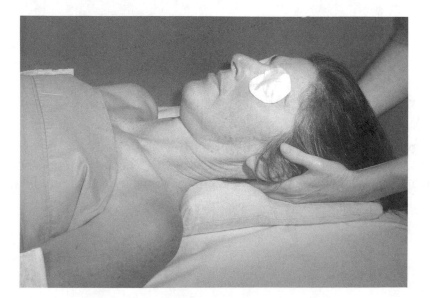

30. Inhale and move away.

   Tell the client that you are going to let them rest for a few minutes.

PHASE FIVE—Closing:

1. Starting with the right arm, remove the mud with a warm, moist towel and pat dry. Then do the left arm, the right leg, and the left leg, in that order.

2. Gently hold the point that is halfway between the medial malleolus and heel until there is a sense of balance. Hold both gently with your thumbs. When you feel a sense of balance, inhale and move away.

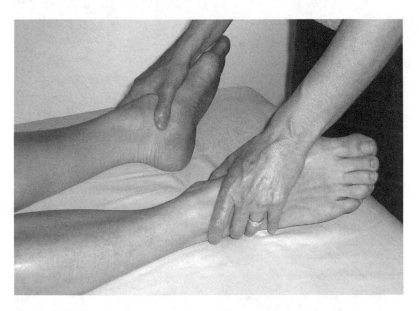

3. Finally, before you remove the eye pads, remind the client to keep their eyes closed. Then slowly take off the pads and cover the eyes with your palms. Have them open their eyes into the darkness of your palms, then slowly draw your hands away.

Suggested Post Ritual Snacks: After the client is dressed, serve them black sesame halvah and the Sorig Tibetan Tea blend with ½ teaspoon of Coyote Smile Ayurvedic tincture or another dosha-appropriate blend.

■ *Tibetan Blissful Sleep*

One of the most common complaints a therapist will hear in a spa is that people have restless, fitful nights or suffer from insomnia. In general, this has to do with an imbalance of the Vata dosha; where irregular lifestyle patterns, stress, and adjustments to becoming old, hence coming into the Vata-stage of life, are all contributory factors. At the same time, the overly active Pitta whose anxiety levels are high will also suffer such problems. Medications tend to aggravate rather than help this situation. Medicines—including sleep medications—impair calcium absorption and paralyze our capacity to dream. Antibiotics, steroids, contraceptives, and thyroid meds are particularly unhelpful.

There are a whole list of suggestions that can be made to help your client sleep and truly rest. These will follow the Tibetan Blissful Sleep treatment ritual. This ritual has three phases. The first is an advanced form of reflexology that adheres to Ayurvedic principles while using commonly recognized reflexology points. The emphasis here is on stimulating the digestive tract and the elimination of toxins. The second phase is the Abdominal Massage that you will find in several other of the treatment rituals. Again, the emphasis is on digestion, but essentially good deep work on the colon, the seat of Vata. The ritual culminates in another of the Tibetan Dzub Nyin sequences, one that is specifically designed for insomnia. As with other treatment rituals, all three of these components can be done separately and included in other treatments with excellent results. The reflexology series offered here will assist any other treatment you do to aid a client's digestion. The abdominal massage can be used towards that end as well and can also be used as a part of any other form of full-body or deep-tissue massage. The Tibetan Dzub Nyin series for insomnia can be done alone with great results, even without the aid of the oils mentioned.

Our experience of the full treatment ritual as laid out here is that clients virtually fall asleep on the table. If they do not, when they leave, they find that their body is so relaxed that when it finally is time to go to bed, they drop very easily into a very deep sleep that often lasts longer than usual. Because of its effects, we usually advise clients to book such an appointment towards the end of their day or, if you have late appointment hours, in the evening.

Suggested Menu Description

Tibetan Blissful Sleep

In Ayurveda sleep is called the "wet nurse to the world". It is nurturing, nourishing, and regenerating. Our Tibetan Blissful Sleep ritual will help to dissolve the stresses and strains that keep you from enjoying sleep's benefits. Deep massage to the feet with special Tibetan relaxation oils will be followed by a soothing abdominal massage to help your breathing deepen. Finally, a simple, gentle, and effective Tibetan marma energy sequence for encouraging sleep will leave you feeling so relaxed that when you go home to rest, your body will sink into an exquisite slumber that you will awake from, hours later, with great vigor and clarity.

Product and Equipment Needs

Massage table

2 sheets

Blanket

Therapist chair

Hot towel cabinet or equivalent

1 warm damp towel

1 warm dry towel

Head and Neck pillow or equivalent

Tummy Warmer or equivalent

Cool Eyes pack or equivalent

Tibetan "Calm and Clear" or Vata-balancing Oil in a dropper or pump-
   style bottle

Nutmeg Tibetan Lotion

Relaxation music (instrumental best. Recommended is Krista Lee Or-
   man's "Deep Sleep")

Vata-reducing tea (Valerian, Chamomile, etc.) for post-treatment

Preparation

Have the Tummy Warmer (or equivalent) wrapped in a plastic bag and placed in the hot towel cabinet. Place a wet towel that has been wrung out in the cabinet is well. If you have an oil warmer, make sure that the Tibetan relaxing or Vata-reducing oil is in the warmer.

PHASE ONE: Reflexology Series

The form of reflexology described here is done with the client lying on their stomach. This has a more grounding effect and allows your client to let go of areas that may be painful when you touch them.

The diagram supplied is a standard reflexology chart that has been turned upside down. In time, you will find that this method of reflexology is much easier and more effective for you as well as your client.

Reflexology Chart

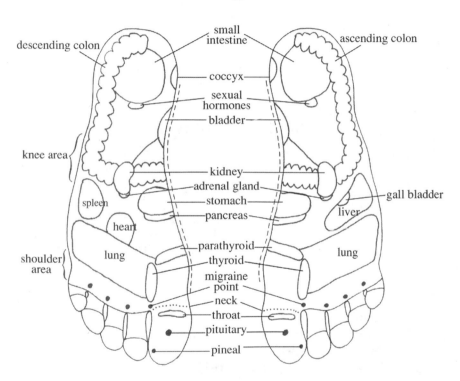

Outside View of Foot

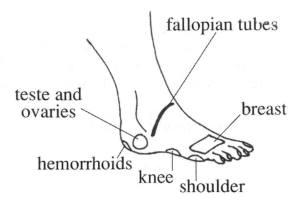

fallopian tubes

teste and ovaries

breast

hemorrhoids

knee shoulder

Inside View of Foot

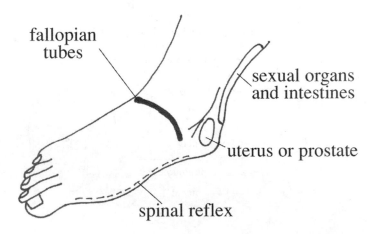

fallopian tubes

sexual organs and intestines

uterus or prostate

spinal reflex

Have the client lie on their stomach on the table. If they need a pillow under the chest to make their neck and/or chest region more comfortable, place it there now. Their feet are facing toes downwards, either over the edge of the table, over a small bolster under the ankles, or both. Cover them with a sheet and a blanket.

Expose both feet and with the warm moist towel, wipe off the right, then left foot and pat dry.

Starting with the right foot:
1. Loosen the ankle by rotating.
2. Pronate and supinate the ankle.

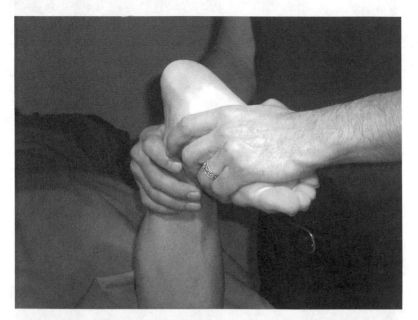

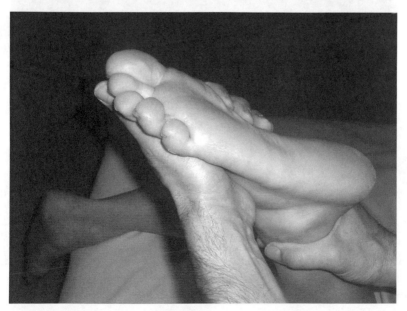

3. Loosen and stretch each toe, starting with the little toe.

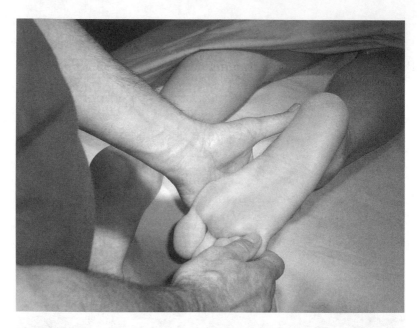

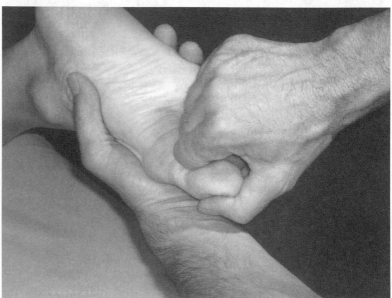

4. Apply a light coating of the "Calm and Clear" or Vata-reducing oil onto the foot. Rub it in for a few moments. Then spend approximately 30 seconds on each of the following reflex points.
   a) Pituitary.
   b) Pineal.
   c) Neck Reflex.

d) Loosen sides of all toes down to little toe.

e) Shoulder.

f) Webs underneath, starting between fourth and fifth toes (marmas).

g) Spinal reflex.

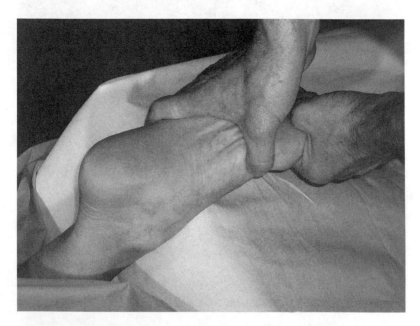

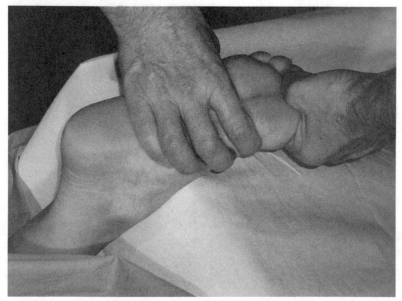

h) Achilles tendon—an excellent way of doing this is by squeezing the tendon out, starting at the base of the gastrocnemius and working your way down to the top of the heel.

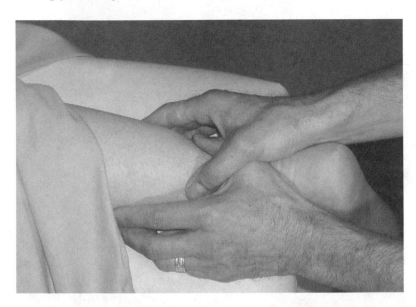

i) Heel compression—clasp your hands and grasp over the entire heel. Squeeze, then release suddenly.

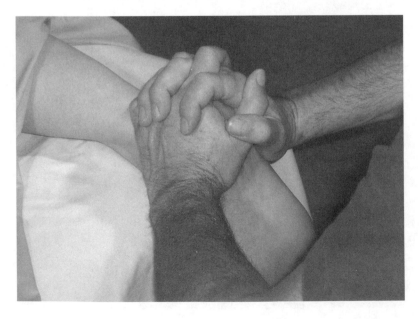

j) Outside of foot—fan using the crease in your palm.

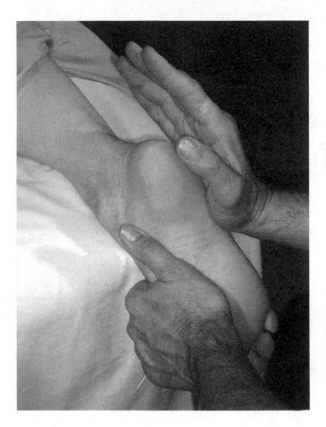

k) Lungs.

l) Stomach.

m) Liver.

n) Gall bladder (when doing left foot, substitute 'n' and 'o' for spleen and pancreas points).

o) Adrenal.

p) Small intestine.

q) Colon (ascending and transverse on right and transverse and descending on left).

r) Bladder.

s) Kidney (gently).

5. Repeat sequence for left foot.

At the end, hold both heels for a few moments, then ask your client
to turn over onto their back. Place a Head and Neck pillow
or equivalent under their head.

PHASE TWO—Work on the Abdomen

(approx. 7 minutes)

Make sure that your client's knees are drawn up and/or that there is a bolster under the knees. This will allow the abdominal muscles to be soft and more accessible. Standing to the client's right side:

1. Check the following points using deep clockwise rotational pressure **(note: As you do this have the person breathe in with your thumb just over the point and as they breathe out, sink your thumb into the point)**.

   a) ½ inch below the xyphoid process—a Kapha dosha diagnostic point.

   b) The point that is halfway between the above point and a point just above the navel—a Pitta dosha diagnostic point.

   c) The point just above the navel—Vata dosha diagnostic point.

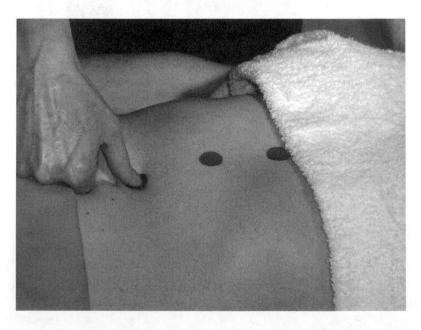

   Ask the client which of the points is most sensitive, then apply clockwise rotational pressure into that point another two times.

2. Take the "Calm and Clear" or Vata-balancing oil, place an adequate amount in your palm, and then tip it into the navel. Spread it over the abdomen in spiral clockwise swirling motions.

3. Roll the abdomen, using the heels of the palms on the right side of the abdomen, pushing gently to the left, then pulling back towards you with the fingers. Do this 7 times back and forth.

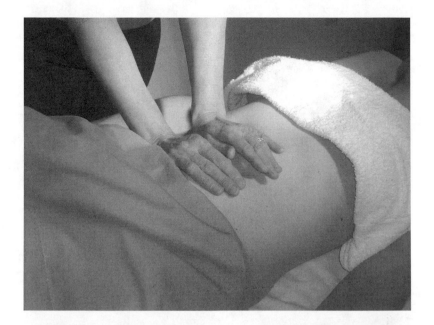

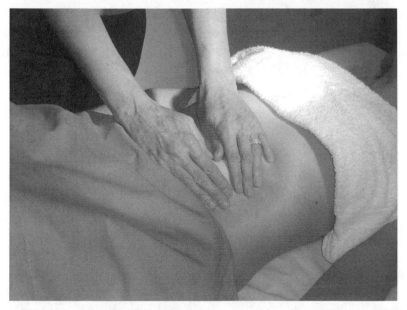

4. Do circular kneading in clockwise strokes around navel region.

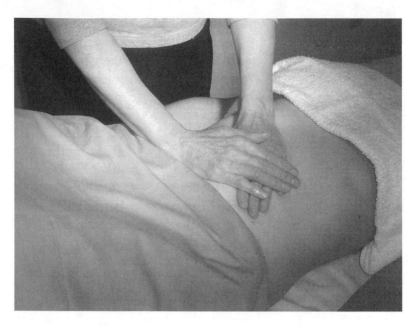

5. Apply circular strokes with the palms and fingertips in a clockwise motion around the abdomen, going deeper and deeper, following along the ascending, transverse, then descending colon. Continue this clockwise motion for at least 3 minutes.

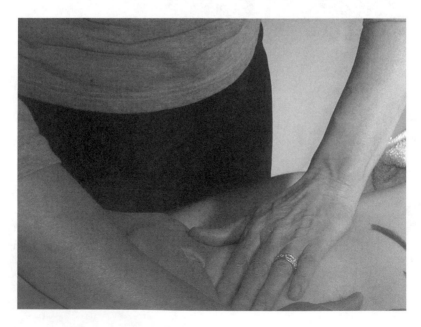

6. Repeat rolling as in number 3.

7. Rest your right thumb about 1.5 inches below the navel (3 finger-widths). Have the client breathe in and as they breathe out, sink your thumb down to the point where you meet resistance, then do 7 clockwise rotational motions. When the client breathes in, lift your thumb out and when they breathe out again, repeat. Do this a total of 3 times.

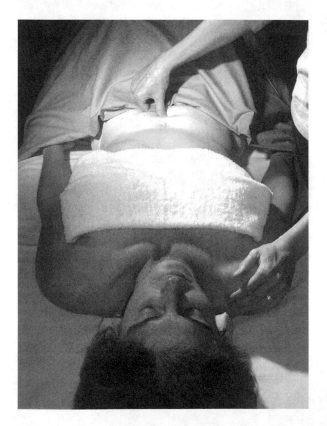

8. Finish with a polarity hold where left hand is under the lower back and the right hand is just below the navel. Hold until you have a sense of balance between your two hands.

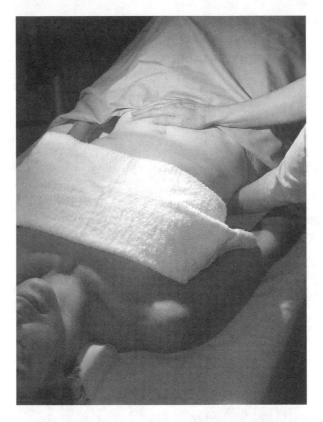

Cover abdomen with a towel and apply a Tummy Warmer or equivalent. Client may lower their legs if they wish.

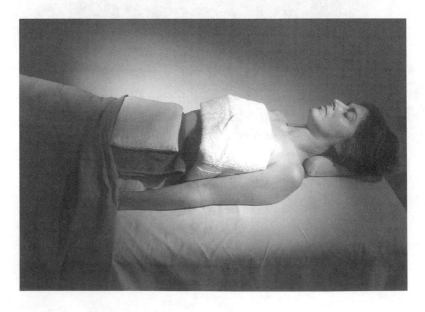

PHASE THREE: Dzub Nyin Series for Insomnia

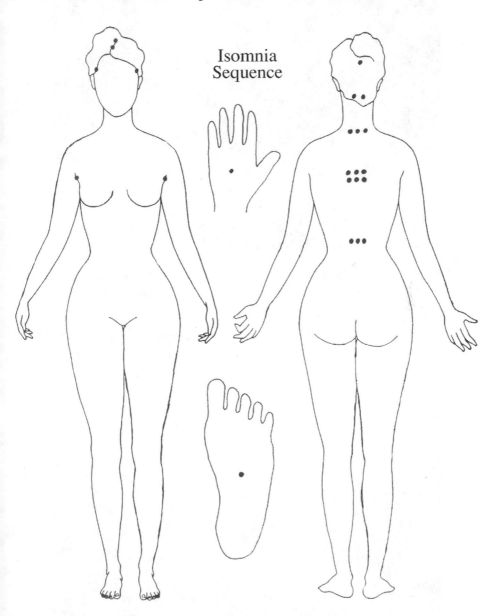

Isomnia Sequence

With the client lying on their back:

1. Turn the client's head to the left and place your left hand around their left ear. Place 3–5 drops of the "Calm and Clear" or Vata-balancing oil blend into the client's right ear.

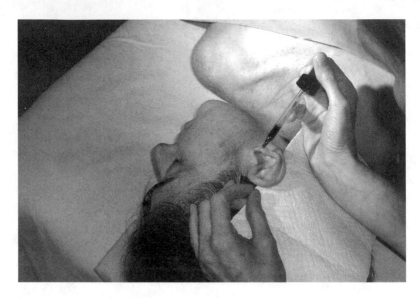

2. Digitally knead the right side of the scalp, starting at the back of the skull and working up over to the forehead. Do this kneading 3 times.

3. Repeat for the left side.

4. Using the Nutmeg Tibetan Lotion (which you will use on all subsequent points mentioned in this ritual), make your fingertips slightly oily, then massage the following points with the recommended hand positions. Do 7 clockwise rotational pressure movements on each point.

   a) Murdhi (central fontanel) Marma.

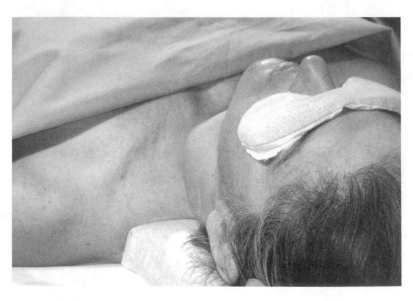

b) Shiva (posterior fontanel) Marma.

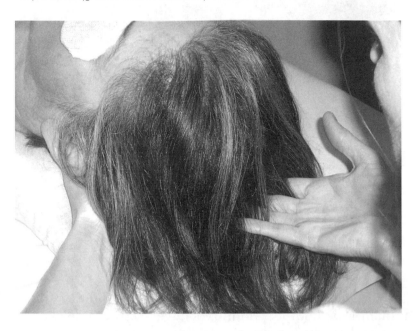

c) Brahma (anterior fontanel) Marma.

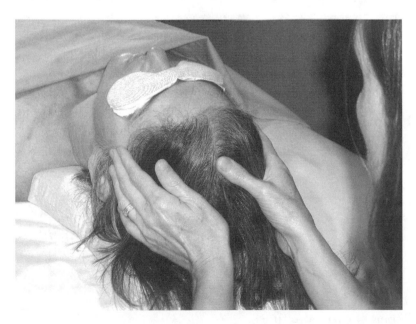

d) Posterior bilateral fontanel Marma (removes tension from eyes).

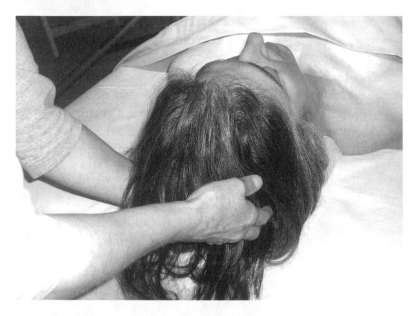

e) Shankhar (temple) Marma—(NOTE: On the third time through, leave both your thumbs or fingers on the temples and think positive thoughts about feeling sleepy or drowsy).

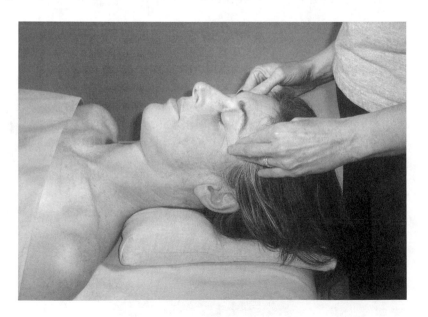

5. Repeat 4 two more times.

Remove the warm pad to the abdomen and ask the client to turn over onto their stomach.

6. Now focus on the spinous processes and points approximately ½ inch to the right of the following vertebral processes, using a small amount of the Nutmeg Tibetan Lotion.
    a) Cervical 7—center, right, then left (Vata marma point).
    b) Thoracic 5—center, right, then left (prana marma point).
    c) Thoracic 6—center, right, then left (heart marma point).
    d) Thoracic 10—center, right, then left (spleen marma point).

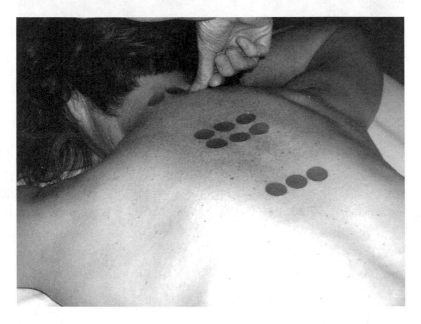

7. Repeat 6 two more times. (Note: use the thumbs on the points to the sides and the three finger "prong" approach to the spinous process itself.)
8. (optional) Apply deep palm pressure along both sides of spine, from the shoulders down to the buttocks. Go slowly. Have the client breathe with you. They breathe in and you do the same as you lift up and move. Then they breathe out and you breathe out and you press your palm deep into the muscles beside the spine. Do the right side first.

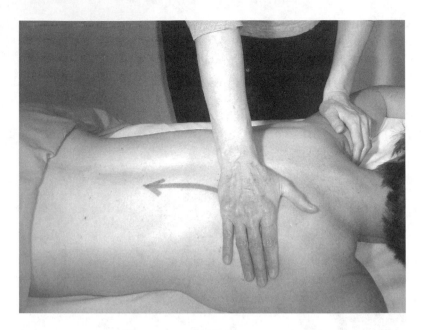

9. Cover the back and gently do meridian stroking, from the shoulders to the buttocks 7 times, then from the buttocks to the heels a minimum of 7 times.

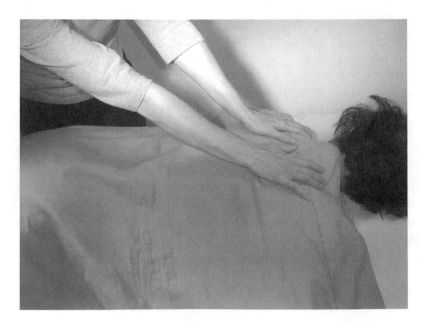

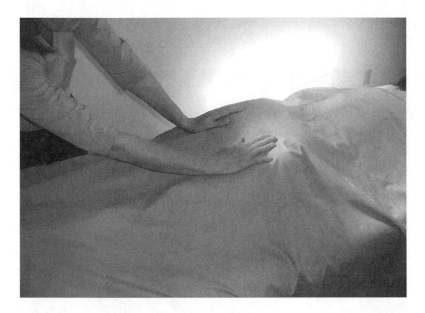

*Have the client turn onto their back again. Place the Tummy Warmer
on their abdomen and a Cool Eyes or eye pack over the eyes.*

10. With a small amount of Tibetan lotion, do the following points in
   sequence, pressing each with 7 clockwise rotational pressure movements (**remember: as you go from point to point, move around
   the table in a clockwise circle**).

   a) Marma in the center of the right hand.

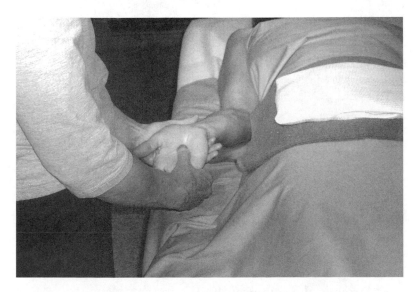

b) Marma in the center of the left hand.
c) Marma deep in the right armpit.

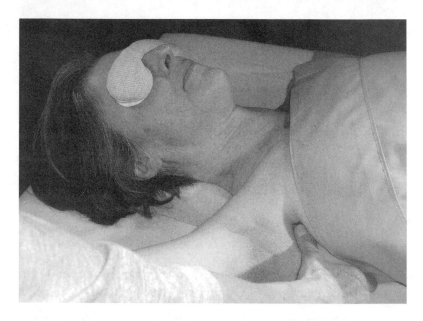

d) Marma deep in the left armpit.
e) Marma in the center of the bottom of the right foot.

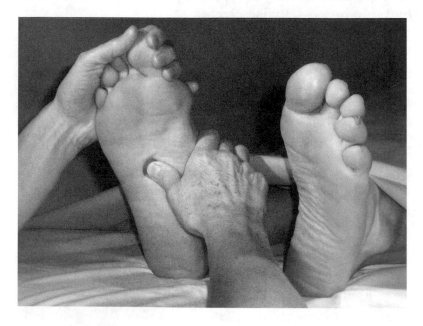

f) Marma in the center of the left foot.

11. Repeat 10 two more times.

12. Finish by holding the points that are midway between the medial malleolus and the edge of the heel. As you hold these points, encourage the client to breathe slowly and in sync with you. Make them aware of the contact they have with the surface that they are lying on. Hold the points until you sense that they are letting go and you feel that the points are balanced.

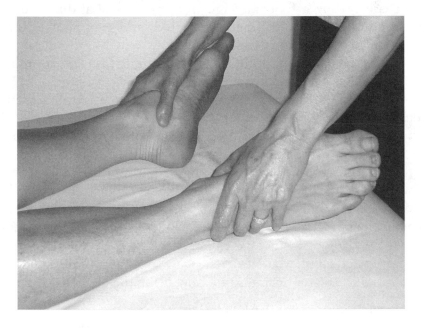

13. Cover the feet up. Breathe in and move away.

When it is time for your client to get up, assist them as they may be very drowsy. Offer them a beverage, such as the hot tea recommended in the products list.

■ *PediKarma*™

Ayurveda has a deep respect for the bathing and massaging of feet. The Padaprakshalana Ceremony is described in the epic Mahabharata, where the Hindu god, Krishna, washes the feet of his childhood friend, a Brahman. The people of the kingdom are stunned to see this and moved by this display of humility. Then there are the classic images of Vishnu, the Lord of preservation, who is always shown reclining in his serpent coil getting a foot massage from his wife, Lakshmi. Also, on many Hindu shrines you will find the sacred sandals of Shiva displayed to represent the presence of the deity.

Foot massage is said to protect people from disease and trouble and is also said to bring peace, prosperity and good luck. Still today in India, in many places, the host washes the feet of his guest with a blend of sandalwood paste and rose water and students wash the feet of their teachers, placing rings on their toes as a sign of deep respect and connection. But more commonly in India, they wash their feet 2 or 3 times a day as part of good hygiene, finishing with a splash of cool water on the bottoms of the feet. This increases blood circulation so the brain gets more oxygen and the spirit becomes more alert.

The healing practices of Ayurveda include a long tradition of understanding the body by being able to 'read' the foot. Beyond the analysis of reflexive points as in what we in the west know as reflexology, according to Ayurveda the foot can also be read using the elements.

- The heel represents the EARTH element.
- The area opposite the arch, the hollow, represents the WATER element.
- The ball of the foot represents the FIRE element.
- The toes represent the AIR element.
- The tops of the toes represent the Space element.

By observing the soles of the feet, the color, tone etc. in the different zones we can gain precious knowledge as to the condition of the client. E.g: hard skin on the fire element area suggests a logical, pragmatic, reasonable personality. This person knows how to balance the fire energy in their body. Dry skin on the heel indicates extra air element or fire element in the earth zone. Water element represents the feelings, affection, the esthetic and artistic sense, tenderness, desire, the intuitive side, receptiveness. Very often artists have a noticeable water zone. A white color to the foot means that there is more air element. A red color to the foot means more presence of the fire element.

The comparison of the right foot and the left is also significant. The left foot represents the feminine (the moon), and the right foot represents the masculine (the sun).

PediKarma™ is the trademarked name we have selected for a treatment ritual that focuses exclusively on the feet and uses three distinct Ayurvedic therapies on the feet. "Pedi" refers to foot and "Karma" in Sanskrit means action. As we see the deep benefits of this ritual, we decided to name it thus in keeping with the treatments of *purva* and *pancha* karmas.

The main action of this treatment is detoxification. Phase One begins with a foot soak as discussed earlier using the tridoshic bath salts. Prior to the feet being placed in water, however, the feet are looked at for where calluses have formed, reflexively indicating imbalances or sluggishness in the associated organs or areas of the body. Where there is a noticeable build up of callus, a foot file is applied to smooth the area and make it easier to work with. Traditionally, Ayurvedic practitioners used rough clay tablets to exfoliate the feet after they have been soaked. We have chosen a more gentle and hygienic method of removal using a metal file. The file that is used is best done prior to the soaking. The benefits of foot filing are:

- Increased absorption of essential oils.
- Allows for a deeper massage.
- Balances the pads of the feet for a more even step.
- Beautifying.

After the filing, the feet are placed in the foot soak for approximately 5–7 minutes. The benefits of the soak are:

- In keeping with ancient tradition it is welcoming, luxurious, and nurturing.
- Relaxing and grounding.
- Calming to the nervous system.
- Thoroughly cleansing in a gentle and comfortable way.

Phase Two involves an advanced Diamond Way Ayurveda reflexology treatment, focusing primarily on the skeletal structure reflexes. As with most standard reflexology, the treatment ends with the organs of elimination, which also means that these are, in turn, being stimulated for benefits. Phase Three is the use of the Kansa Vataki treatment as used in the Marma and Mud Magic ritual. However, at the end of this phase, ubtan powder is used as a way of removing the toxic oil.

Therapists who perform this treatment ritual with clients report excellent results. Clients feel lighter and relaxed. Stimulation to the feet helps with posture, digestion, and facilitates greater ease of movement.

This is a wonderful introduction for clients into Ayurvedic bodywork as well as massage in general. This can be especially effective for the older client. For therapists new to Ayurveda, as many already have some experience with standard reflexology, this treatment builds on skills and adds an Ayurvedic treatment to their service menu. Also, note that like all previously mentioned treatments, each phase can be done by itself or added to other treatment rituals or regimens.

Suggested Menu Description

PediKarma™

Your PediKarma™ experience begins with a balancing aroma-therapeutic foot soak. Then while comfortably resting you will receive a rejuvenating marma point and reflexology foot massage using customized oil followed by a rare foot massage with a Three Metal Bowl from India. Finally, your feet are dusted with a scented herbal powder and wrapped in warm towels.

Products and Equipment

Large foot bath

Massage Table

2 sheets and a blanket

PediKarma™ Foot Soak Salts

Ghee or Anise Tibetan Foot Lotion

Ankle support pillow

Kansa Vataki Foot Massage Bowl

Sandalwood Ubtan

'Checi' Foot File or equivalent

Optional:

Glass marbles for the bottom of the foot bowl

Pure Water Spray—super oxygenated water to spray off the feet after the soak in the salts

Warm Neck Pillow or equivalent

Nutmeg Lotion

PHASE ONE: Ayurvedic Tridoshic Bath Salts Foot Soak

1. Before soaking the feet, look at the calloused areas of the feet, observe foot coloration and refer to the reflexology chart to identify areas of congestion. Then use the Checi callous file and clean off some of the extra calloused skin.

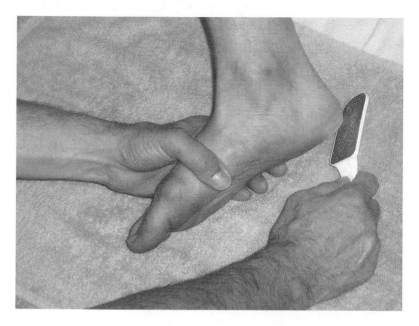

Prepare approx. 2 gallons of comfortably warm water in a footbath with 2 rounded tablespoons of the appropriate Ayurvedic Tridoshic Bath Salts blend. Placing small stones or glass marbles in the footbath provides added stimulation and stress relief. Decorate the bath with herbs or flowers if you have them.

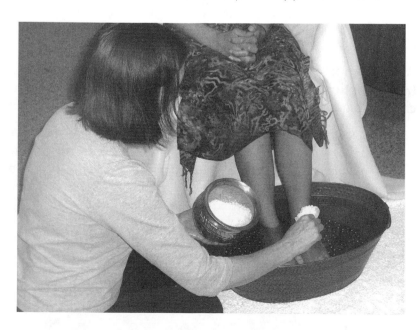

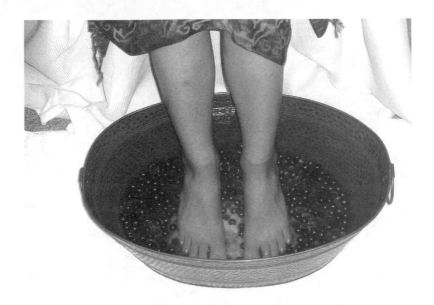

2. With the client sitting upright or in a chair, place both feet in the water and allow them to soak for 5 to 7 minutes.

3. While the client's feet are still soaking and for an *additional extra*, apply nutmeg lotion to the neck and tops of the shoulders, massage in, apply a warm rolled dry towel and, if available, a heated neck pillow. Use this time to discuss with your client ways in which they can help to balance their body and improve their health through foot care. Provide some ideas, products, etc.

4. After this, remove feet from water and pat them dry, right foot first. (As an option in the summer or for more pitta clients you may choose to quickly spray the feet with pure water.)

> *Bring the client to the massage table and direct them to lie down on their stomach. They may have their feet over the edge of the table or up on a bolster. (The primary consideration is the client's comfort. But make sure that your chair is at a good height so as not to put stress in your own shoulders.)*

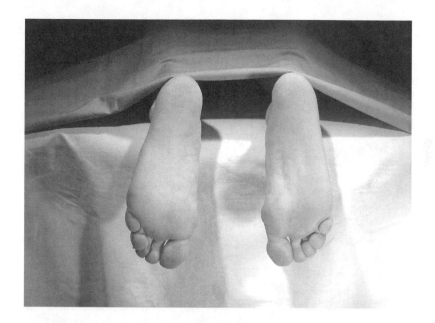

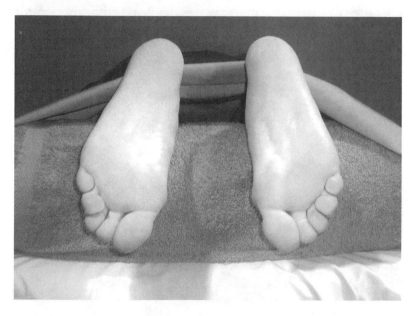

PHASE TWO: Marma/Reflexology Series

Most actions will be done with clockwise circular motions. However, marmas will just be pressed relatively firmly a minimum of 6 times. Starting with the right foot:

1. With knee bent, loosen the ankle by rotating.
2. Pronate and supinate the ankle.

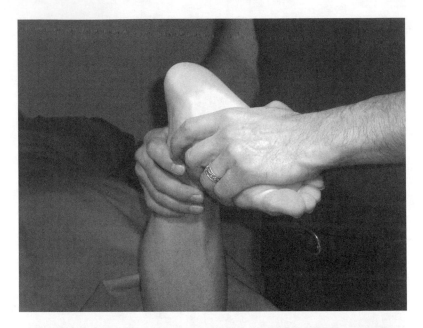

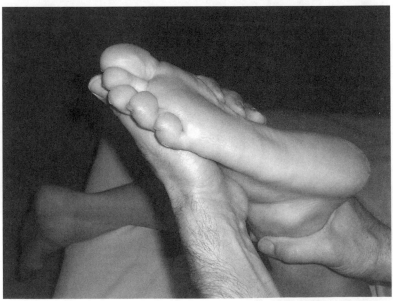

3. Loosen and stretch each toe, starting with the little toe.

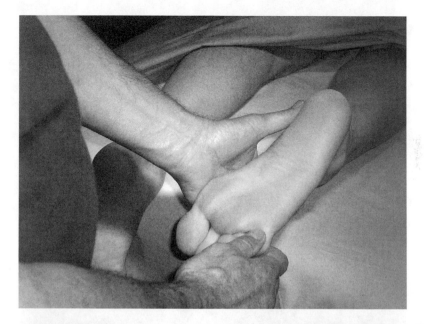

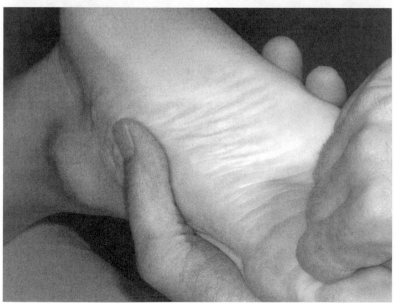

4. Onto the foot, rub (in winter) Ghee or (in summer) Tibetan Anise Lotion (NOTE: use the Tibetan Anise Lotion if the client tends to get tired or hot eyes).

5. Pituitary reflex.

6. Pineal reflex.

7. Neck Reflex.

8. Loosen the sides of all toes down to the little toe .

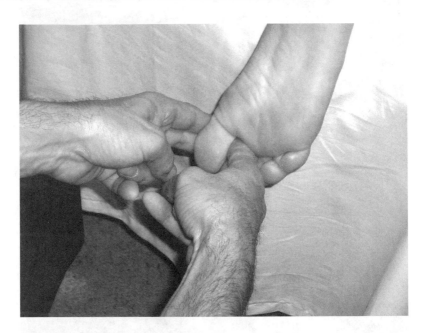

9. Shoulder reflex.
10. Webs underneath, starting between fourth and fifth toes (marmas).

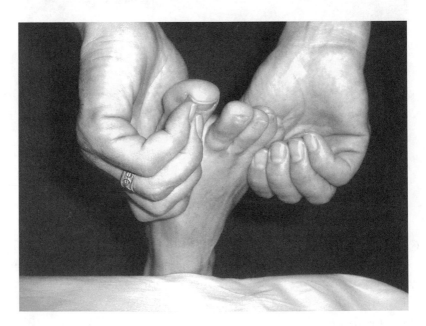

11. Spinal reflex, using one finger and going down from the base of the

big toe to the heel, or using the method with all fingers as shown in picture.

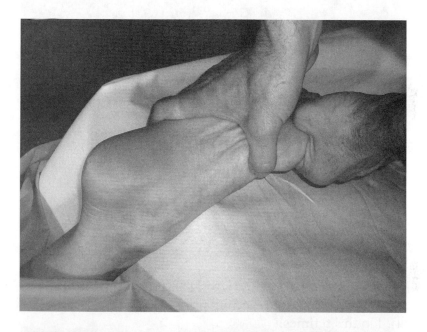

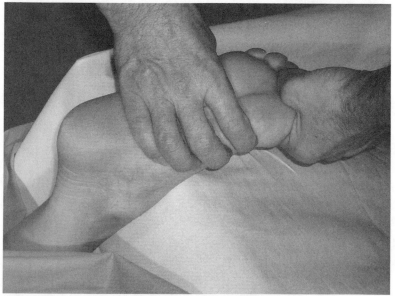

12. Achilles tendon, using the butterfly-type squeezing method.

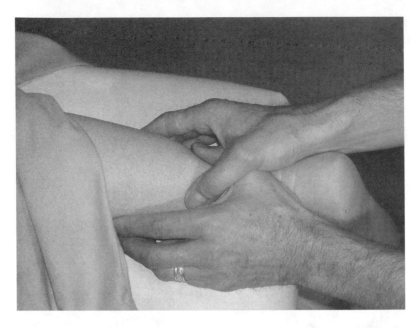

13. GULPA marmas (below the lateral and medial malleolus)—to tone genitals (NOTE: avoid during pregnancy and if menstruation is full). Do this 6 times.

14. Heel compression—squeeze, with quick release.

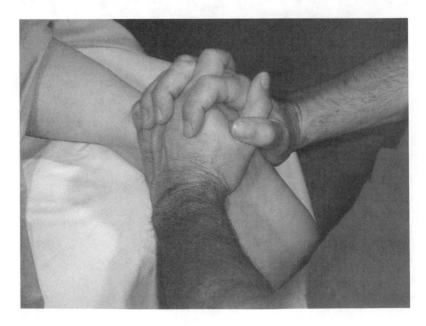

15. Outside of foot, fan.

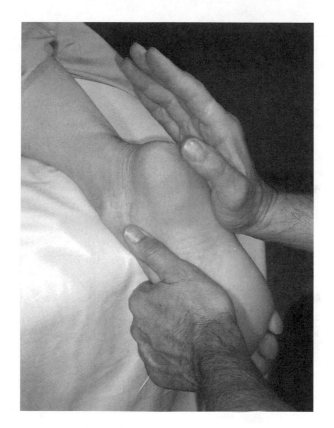

16. KSHIPRA marma (between base of big and 2nd toe)—for increase of prana and lower limb strength. Do this 6 times.

17. KURCHA (KURUCHCHA) marma (lateral edge of stomach reflex)—to calm the body and increase mental acuity. Do this 6 times.

18. KURCHASHIRA marma (middle of small intestine reflex)—for digestion. Do this 6 times.

19. Colon reflex (ascending and transverse on the right and transverse and descending on the left).

20. Bladder reflex.

21. Kidney reflex(gently)—same as TALHRIDAYAM marma.

Reflexology Chart

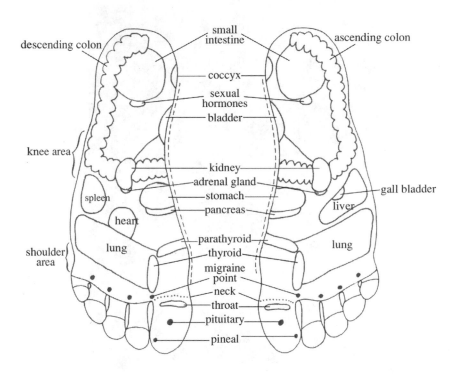

Outside View of Foot

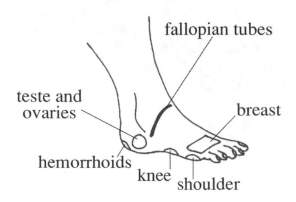

Inside View of Foot

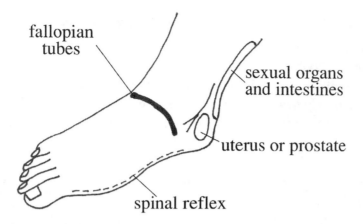

fallopian tubes

sexual organs and intestines

uterus or prostate

spinal reflex

Marmas on the Bottoms of the Feet

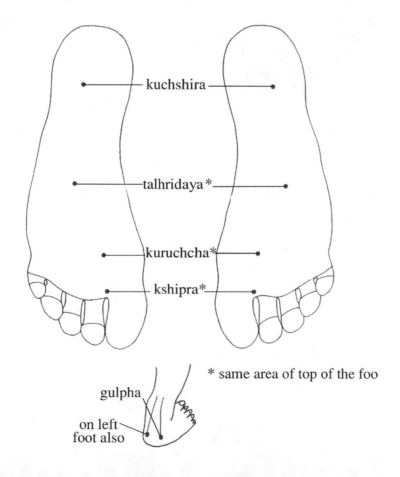

kuchshira

talhridaya *

kuruchcha*

kshipra*

gulpha

on left foot also

* same area of top of the foo

22. Repeat sequence for the left foot.

23. At the end, hold both heels for a few moments.

PHASE THREE: Three-Metal Bowl Foot Massage

1. Starting with the right foot, apply more of the Ghee or Tibetan Anise Lotion, coating the entire foot.

2. For 5 minutes, take the three-metal foot massage bowl and with slow, relatively firm movements, massage the entire right foot:

    a) The bottom: rub back and forth along the entire length of the foot at least 21 times.

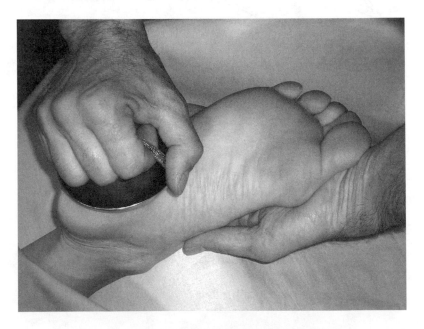

    b) The ends of the toes, starting with the big toe: perform 7 clockwise circles on the very tips.

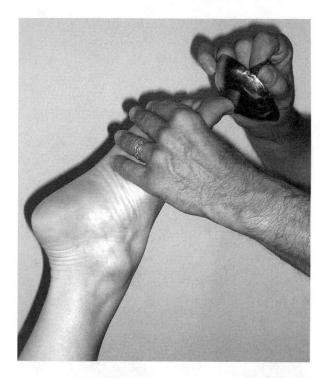

c) Starting at the edge of the big toes, make small clockwise circular strokes along the inner side and arch of the foot, around the back of the heel, and finally up along the outer edge of the foot up to the toes. Go around like this 3 times.

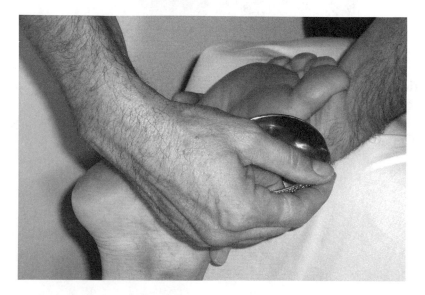

d) The top of the foot: as the area is bonier with less dense tissue, use lighter pressure. Go up and over both medial and lateral aspects of the ankle joint. Strokes back and forth along the metatarsal lines.

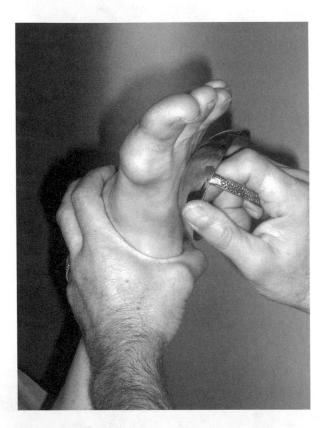

e) Do the bottom again, this time doing clockwise circular motions, followed by figure eights over the entire bottom, then deep rotations into the arch.

f) Three spins on the tips of the toes, starting with the big toe. The motion is like trying to untwist a lid off of a can.

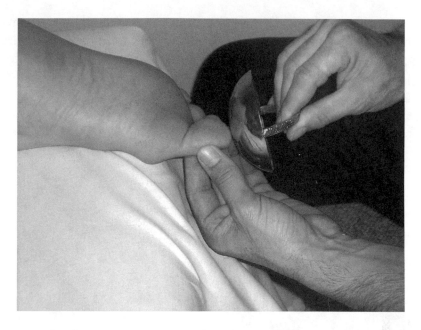

3. Wrap the foot in a warm towel and repeat Step 2 on the left foot.
4. After completing the left foot, wrap it and allow the client to rest for 2–3 minutes.
5. Apply Sandalwood Ubtan to the right, then the left foot. Cover the feet with warm towels and allow the client to rest another 2–3 minutes.

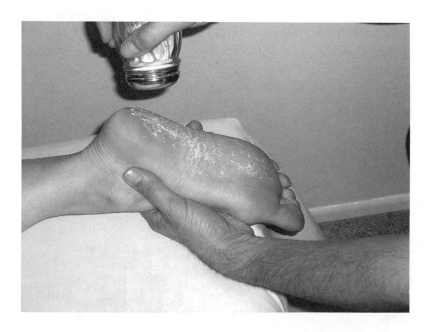

6. Clean off the right, then the left foot, first with a dry towel to remove the excess dust , followed by a warm, moist towel. Pat dry.
7. Hold the marma that is halfway between the medial malleolus and the edge of the heels. Hold these points until you have a sense of balance. Inhale, then move away.

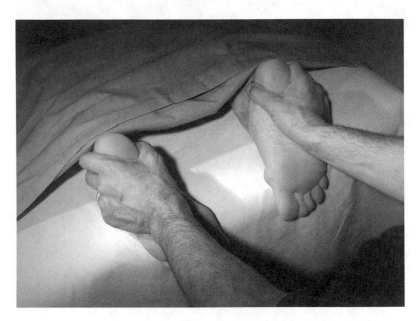

Allow the client to rest another few minutes before you have them get up.
As they have been on their stomach, if their head has been turned
to one side or the other, you might want to have them turn over and
loosen their neck. The Nutmeg Tibetan Lotion can be helpful for this.
Offer a warm beverage such as hot tea.

As there is a home version of the foot soak, Kansa Vataki, and reflexology mentioned with previous treatment rituals listed, refer to those. At the same time, your client may wish to purchase a foot file or know where they could get something similar.

■ *Special Techniques and Add-on Services*
Nadi Swedana: The Use of Gentle, Penetrating, Moist Heat

NADI (nah-dee) means tube or channel. SWEDANA (sway-dahn-nah) means the use of herbal steam. Literally swedana means sweat but the goal here is not necessarily to produce sweat but to warm the skin. Thus, Nadi Swedana treatment is the application of herbal steam to a particular part of the body.

In ancient times herbal tea was simmered in a clay pot over a fire and the steam directed into a bamboo pipe. In recent years, western Ayurvedic practitioners have tried to create variations on this theme using pressure cookers set upon hot plates with a heat-resistant hose attached as the steam delivery device. This has often proved precarious and looks very much like the kitchen equipment that it is. In today's spa, or even for a serious Ayurvedic clinic, we have found that a portable facial steamer is capable of delivering the same benefits, is more hygienic, and is also aesthetically pleasing.

Localized steaming using the facial steamer/nadi swedana equipment differs from a generalized steam bath in that the steam is a little hotter, more forcefully delivered, and specific. The aim is to direct heat, moisture, and herbal compounds deep into small areas to open up the tiniest channels in the skin to allow cleansing and re-balancing of subtle energy. This type of application is best suited to thicker or denser tissues as well as over the spine and other joints of the body.

What does Nadi Swedana do exactly? In Western terms we would say it moistens, stimulates, and increases the circulation in the tissues that are being touched by the jet of warm steam. In Ayurvedic terms we would say it decreases the Vata and Kapha qualities of the body and increases Pitta qualities.

It is the Vata or wind-like quality of the body that is increased by high stress levels, travel, fast paced living, lack of routine, and just by getting older. It is this increased Vata that makes our mood variable, our jaw tight, our back ache. Eventually, as this wind-like energy dries out our body, our face wrinkles and our posture erodes. Nadi Swedana keeps this Vata quality in check by warming and moisturizing the joints. In this way Nadi Swedana reduces pain and stiffness in the body, and helps maintain a youthful posture and flexibility. The feeling is one of being gently eased into a space of relaxation and deeper connection with your body.

Nadi Swedana also reduces Kapha qualities. These qualities get the chance to increase when we don't exercise regularly and eat a diet high in fats and carbohydrates. Typical symptoms are like feeling a little hungover, lethargic, sluggish, sticky, and depressed. Increased Kapha means the body gains weight, retains liquid and blocks the natural channels through which toxins leave the body. Nadi Swedana uses herbs and pressurized steam to stimulate tissues, allowing toxins to move freely. The result is that our bodies feel lighter, fresher, and happier.

Pitta qualities are increased by Nadi Swedana. That means heat is increased by this process. This is beneficial unless there is already heat from inflammation or infection in the area being worked on. Nadi Swedana should not be used on rheumatoid arthritic joints, on infected skin, over the head, eyes, heart or genitals. **Extra heat on these conditions or over these areas could cause health problems.**

The Benefits of Nadi Swedana:

Nadi Swedana is used in pancha karma when it is deemed appropriate by an Ayurvedic practitioner. However, it is a perfectly safe treatment to be offered by most therapists or spa technicians, once trained with respect to technique and appropriateness. To determine whether it is an appropriate and/or useful add-on service in a spa, the length of which can be anywhere between fifteen minutes and half an hour, you should consider offering Nadi Swedana for the following conditions:

- To help release muscle spasms in the back and neck.
- To reduce pain and stiffness in the joints.
- To improve posture.
- To help the body feel lighter, fresher, and more flexible.

What to Say to Your Client:

If you wish to offer Nadi Swedana as a 15 or 30 minute add-on, you can explain this treatment in the following way to your client.

Nadi Swedana is an excellent way for me to be able to get beneficial oils and herbs to go deeper into areas where you feel discomfort. It is very gentle and relaxing, and it makes it easier for your body to let go without me applying any unnecessary deep pressure.

What you need to do the treatment:

Portable, hand-held facial steamer/nadi swedana equipment

Dosha-appropriate massage oil

The following herbal preparations, excellent for all doshas

- Raw herbs of Bay Leaf, Eucalyptus Leaf, and Ginger—in equal parts, this herb decoction is *Tridoshic* in its benefit.

• (optional) essential oils of ginger, bay, and eucalyptus that can be placed on a cotton ball and placed in the wick compartment on the arm of the facial steamer.

Procedure:

1. If you are using the facial steamer, fill with cold tap water to the level recommended (see red line in the clear portion of the tank).

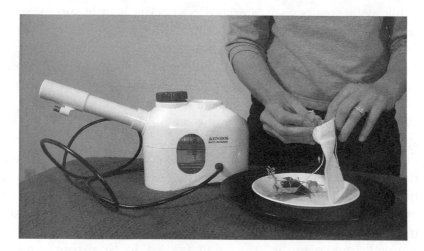

Take a small muslin or cloth bag or pouch, place the herbs into the pouch, and place the pouch in the herb receptacle at the top of the steamer. Alternatively, you can take a ball of cotton and put a few drops of each essential oil on the cotton and place in the steel compartment near the opening of the steamer arm.

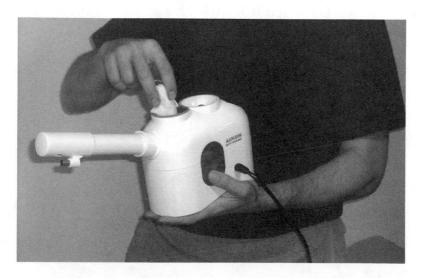

2. Turn on the facial steamer and bring it up to the point where a good forceful stream of steam is pouring through the opening of the arm. If you are using a pressure cooker variety of nadi swedana equipment, fill the cooker and place the oils or the herbs in the water. Turn your hot plate up to maximum (you will need a hot plate with a minimum of 1000 watts capacity to bring your pressure cooker up to pressure).

3. While your steamer (or pressure cooker) is heating up, apply and massage in warmed organic sesame oil or dosha-appropriate oil to the area you are going to focus the steam on. Then massage the area, using enough friction to work the oil into the skin. The procedure offered for the back, which follows below, mentions specific marma and acupressure points onto which medicated oils can be placed.

4. When you are ready to apply the steam, if you are using a facial steamer, hold it so the base or body stays parallel to the ground. In other words, don't tilt it. Also, the opening of its arm should be turned to the side, rather than pointing downwards. It can be slightly downwards, which can be good to reach the back. However, it is even better and safer if you have the client turn on their side to get these areas. The steam should feel pleasantly warm and as if it is evenly flowing over the area being worked on. **Scalding can occur if you hold the nozzle too close or hold it in one place too long.** Do check with your client for comfort, as everyone experiences heat differently. To do this follow the next step.

5. Before playing the steam directly on the desired area, place one hand directly on that area and aim the steam at your hand. In that way, you will know approximately how warm the steam will feel to the specific area.

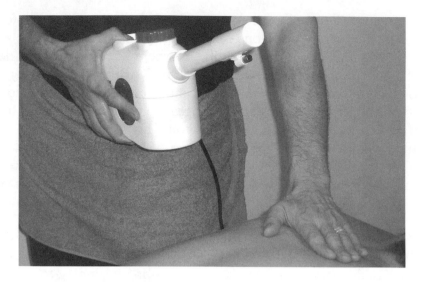

6. Gently play the steam over the area needing attention e.g. back, hips, shoulder, or other joints for five minutes or until the skin feels moist, warm to the touch, and looks slightly pink. Move the steam over the area, back and forth, like you were painting the area with the steam. You can even use clockwise circular movements to pacify and ease the tension out of the area. **Don't keep the steam focused or stationary as this can create the risk of scalding.**

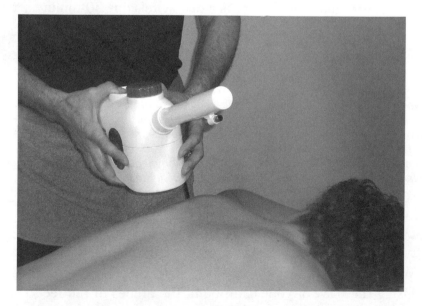

7. Pat the skin dry with a warm towel. Alternatively (and more traditionally), apply an Ayurvedic herbal cleanser, or *ubtan*, to the area.

Steaming will drive the oil into the skin. Although a doshic appropriate oil is recommended, one can also use plain sesame oil which can penetrate into the joint lubricating it rather like oiling a creaky door. (Sesame oil is mostly useful for VATA or KAPHA complaints.) The oil that remains on the skin surface must be removed. If it is allowed to remain it will act like a toxin, congesting the area, and it can make the client feel achy and sluggish later on. This is why the oil and moisture should be patted dry or removed with an ubtan. Sprinkle the ubtan on dry and rub in. Cover the area. Alternatively, one can also mix the ubtan with warm spring water to make a fine paste that you wipe on. Leave for a minute and wipe off with a warm moist towel.

How often can this procedure be offered?

This treatment is safe to do as often as once daily. It makes a luxurious add on to full-body massage or an unusually nurturing beginning to any one-hour service to help the client feel extra comfortable in areas where there is extra tension or stress, such as the neck or any region of the back. For those in a hurry it makes a deep-acting, long lasting half-hour unique service.

Nadi Swedana Relaxed Back Ritual: A Suggested Series

The following is a back treatment ritual that can be done by as either aestheticians or massage therapists a deeply relaxing 30-minute service.

Spa Menu Description

Nadi Swedana Relaxed Back Ritual

Nadi Swedana is a unique Ayurvedic treatment that delivers a soothing blend of healing herbs to those areas where you feel your greatest stress and tension. In just 15 to 30 minutes, feel how your tissues are softened, hydrated, and relaxed. As a wonderful 30 minute treatment for back tension and tightness, as the start to your other services or done with Abhyanga or Ayurvedic Massage, Nadi Swedana will provide you with a sense of lightness and ease.

Start with Steps 1–3 in the above mentioned Nadi Swedana general protocol. Where it mentions to do massage, do the following:

1. With the client lying on their front, apply oil to the back in general.
2. Using the back of your fist, pound the arches of the feet, starting with the right. This has a deeply relaxing effect on the entire back.

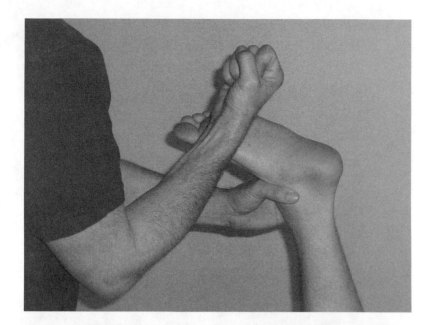

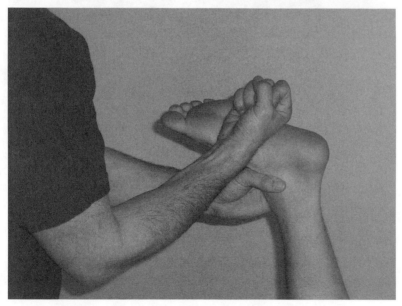

3. Using the thumb and 3-finger methods of Dzub Nyin, do the fol-
lowing marma points with clockwise, rotational pressure:
   - Cervical 7 (VATA point), center, right, then left.
   - Thoracic 5 (Chi point), center, right, then left.
   - Thoracic 6 (Heart point), center, right, then left.

- Lumbar 1 (Kidney point), center, right, then left.
- Lumbar 3 (Large Intestine point), center, right, then left.
- Lumbar 5 (Urinary Bladder point), center, right, then left.
- Marma point that is midway from bottom of buttocks and back of knee.

4. Repeat Step 3 two more times.

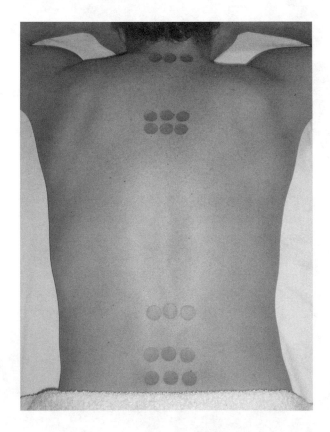

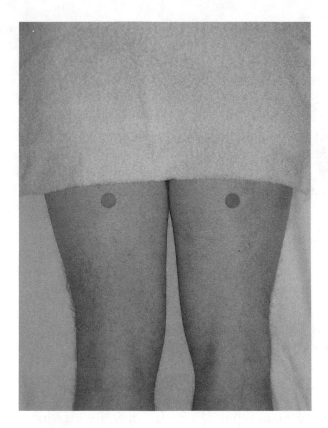

5. Have person roll to either side and continue on with Steps 4 through 7 as mentioned above. The steaming of the back should go for approximately 5 to 7 minutes.

Nasya—Ayurvedic Sinus Treatment

Have you ever had a client ask if there was anything you could do for a persistent feeling of congestion in the head? What about a treatment to banish those deep, dark circles under their eyes? And of course, there's always a bit of neck pain and stiffness that most clients wouldn't mind seeing less of.

In the vast repertoire of Ayurvedic treatments, there is one treatment that can address all of these health and beauty concerns: **Nasya**.

Nasya (also known as Najong in Tibetan) is a sinus treatment that delivers herbal preparations into the sinuses in a variety of ways for a number of purposes. Treatments that focus on the cleansing of the nasal passages are one of the five karmas in Pancha Karma and Nasya is featured as one of the primary methods to do this.

Nasya can be done with herbal oils, decoctions, juices, powders (as in snuffs), even the smoke of herbs and incense inhaled nasally. Tibetan doctors will recommend that incenses with calming herbs are strongly inhaled by those under stress. However, the most common type of Nasya used by itself or as a part of the practice of Pancha Karma, is the use of drops of herbal solutions and preparations that have as their base sesame oil or clarified butter (ghee).

Within the context of a spa service, if one has medical backing or has training and feels both competent and confident to offer Nasya as a service, there are a number of reasons why it is a beneficial service to offer. Using the Nasya treatment ritual provided below, we have seen the following benefits:

- clearing the head.
- banishing dark rings and/or puffiness from underneath the eyes.
- relieving chronic neck pain, especially as in the case of whiplash injuries.
- facilitating a full night of restful sleep.
- increasing vitality.
- looking younger.
- freeing the mind to connect with its joyful nature.

There are three main types of Nasya. They are classified according to their action: 1) *Shodhan*, or cleansing Nasya, 2) *Shamana*, or pacifying Nasya, and 3) *Bruhan*, or nourishing Nasya.

For general purposes and within the context of spa, we recommend simple forms of *Shamana* and *Shodhan* Nasya, both done as 15-minute add-on services. The warm oil Nasya is *Shamana* or pacifying in nature. A simple home version of this treatment ritual can be given to clients. The form of *Shodhan* Nasya that we recommend uses diluted fresh ginger juice and raw sugar. It is an entirely different experience and has the most dramatic effect on the client's appearance. Traditionally, it is given as one of the five cleansing processes of Pancha Karma. However, it may be used outside of this context with excellent therapeutic results for those with either chronic or intermittent sinus congestion, dark circles under the eyes, and/or stiffness or pain in the neck. **It is best administered by a therapist.**

The following descriptions for your menu will help both you and your client in deciding whether or not this treatment ritual should be offered.

Spa Menu Descriptions

Shamana Nasya

Warm herbal oil Nasya is a Shamana, or pacifying, treatment that is gentle and soothing. After your sinuses are warmed, drops of medicated herbal oil are administered to one nostril at a time. This form of Nasya will lubricate the sinus passages and then go deeper to penetrate the bony joints of the face. The result is greater freedom to breathe from the nose. With the breath travels prana, the subtle life-force energy that makes us feel joyful and alive. Stress and tension in the face are relieved. It is a very useful treatment for anyone that flies frequently, lives in a dry climate, or suffers from general dryness.

Ginger Shodhan Nasya

Shodhan Nasya is intended to cleanse your nasal passages. After warming up the forehead and cheeks, a mixture of freshly grated ginger juice and raw sugar are administered to each of your nostrils. This is a very effective treatment for chronic or periodic sinus congestion, puffiness or dark circles under the eyes, and pain and/or stiffness in your neck.

General Precautions

Regardless of the form of Nasya administered, avoid offering or doing Nasya

- after a hot bath.
- after eating a meal.
- after having sexual intercourse.
- after drinking alcohol.
- during menstruation or pregnancy.

Products and Equipment Needed

There are some products and equipment that are common to both forms of Nasya. These are:

- glass eye dropper with a rubber end.
- hot water and wash cloth or hot water bottle.
- facial tissue.
- head and neck pillow or neck support equivalent.
- quarter cup of sesame oil.

If you are doing the pacifying or *Shamana* Nasya, warmed sesame oil, ghee, or a commonly available Ayurvedic oil called *Vacha* or *Sidda Soma* oil can be used for the nasal drops.

If you are doing the Ginger *Shodhan* Nasya, you will need the following:
- fine grater or blender.
- 3-inch-long piece of good, fresh ginger root.
- a small amount of purified water.
- strainer or muslin cloth.

Preliminary Preparation for performing Ginger Shodhana Nasya:

Here we use liquid drops of diluted ginger juice to create a cleansing action. By cleansing we mean cleansing the sinus cavities but also clearing the head and neck area of excess Vata energy—that which causes pain and tension. Vata energy in the head is known as "prana". Prana energy relates to higher cerebral, sensory, and motor functions and movement in the kidneys.

Classically, this type of treatment is used for clearing the sinuses, reducing pain in the face, head, and neck, and helping kidney function. From the beauty point of view it definitely reduces dark rings under the eyes, a pinched look in the sinuses, and/or a sunken or puffy look around the eyes. It is a simple technique, but its effects run deep, both physically and emotionally. **More than the Shamana type of Nasya, please always observe the contraindications listed above for Ginger Nasya.**

PHASE ONE: Prepare the Ginger Solution

1. Grate the ginger using a fine grater or blender. Squeeze out the juice from the pulp into a small bowl (if you have a juicer, this will also work). Strain juice through a fine meshed strainer.
2. Add a pinch of raw or brown sugar and a dash of water per 2 tablespoons of ginger juice. The sugar stops the ginger from burning. Place in the dropper bottle (if you make a large quantity of the solution or if it is to be used much later on, store it in a refrigerator). Otherwise, place the bottle of ginger solution in a hot towel cabinet or a cup of hot water to warm. When you are ready to use the solution, it should be just above body temperature. Test this by putting a few drops on the back of your hand before you administer it to the client.
3. Wrap the hot water bottle in a towel to keep it warm, or prepare the hot water with a wash cloth so that it is ready for use.
4. Warm the sesame oil.
5. Arrange all the equipment to be within easy reach. Make sure the room is quiet and warm.

PHASE TWO: The Nasya Procedure

If you are performing the *Shamana* Nasya with warm oil, follow the above from Step 2 with respect to getting the oil warm and prepared for the client. Then follow with Steps 3 through 5 as described. After this is done, for either form of Nasya, do the following steps:

1. With your client already on their back on the table, be sure that their head and neck are supported by the head and neck pillow, a towel roll, or equivalent.

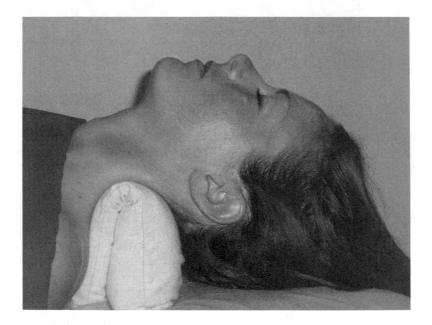

2. If you have not already given your client some form of face massage, you can do the Opening Sequence of the Ayurvedic Face Rejuvenation followed by a vigorous facial massage with warm sesame oil. Clockwise circular motions will relieve stress in the facial tissue. However, the main purpose of the massage, at this point, is simply to increase circulation and work the oil into the skin.

3. Place a wet, hot face cloth on the forehead and both sides of the face so that the nose is the only exposed area. Keep applying heat in this way until the face, especially the forehead and cheeks, is really rosy and the oil is absorbed.

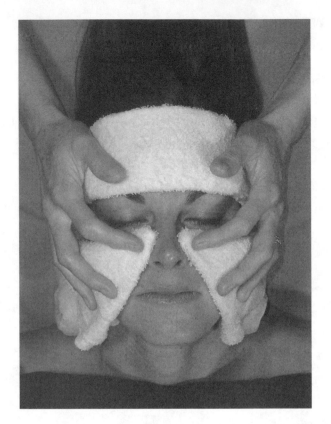

4. Adjust the position of the head so the neck is supported and slightly cocked back, the nostrils pointing upwards.

5. Block the left nostril with your left fingers so that the right nostril is the only one open. If you are doing the warm oil *Shamana* Nasya, drop 3 to 5 drops of oil into the right nostril with the eyedropper. If you are applying the Ginger solution, do the same with 3 to 5 drops of the ginger juice solution (if you are going to offer this treatment as part of what you do with your client over a period of weeks, you can increase the amount by two drops per week. For example: week 1, 3 drops; week 2, 5 drops; and so on up to a maximum of 9 or 10 drops per nostril).

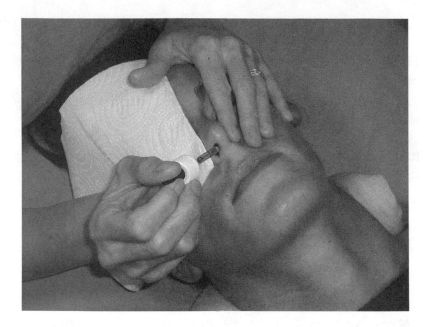

Nasya

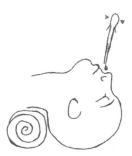

6. Encourage your client to breathe normally.
7. Massage the sinus area above and below the right eye. The eye may tear, especially with the ginger solution, indicating some emotional release. The client may also feel energy dancing over their face (they may also gag a bit as the spicy ginger or oil hits the back of their throat). Use smooth massage strokes around the sinus area to ground this energy.

8. Ask when they are ready for the application to the left nostril. Proceed in the same manner as you did on the right side.
9. Have your client rest briefly after the procedure, especially if you are then going to go on to any other treatment.
10. Take your time. If this is the end of the treatments to be offered, when the Nasya is complete, support your client's shoulders as they sit up. Support the sternum with one hand and use your other hand to stroke down their spine. Have them move slowly and suggest that they take their time with things over the next hour.

Netra Basti: Bathing the Eyes in Clarified Butter (Ghee)

There are many sense-oriented therapies in Ayurveda that use oil. Although each sense is associated with a particular organ and specific body energetic (i.e. dosha, i.e. Vata, Pitta, or Kapha), in general the nervous systems of the body are associated with Vata, where a stimulation moves into the body through a sense organ, is interpreted, and then acted upon. As such, all senses can be nourished or traumatized, leaving impressions in the mind that will, in turn, be acted upon in one way or another other in the future.

Netra Basti is a technique that has as its focus the eyes. *Netra* means eyes. The word *basti* is Sanskrit and implies a cleansing action. Netra Basti is, therefore, a technique that has a cleansing effect on the eyes. The eyes are bathed in plain or medicated warm ghee. A ring of dough is built up around the eye to create a well, into which the ghee solution is poured. It is allowed to sit on the eye for approximately twenty minutes. Dust, dirt, even substances trapped in the eyes that a person has been unaware of can surface in the liquid ghee. Besides this cleansing aspect, Netra Basti is also nutritive. Gazing through a warm ghee solution has a directly nourishing effect on the optic nerve and the nervous system. It is used for any number of eye complaints.

Beyond specific eye conditions themselves, there are other medical, therapeutic, and aesthetic benefits. Netra Basti is used for a number of conditions with psycho-social factors involved. For example, it is considered one of the treatments of choice for hyperactivity or Attention Deficit Disorder. According to Ayurvedic theory, the cause of such a condition is that not enough light is getting to the brain. As Netra Basti nourishes the optic nerve, peripheral vision is improved and vision become more acute and, at the same time, relaxed. We have seen cases where a child's focus as well as their ability to use language has been dramatically improved following both individual and series of Netra Basti treatments. We have also seen and used Netra Basti as a gentle means of helping clients in counseling to retrieve painful visual memories which are not only psychological issues, but have also have been a contributory factor in their vision impairment. As such, as a social worker, I have recommended the use of Netra Basti in conjunction with such therapies as EMDR (Eye Movement De-sensitization and Reprocessing).

All of these examples convey the depth to which Netra Basti can benefit clients. It should also make it clear why, beyond the orifice issue in providing insurance for this treatment, Netra Basti is best done within the context of a medi-spa or place where the therapist is either medically licensed or working under someone else's license umbrella. That being said, the spa therapist in such an environment may want to consider offering Netra Basti for purely aesthetic reasons, provided they understand that along with such benefits as relaxing the entire area around the eye sockets, which can alleviate dark rings and puffiness around the eyes, and gives the eyes a lustrous quality, there will also be some psychological and emotional benefits. Like Shirodhara, Netra Basti opens up the sense fields, making the client more impressionable. Consequently, **if Netra Basti is to be offered, it should be offered as the last in any series of treatments. Also, the client should be provided space and time to ground themselves and be instructed to not go straight into any stressful situations afterwards.** Encourage your client to give themselves a minimum of two hours quiet time away from the stresses of bright lights, loud noise, crowds, or emotional confrontations. This process opens the field of vision allowing impressions to flow deep into your visual memory banks. Let these impressions be pleasant ones.

Spa Menu Description

Netra Basti: Bathing the Eyes in Clarified Butter

Netra Basti means to bathe the eyes with medicated oils. In both Indian and Tibetan Ayurveda, it is used to relieve the tensions trapped in and around the eyes and their socket. A deceptively simple, but deep-acting treatment, Netra Basti eases stress lines and puffiness from around the eyes, brings back your eyes' natural luster, and enhances depth and color perception. It promotes a deep calm and contentment.

Beyond this description, the list of benefits we have seen and are described of Netra Basti include:

- improved memory.
- greater ease in seeing.
- relief of sunburn on the eyelids.
- easing of dryness and discomfort from allergic reactions around the eyes.
- softness of appearance.
- a release of tension throughout the body.
- remembering visual trauma in a way that is gentle and supported through the process.
- increased ease in speaking a foreign language.

Contra-indications for offering Netra Basti include:

- client has an active eye infection.
- recent eye surgery.
- active use of other eye medications.
- situations where the client may have had other medical procedures which have affected vision or the structure of the eye (i.e. scleral buckles. We have no data on the effect of Netra Basti after someone has had laser corrective eye surgery).

Netra Basti is often used in conjunction with Pancha Karma. At the same time, as mentioned earlier, it can be used at the end of a series of aesthetic or body treatments, or by itself. The following procedure has Netra Basti offered on its own.

Product and Equipment Needs

- ½ cup of pure ghee or clarified butter. (This is easily made or purchased at an Indian, Oriental or natural food store. See description on how to make ghee in the Appendices.)
- 1 cup whole wheat flour, mixed with warm water to form a dough of earlobe consistency, but slightly sticky, formed into a round doughnut-like ring big enough to encircle the eye. (NOTE: We have also found that some people with allergies to wheat react to the dough. If you know that someone is wheat intolerant, we suggest the use of spelt flour.)
- head and neck pillow or head support equivalent.
- small wash cloth.

- small face towel, rolled.
- facial tissues.
- 2 small bowls.
- hot towel cabinet, food warmer, or a small bowl of hot water in which the bowl or bottle of ghee ca be kept warm.
- a quiet, warm, and tidy room that is pleasant smelling and pleasing to the senses.
- available blanket.

Preparation

Set up the equipment on a small tray for easy access. The temperature of the ghee should be just warm to the touch. **Like Shirodhara Oil**, the ghee for Netra Basti is an oil and you cannot tell its exact temperature by just sticking your finger into it or placing it on your wrist. The ghee will just coat your finger like a tiny glove and give you a false impression. **The safest means of testing the ghee temperature is to place your finger into the ghee and** swish your finger back and forth. **Your finger's movement in the ghee will give you the exact temperature of the ghee.**

The Treatment Ritual

1. Check that your client has removed their contacts if they wear them. If they have eye makeup on, including mascara, have them remove it as these can mix with the ghee and cause eye irritation.
2. Have your client lie down on their back. Place a head and neck or other supportive pillow under their head so that their head and neck are well supported. Make them warm and comfortable. You may even want to offer them a knee bolster. A tummy warmer or equivalent can also be a nice touch.
3. If the treatment is being performed outside of the context of Pancha Karma preliminary therapies or if the client has not already received some massage or aesthetic work to their head or neck, offer them the Opening Sequence of the Ayurvedic Face Massage Sequence. At a minimum, loosen their neck and scalp, and apply gentle rotational pressure on the Murdhi, Brahma, and Shiva marma point on the top of the head,

Side Face

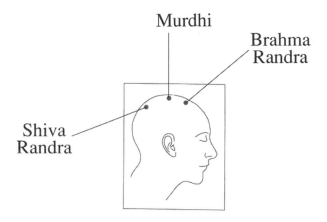

Murdhi

Brahma
Randra

Shiva
Randra

then follow with a short, gentle massage to the face using stroking motions from the chin to the temples and then from the center of the forehead towards the ears.

4. Next, have the head slightly turned towards the left so that the right eye socket is facing the ceiling. If there is any oil or lotion around the right eye socket or on the lid, use a dry tissue to thoroughly wipe all residues off. Place the small rolled towel so that it is butt up against and slightly under the client's head to support the left side of their face.

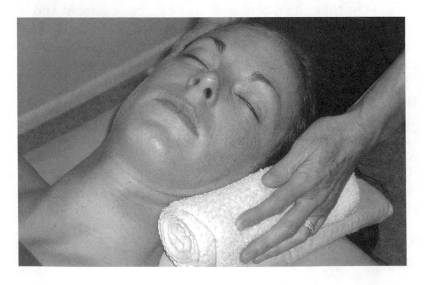

5. Take about a golf-ball sized piece of the whole wheat/spelt dough and form it into a donut ring around the right eye socket. Press this donut firmly around the entire right eye socket to ensure that there is a good seal to the skin and that the eye within the ring is able to open and close freely. You are basically creating a dough well around the eye into which the ghee solution will be poured.

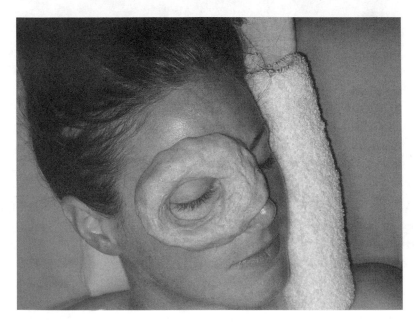

6. Have the client close the eye that is inside the dough well. Pour ½ teaspoon of the ghee (that feels barely warm to your finger) onto the outer corner of their closed eye.

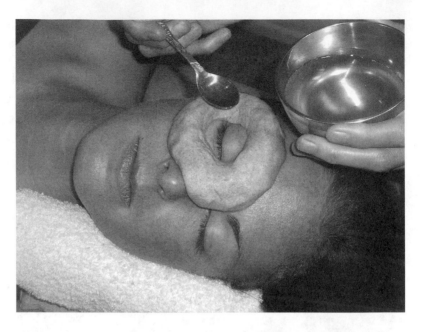

Ask if the temperature is comfortable. (This is relative and will vary from person to person. If they report it seems a bit too warm for their comfort, allow the ghee to cool for a few moments. Pouring it between two containers will make this happen faster.) If it feels cool, you can always warm it up relatively quickly. Add a bit more and check again. When they report it as being warm and comfortable, spoon another 4–5 teaspoons of the ghee into the well or until the eyelashes are completely submerged. Some people like the other (left) eye covered to block out light and visual distraction. Use a small face cloth, drape, folded tissue, or eye pad and place over the eye. Some people even like the feeling of you holding their eye gently closed with the tissue and your fingertips.

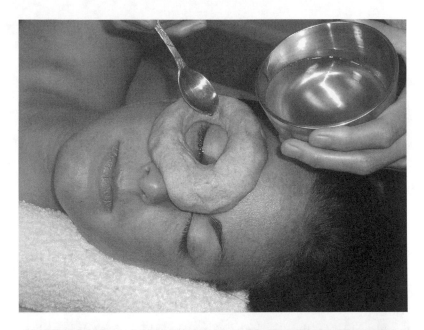

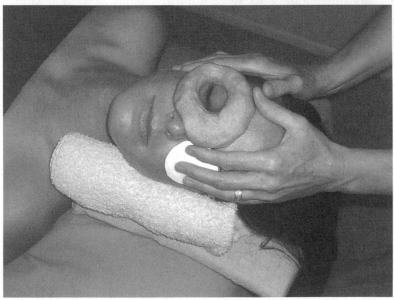

Netra Basti

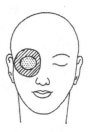

7. Encourage the client to open and close their eye gently and in their own time. **The ghee should remain like clear amber liquid.** If it begins to cloud or harden, it means that you started at too low a temperature or that the room temperature is effecting the solidification.

8. One should ideally aim at keeping the ghee as a clear solution for between fifteen to twenty minutes. It has been our experience that it is best to hold or at least make gentle contact with the head and neck during the treatment.

9. As the ghee remains on the eye, physical and psychological changes can occur. The ghee can sting for a while as the eye releases tears and toxins, so the person should be re-assured that this is a normal part of the process should it occur.

10. Remove the ghee by making a small indentation on the outer edge of the dough well so that it will act as a spout. Placing an empty bowl just at the outer edge of the well, have the client tilt their head towards the right to allow the ghee to drain into a bowl (this ghee should not be used again). Wipe the eye and the skin around the eye thoroughly with a tissue.

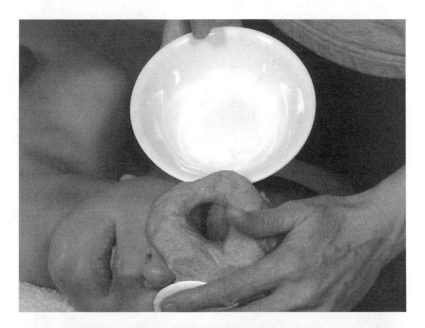

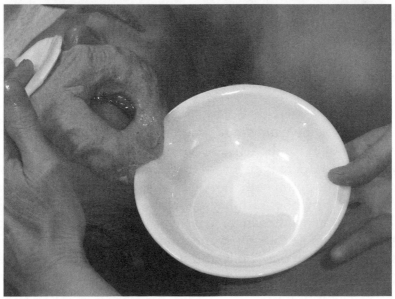

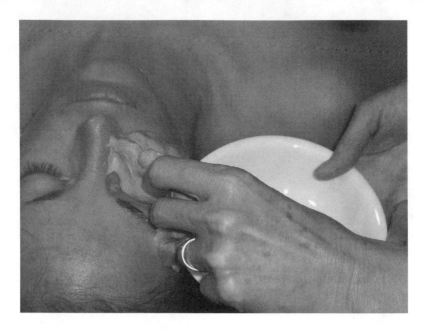

11. Repeat the process for the left eye.

At the end of the session, it is also normal for the person to experience some blurriness of vision. If they are planning to drive soon after the treatment, encourage them to wait about fifteen to twenty minutes.

Karna Purana

The cleansing of the ears is not only important for maintaining good physical conditions for the sense of hearing. In the orient and especially notable in China, there is an entire tradition of *auricular* therapy where conditions for the entire body can be treated through the massage, acupuncture, and a number of other methods relating directly to the ear. For daily health maintenance, ear massage is encouraged. And in Ayurveda, to promote the proper functioning and health of the ears, oils are used. In fact, the use of oils and hydrogen peroxide and the gentle wiping out of the ears with soft cotton are preferred over soaps or the flushing of ears with water.

The practice of using oil in the ears is the basis of Karna Purana. This is another Ayurvedic treatment that is often done with Pancha Karma, but can also be done in conjunction with other treatments, or on its own. The most basic aspect of it is filling the canal of the right, then left ear with warm sesame or medicated oils for a period of ten to twenty minutes. The treatment gets its name from the significant marma point known as *karna* that is just behind and slightly below the earlobes. Stimulating this marma helps with various ear conditions, tinnitus, jaw and neck tension, even anxiety. Karna Purana uses the energetics of this marma by stimulating it directly and through the presence of the oil. The **benefits** to the client are:

- relieves itching and dryness in the ears.
- helps to dissolve wax build-up.
- reduces Vata dosha excess to clear the sense of hearing.
- is useful in relieving ringing in the ears.
- helps with TMJ.
- generally loosens jaw and neck tension.

Although this is another treatment that focuses on a body orifice, i.e. the ear canal,

Karna Purana is less invasive and potentially troublesome than Netra Basti. Therefore, although this treatment is best done under medical licensing or supervision, we leave its practice up to the expertise and discretion of the therapist.

Karna Purana can be given as a single treatment. If the above conditions are chronic, a series of three treatments in one week may be offered, then weekly for maintenance. Some therapists will offer this treatment with ear candling. This can help to remove excessive earwax. In some rare cases, if the person has a history of very waxy ears, the amount mobilized will require the attention of a medical practitioner for it to be removed. One should check with your client to find out if they have this tendency. Other **precautions** include:

- an active ear infection.
- abscesses in the ear canal.
- perforated eardrum.
- pain in the ears.

Karna Purana can be done at any point that seems appropriate in the context of other treatments. It can be a wonderful preliminary to scalp or Ayurvedic *champissage* or head massage or at the completion of a facial or the Ayurvedic Face Massage Sequence.

Karna Purana

Karna Purana is a gentle and effective way of cleansing the ears and, as a result, improving the sense of hearing. It is also an effective way of helping with jaw, neck, and face tension. Warm packs are placed over your jaw and your ears are, one at a time, filled with warm sesame oil. In the warm silence, feel the tension in your jaw and face melt away.

Products and Equipment:

- organic unrefined sesame oil
- small dropper or squeeze bottle for the oil
- heat source: hot towel cabinet, food warmer
- pot of hot water
- cotton face cloth
- tissue
- cotton balls
- Dixie cup or equivalent
- *head and neck* pillow or equivalent (rolled-up towel)

Treatment Ritual

1. Have your client lie on their left side with a *head and neck* pillow or rolled-up towel under the left side of their neck for support. Arrange them so that their arms are comfortable. Have the left leg straight and the right leg bent. Use a cushion or support bolster under the bent knee or make adjustments to their posture. The aim here is for the body to be as comfortable and relaxed as possible. Also, their right ear canal should be easily accessible so that oil can be poured into it.

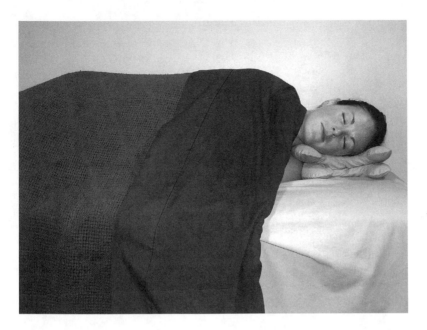

2. Take a small amount of warm sesame oil and rub it along the entire right jaw line, from below the KARNA marma point below the ear-lobe to the tip of the chin. Then take a warm, folded face cloth and lay it over the jaw. Lift after a few moments, then replace with a refreshed warm cloth. Do this a few times, then allow it to lie on the jaw.

Karna Purana

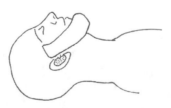

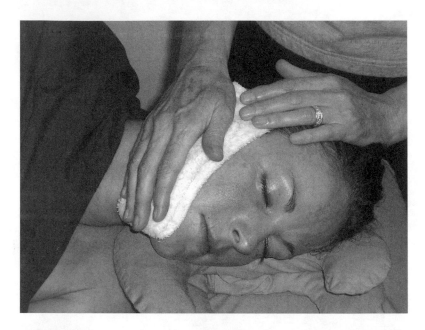

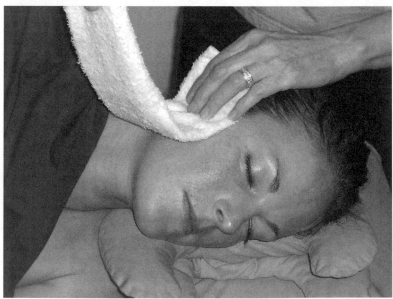

3. Fill the dropper or sq.ueeze bottle with a small amount of warmed sesame oil (**note: Like with the oil for Shirodhara and Netra Basti, check the warmth of the oil by the "wagging" of the finger method**) and fill the right ear as full as possible without spilling.

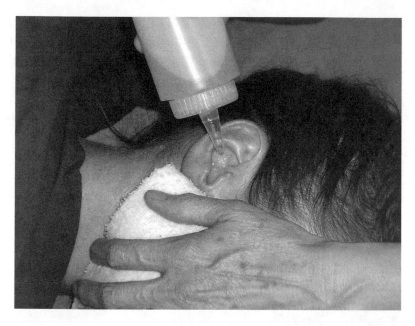

4. Using your index finger, massage behind the ear, from top to bottom with clockwise circular motions, finishing directly on the *karna* marma. Then massage in front of the ear, from the top to where the jawbone hinges.

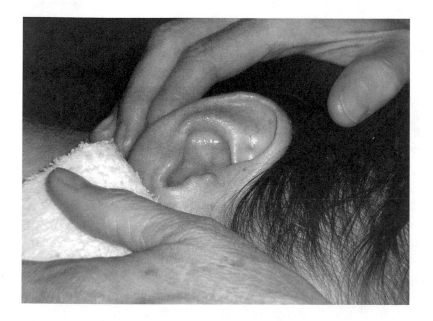

5. Allow the oil to remain in the ear for a minimum of 10 minutes (maximum of twenty, **which will change your treatment time**). Continue to massage as in Step 4, and re-warm and replace the face cloth periodically as well.

6. Remove the cloth from the jaw. Then empty the oil out of the ear into a bowl or Dixie cup by having your client turn their head and slowly roll onto their back. Wipe away excess oil from the ear with a tissue. Place a cotton ball in the ear.

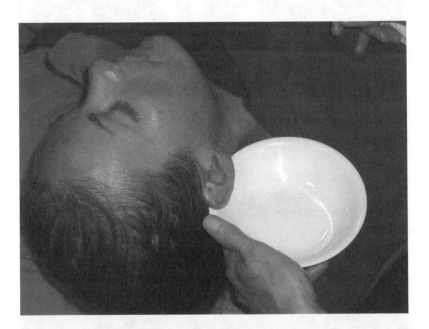

7. Have your client turn over and reverse all body positions as in Step 1. Repeat entire procedure for the left ear.

A Final Point: Useful Tips on Cleaning Your Linens

There is no getting around it, Ayurvedic treatments use oil, and in greater quantity than other types of spa treatments. With practice and care their beauty and simplicity will shine through and your room and linens will not be trashed but no matter now mindful you are, oil will get on the sheets and into the towels.

We have tried many of the products suggested for easy oil removal and have found any of the citrus-based detergents to be the most economical and effective for both de-greasing and deodorizing linens. They are also great for cleaning surfaces and oily equipment. They are not harsh but do dry your skin, so use gloves. They are also septic system safe, biodegradable, and compatible with all kinds of bleach.

Here are a few hints that will make your laundry easier.

- If the sheets are generally oily, sprinkle cornstarch powder on them and rub it in with your fingers. The cornstarch helps to lift the oil out of the fibers so the detergent can get in and go to work.

- If you just have spots of oil on the sheets, spray them with undiluted citrus detergent before you take the sheet off the table. Wipe the table with a warm damp cloth right away so there will be no risk of the table vinyl being damaged over time.

- Always try to wash linens within one day of use.

- Before washing, store linens in a black plastic trash bag. Keep the bag tied shut so air and light cannot get in as these are the two things that will turn the oil rancid.

- Wash in lukewarm water. Surprisingly, hot water will set oil into linens instead of washing it out.

- If linens are very oily, allow them to soak, the launder them twice without drying to completely remove the residue. If there are stains add bleach after the first wash so the bleach can penetrate better.

- Do not over-dry linens; the heat of the dryer will also set oil stains. Don't despair; pure orange detergent will remove even dried in oil stains! It has been known for oily sheets to ignite in a dryer so be cautious about leaving them unattended.

- Use a small towel for wiping off excess oil and wash these linens separately. This way the extra oil is contained and will not get spread throughout the wash.

- Use 100% cotton linens. They release the oils more completely than polyester-cotton blends. They also feel better on the skin.

CHAPTER 10

Marketing the Experience

When we first started to offer classes, our sole focus was on education. We had no products, no professional marketing skills, and no real interest in developing them, either. We were teachers and some thought of us as 'healers'. But it became apparent to us that if people want to practice the Ayurvedic treatments that we offer, they need products and equipment to work with. Although Ayurvedic products and oils are becoming more readily available in the west, we found that the quality and availability varied tremendously; that is, they were unreliable. Furthermore, many of the products had scents and tastes unfamiliar to western noses and palates. And so, reluctantly and at the imploring of our students, we found ourselves in the business of manufacturing a good many of the products for our treatments. Like many small specialty businesses the arrival of the internet has made it easy to reach clients and serve our students. This has been true for a number of our friends as well that you will find in our Resource Guide.

If Ayurveda is to become an established approach in the spa industry, it has to make sense on all levels, including making money. In the west there is a prevalent belief that being successful and making money is somehow wrong for people who are trying to lead a life focused on serving others and developing spiritually. However, ancient Tibetan wisdom reassures us that there is nothing wrong with money itself. In fact, people with money can do tremendous good in the world and many spiritual traditions encourage the donating of money or means to worthwhile projects that benefit people. The questions really are: 'How do we make the money?' 'Do we understand where the wealth comes from, and how we can continue to make it manifest?' and finally, 'Can we keep a healthy attitude about the wealth we gain?' We should try to make our money in a clean and honest way.

In this respect, we have tried to live up to the following consider-

ations. With respect to the manufacturing or marketing of products and packaging, we should strive to have products and packaging that are
- designed to have no harmful side effects.
- made from renewable resources.
- manufactured in places where workers are treated fairly.
- environmentally friendly.

We should treat our co-workers well by
- rewarding behaviors that show kindness and respect.
- offering benefits such as health insurance, workmans compensation or access to services as trade or at reduced rates.
- providing space to sit peacefully in breaks.
- providing time for lunch.
- offering incentives for on-going education.
- being flexible to the needs of working mothers.
- providing a generous maternity leave.

We should try and understand why we are successful, appreciate and share our success, and keep a healthy relationship with our wealth while we have it. We feel blessed to be involved in an industry that does do that in so many wonderful ways. We have worked with spas that
- donate much of their profits to women's AIDS relief in India.
- offer free makeovers to welfare mothers going on their first job interview.
- provide free services to others giving valuable service such as police officers and firefighters.
- have acted as official safe havens for people in marital conflict.

If we can do some of these things or even aspire to doing some of them as the opportunity arises, then making money is completely consistent with a life devoted to higher goals.

We should also enjoy the money we make and keep our minds and bodies happy and healthy while we earn the money. Our work should not exhaust us. Far too many spa owners do not walk their talk. Few receive services even at their own spas on a regular basis. Burn-out is extremely high for massage therapists. Someone who is ruining their health to make a good living is defeating the purpose of being in business in the first place and people in the spa industry should understand that more than most.

At the end of the day, we should be able to look back on our work life and feel we have indeed done something useful and meaningful. That is, we have used our minds and bodies to create something that leaves a good mark in the world. This we can call success. In the words of Emerson, "To laugh often and much, to win the respect of intelligent people and the affection of children, to earn the appreciation of honest critics and endure the betrayal of false friends, to appreciate beauty, to find the best in others, to leave the world a bit better, whether by a healthy child, garden patch . . . to know even one life has breathed easier because you have lived. This is to have succeeded."

If you find that these ideas move your heart you maybe interested to read *The Diamond Cutter—the Buddha on Strategies for Managing your Business and Your Life* by Geshe Michael Roach.

ANYWAY

People are unreasonable, illogical, and self centered.
LOVE THEM ANYWAY

If you do good, people will accuse you of selfish, ulterior motives.
DO GOOD ANYWAY

If you are successful, you win false and true enemies.
SUCEED ANYWAY

Honesty and frankness make you vulnerable.
BE HONEST ANYWAY

What you spent years building may be destroyed overnight.
BUILD ANYWAY

People really need help but may attack you if you help them.
HELP PEOPLE ANYWAY

Give the world the best you have and you'll get kicked in the teeth.
GIVE THE WORLD YOUR BEST ANYWAY

From Shistu Byayan, Children's home Calcutta
Adapted from words by De Wijngaard te Brugge

Marketing

The basics of a spa are to have a well-trained staff that offers great services, a clean, efficient, pleasant setting, and a good support team that will take your business to the next level. But you also need to be able to market yourself. We do not feel this book would be complete without offering some thoughts on marketing.

I personally have never focused on "selling", but I have always been curious as to why people buy and what they are happy to spend money on. Ayurveda is all about what makes people healthy and happy, and what inspires them. It is about meeting these needs today in connecting people to what will benefit them. In the modern world we call this marketing. So how do we make this connection in a natural and graceful way?

To address this from the most cutting edge of the marketing industry, we have been fortunate to meet an expert in experience-based marketing, Uta Birkmayer, who has been gracious enough to contribute some great answers in this chapter. We believe her approach will be key not only to those wishing to offer Ayurvedic services but anyone wishing to provide any genuine, heartfelt rewarding experience for their clients and staff.

Experience Management—The New Marketing
by Uta Birkmayer

How does one sell the unique offerings of a spa, which are very personal and special for those who have experienced them but a figment of the imagination to those who have not? According to ISPA's 2004 Consumer Trends Report, "spa services are primarily evangelized through informal social networks (i.e. family, friends, and co-workers). Yet, most spa advertising and promotion does not utilize these networks".

These word-of-mouth networks are best utilized when you give spa patrons a compelling story to tell about your business—a story they cannot wait to share with others about their own spa experience. In other words, if you do your best to manage your customers' experiences at your spa in the most luxurious and professional way, they will in turn do the marketing for you via these word-of-mouth channels. Creating a story about your spa is your first task, and is achieved by being honest about who you are and concentrating on authenticity so that your story can never be confused with a competitor's. A story will "stick" with the customer when he or she is connected with the spa on an emotional level through education, entertainment, aesthetics, or by giving them an escape from everyday life. In the end a good, authentic story lends your spa an emotional offering far above the interchangeable nature of products and services—and one that customers are going to want to tell others about.

Of course, any business is only as good as the employees who work there. So the final, but certainly important, task of a spa owner is to make the spa one that not only customers love to be at, but that employees do, as well. When a spa is a place employees love to work at, you will continue to attract the best employees in the market, and the best will continue to satisfy customers to the highest extent.

While this all sounds pretty straightforward, this new and experiential way of management and marketing requires a good understanding what a spa is today, who the spa customer is, and how they spend their money. It also requires a spa business to embrace the concept of authenticity and learn how to apply experiential principles throughout your operation. This chapter will cover all of these points.

What is a Spa?

Firstly, let's make sure we all agree on what a spa is today. The definition of a spa seems to change with every generation, from the Roman baths to the Fat Farms of the 1960s. However, today "spas are entities devoted to enhancing overall well-being through a variety of professional services that encourage the renewal of mind, body and spirit" (International Spa Association, ISPA, definition). Spas, like other businesses, adapt to the needs of the market and cater to the changing consumer.

Understanding Today's Spa Consumer

In order to market to today's consumers, we must understand them. In these times, the American consumer is looking for a way to slow down, simplify, and feel connected, and the spa experience is helping them achieve this, therefore becoming a more sought-after and relevant lifestyle experience. As the ISPA 2004 consumer trends report revealed, the American spa consumer is divided into three groups: a small percentage, the "core" group, who believe that spas are an integral part of health and wellness (physical, mental, emotional and spiritual); a broader, mid-level group, who regularly visit spas, but less frequently; and a large peripheral group of people who are toying with the idea of going to a spa, but are still not very familiar with services beyond the basics (massage, facial, manicure and pedicure). Most spa goers are still infrequent spa goers, interested in indulgence and escape, and specific quick relief from aches and pains, without a long-term perspective on health and wellness. While there are still those who view spa experiences as an unnecessary indulgence, others interpret it as a much-needed relief in a stressful and time-famined life, and assistance in the pursuit of balance and emotional stability.

The 2004 ISPA trend study revealed several other core findings:

- *The U.S. spa industry appears over-developed towards the "core" of the spa world, especially in terms of high-end services and treatments available. This is especially true in terms of advanced hydrotherapy, Ayurvedic and other advanced treatments based on foreign, folk-healing traditions.*

- *Consumers generally want "bread and butter" services (facials, manicure/ pedicure and basic massages) at day spas.*
- *Consumers experiment more at spas when on vacation and expect a broader array of "authentic", indigenous, as well as health and wellness-oriented services.*
- *The best long-term growth opportunity lies in transitioning peripheral customers to more regular users.*
- *Spa consumers appreciate highly refined entrance and transition experiences in spas. Interior design and ritual are the keys to driving the loyalty of all spa goers.*
- *Peripheral customers are price-sensitive when considering services beyond the basics. Price is also a barrier for them when considering "bread-and-butter" services.*
- *Consumer visits to spas incorporate one or more of the following drivers:*
  - *Indulgence (pleasurable, fun, appealing to the senses).*
  - *Escape (relief from the pressures of social life).*
  - *Work (largely related to self-improvement on some aspect of their body, their emotional state or their long-term spiritual and personal dispositions).*
- *Consumers are primarily motivated by and interested in indulgence or cosmetic work of their bodies (face, hair, nails)—areas where improvements are immediately visible.*
- *The spa industry generally has few threats in the eyes of the consumer, but several areas in the spas should be monitored:*
  - *There is an explosion of personal care products, but it is not capturing the attention of the spa goer while in the spa environment.*
  - *Men largely perceive spa visits as indulgence and escape, but the primary driver for them is to get bodywork done.*
- *The most effective introduction to spa services is through word of mouth, yet spas do not utilize this network.*
- *As the industry continues to grow and expand to the mainstream consumer, therapists' credentials and the overall effectiveness of the treatments will come under greater scrutiny.*
- *Human interaction, personalization, and customization will become important for consumer decision-making.*
- *Identifying the consumer's involvement with spas is important. Are they "core" spa customers, mid-level, or peripheral users? This is critical in deliv-*

ering the most appropriate, relevant information. Most spas have no system to gauge their customer's experience level.

- *As more and more treatments become available for home use (facials, manicures, pedicures, etc.), customers are having more and more difficulty justifying having these treatments done at a spa.*

To help meet the conscious and unconscious needs of the customer in the Ayurvedic spa, it is imperative to think through the spa's offerings and customize them for the core, mid-level and peripheral customer groups.

Spa: Still Considered A Luxury?

There are 47 million households in the United States with incomes of more than $50,000. With an average household size of 2.6 people, that is nearly 122 million Americans with the means and the desire to afford products and services above the basic necessities of life. Consumers with very high incomes, $150,000 and above, can afford luxury in many categories. Those with lower incomes selectively afford luxury treatments in some categories and trade down to mid-market or mass-market in others. Many consumers spend a disproportionate amount of their income in one or two categories of great importance to them, a practice known as rocketing.

But what kind of luxury are consumers looking for today? "Old Luxury" goods are typically products associated with a status symbol brand such as Chanel, Cadillac, or Brooks Brothers. They are simply more exclusive, expensive and elitist—often aloof and handmade. Today's consumer, however, is looking for engaging, value-driven offerings at a premium price to fill their emotional voids. The Boston Consulting Group researched this phenomenon in great depth while looking for the common success factor of modern brands such as Aveda, Victoria's Secret, BMW, Canyon Ranch, Kendall Jackson, Panera Bread and many more. They call this new consumer the "New Luxury" consumer and the products "New Luxury" products.

New Luxury is a distinct genre of products and services. Unlike Old Luxury items, intended only for the very wealthy, New Luxury goods are meant to be accessible and appealing to a much larger audience. Unlike conventional goods, which compete primarily on price, New Luxury goods command a premium because of their superior quality, performance and emotional appeal.

The spa industry meets many of the needs of the New Luxury consumer and has therefore enjoyed phenomenal growth in the last decade. Spa treatments, no longer an Old Luxury reserved for the wealthy, have become a lifestyle staple for many urban and suburban Americans. The spa industry generated revenues of $11.7 billion in 2003, up from $10.7 billion in 2001 (WSJ, Nov. 2004).

To understand how New Luxury offerings touch the customer, we have to find a way of looking at emotions so they make sense to the business world. Silverstein & Fiske defined these emotional spaces in the chart below. There are four main areas of emotional needs—Taking Care of Me, Connecting, Questing, and Individual Style—with three sub-categories for each. Below the sub-categories are some interesting examples from all industries, and we have added a further section below, giving examples of how the Ayurvedic spa can fill the above-mentioned emotional spaces.

Let's look at the emotional spaces of today's consumer in more detail:

Taking Care of Me	Connecting	Questing	Individual Style
Time for myself	Attracting	Adventure	Self-expressing
Convenience	Nurturing	Learning	Self-branding
Renewal	Belonging	Play	Signaling
Examples			
Personal care, spas, health care, gourmet in-home foods, linens and bedding are typical categories. This category helps ease the stresses of life and offers reward for accomplishments or solace for disappointments	Clothing, dining out, pet food, home theater and cruises are typical categories. These goods help people build, maintain, and enrich their relationships with family, lovers, friends and colleagues.	Travel, cars, sports equipment, computers and wines are typical categories. These products provide a way for consumers to try new tastes and experiences, learn about ideas and cultures, and expand their horizons.	Accessories, lingerie, watches, cars and spirits are typical categories. These products help them express their individual style, associate them with brand values, and signal their interests and passions to others.

Taking Care of Me	Connecting	Questing	Individual Style
How Ayurvedic Spas Can Fill These Spaces			
Ayurveda demands that you spend time thinking about yourself. It makes you think about yourself in different ways. Refocusing your life in Ayurvedic ways is the basis for renewal. Time to reassess lifestyle choices, gain help with new choices, and feel support for those choices. Provision for Ayurvedic home care products and protocols. Ayurvedic teas and snacks.	Meeting and bonding with people with similar interests and goals. Learning Ayurvedic techniques that are fun to do at home for friends and family. Spa membership that includes community events such as vegetarian potluck, uplifting movie night. Bringing Ayurvedic elements into the home life.	Becoming an Ayurvedic "insider" and therefore choosing Ayurvedic spa services over more usual treatments. Enjoying the idea that treatments go deeper or work on the level of body, mind and spirit. Having fun explaining Ayurveda to outsiders and discussing it with insiders. Learning about your dosha balance and how to better care for yourself. Indian retail items that are pretty and unusual.	Items of organic, natural fiber clothing. Bindis, temporary Indian style tattoos, henna products. Ayurvedic deodorant herbs. Books on Ayurvedic beauty and home care. Ayurvedic cookbooks. Ayurveda-inspired home décor, clothing, scents, make-up, music.

So when developing your own spa experiences for customers, look at the emotional spaces above and see just how many you can fill for your client at your spa. The more spaces you fill, the richer and more meaningful the spa experience will be for the customer—and the more compelling the stories they tell about your spa to others.

We have taken a good look at how today's consumer is choosing to spend his or her disposable income and how the spa industry can partake in filling the emotional voids this new consumer chooses to fill. Not only has this new consumer made the phenomenal growth of spas possible, understanding this consumer even better will enable further growth and increase customer satisfaction. This satisfaction, of course, also comes from the consumer feeling like he or she can trust the spa business, and in order to gain our customers' trust, we need to truly be who we are. We need to be authentic.

Being Authentic

We have learned what spas are, what today's spa consumers want, and how to best fill the emotional voids in their lives. But you may still be wondering, "why do some spas get all the glory, with continual listings among the world's top 10"? "Why do their repeat clientele not hesitate to pay premium prices and talk about them again and again to their friends, providing excellent free marketing to these already flourishing facilities"? And "why, if one were to copy their very concepts exactly, would this not work for other spas"?

Well, what truly separates Bliss Spas, Canyon Ranch, Miraval, The Golden Door, The Oaks, The Greenbriar, The Oriental in Bangkok, Chiva Som and many of the other celebrated destination spas from others that may have superior facilities and services is that they are original ideas—authentic concepts. They have all developed a business around their beliefs, rather than copying someone else's concept, because they know who they are and what they are about. They are powerful and unbeatable spa businesses because of their striking authenticity.

Authentic businesses have a central core belief or story, which initiates an abundance of original ideas that touch customers in unforgettable ways. This, in turn, becomes priceless word-of-mouth marketing by these spas' clients—the best kind of free PR—which has made these spa businesses long-term success stories.

To augment authenticity for maximum effect, one must take a spa's carefully chosen authentic theme or story and apply it to all of the customer touchpoints (every element of your spa the customer sees, hears, feels, smells and touches). Take the Hershey Spa, for instance. Naturally, a Hershey Spa should stick with the unquestionably authentic chocolate theme of Hershey. But where do you go from there? First, you must create the best technical and functional basis. This means that the space, the staff, the treatments, and so on should be of the best possible quality. Second, make sure there is an authentic application of the Hershey chocolate theme to the Hershey Spa. In this case, Hershey researched the health and beauty aspects of chocolate and found unique connections that they implemented into their treatments. Finally, they applied the Hershey Spa chocolate story to every customer touchpoint—the architecture/interior design, treatment ingredients, treatment rooms, treatment props, treatment names, staff uniforms, "scripts" and demeanor, retail products, and so forth. In doing so, they were able to easily see that thalassotherapy, for instance, or shiatsu (and many other treatments available today) had no place in the Hershey Spa theme. However, obviously treatments like a chocolate bath or chocolate body wraps were a perfect fit.

So how do you apply these concepts when adding Ayurvedic treatments to your spa, or when transforming your spa into an Ayurvedic spa? First, find your uniquely authentic story. You can start by looking at the non-spa elements around you that no one can change because they authentically belong where they are, such as:

- The history of the area, the building your spa is in, or historical figures of the area—like Greenbriar Hotel & Spa, a refurbished old grand hotel.
- Natural resources, natural setting, vegetation, a healing plant, healing earth and minerals, mountain air, hot and cold springs, animals—like Terme Saturnia in Italy, centered around sulfurous hot springs.
- Culturally unique elements—like Mii Amo in Sedona, a Native American-inspired resort and spa.
- The story of the owner—like the transformative story of Mel Zuckerman as he created Canyon Ranch.
- A uniquely different proprietary concept—like Bliss Spa, where every element of the experience is uniquely bliss, from the music to the visuals, based on the owner's quirky style.

Also important, of course, is that how Ayurveda fits into your authentic story must be unique (and it can be!). This entire book is, after all, about adopting an authentic Ayurvedic approach. And while Ayurveda has its roots in Indian culture, we would never recommend that the method of integrating it into your spa be anything but authentic (for instance, you shouldn't make your spa look like little India and have your staff in Indian dress just to add Ayurvedic treatments). Of course, if you are indeed Indian or feel passionate or connected to India, you might very well indeed take a successful and authentic traditionalist approach to implementing Ayurvedic principles into your spa. What is most important is finding where your heart is, what your core beliefs are, and what your authentic story is, and then fill in the skills and services and treatments to fit. If it is authentic, it will be nothing but satisfying, even when it is hard work.

Aligning With the Touchpoints

All customer touchpoints are aligned around the authentic story of your spa. Customer touchpoints are all the elements of a business that touch the customer in a sensory (sight, sound, scent, audio and touch) way—from the first phone call, brochure or website contact to the architecture and design, names of treatments, and in-person interaction with staff. Every element ties back to the authentic story, thus following a sort of theme.

For example, say your spa site is located in an old soap factory, and you decide to bring the authenticity of this place back to life with the spa concept.

This starts with the name, perhaps "Ye Olde Soap Factory Spa", and is anchored in a specific period in time, perhaps the 1930s. From there, when working with architects and designers or when working out treatments and procedures in the spa, you will want to tie everything back to this authentic core theme or story. You will therefore need to become creative within the parameters you set for yourself and this unique creative direction will help you develop something that is so unique and impossible to copy that it becomes your entire marketing effort. You will probably develop your very own soap bar (you could even offer soap-making workshops as educational elements), and find ways to use soap bars for a variety of treatments ranging from manicures, pedicures, facials and soap massages all the way to old-fashioned (men's) shaving treatments, soap baths, and more. Instead of tubs, your spa may feature vats that were once used in soap making, and the treatment menu may be built around the story of the woman that stood behind the original soap formulation. The possibilities for creativity are virtually endless.

Below is a customer touchpoint graphic, which shows, again, how all the elements of a business tie back to one core story and how this creates a comprehensive, authentic memory for the customer.

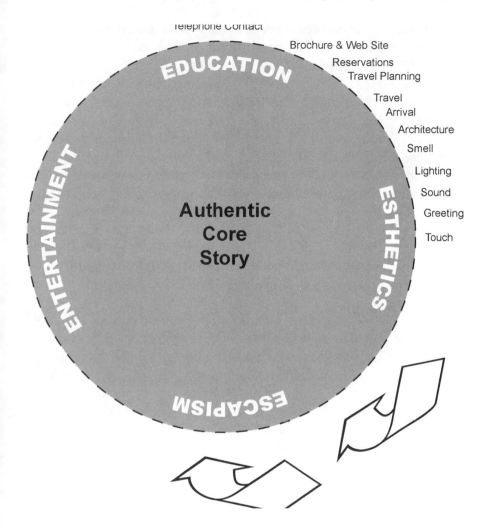

The Economic Value of Experiences

So, we understand the consumer and their need for emotions. We have also grasped the idea of an authentic story and how all elements of the spa should tie back to it. Now, let's look at how we create a story that touches the customer in the way they need to be touched.

Ten years ago, we would have said that the spa industry, along with hotels, restaurants and any other high-touch industries, is part of the service industry. It was common theory that there were three types of things you could sell—commodities, products and services (with many unique combinations thereof). Up until the late 1990s, economical offerings were differentiated by the level of service perceived, such as "good service," "really good service," "excellent service" and so on. But that is not the case any longer. According to today's service definitions, those who provide a service simply deliver an intangible activity that is easily interchangeable, with no difference between providers (Pine and Gilmore, 1999). This means there is also no bursting to tell others about the services you experience—so let's hope we are no longer in the service industry! Today, rather, we are in the Experience Economy. While the term "experience" is used as freely as "service" these days in business, owners may still wonder what it is exactly, how to manage it, and how it can add to the economic value of one's business.

Let's look at a basic, non-spa example to visualize the essence of an experience. Most of us have ordered and consumed a cup of tea at a restaurant. We are given a selection of tea bags with hot water, and choices of sugar, milk or lemon. End of story. The product is tangible (the tea bag and hot water) and the service is intangible (being served, getting cups and a seat), and both are very standard, thus interchangeable at most any restaurant. The proof that this is not a memorable event is that you do not burst out telling people about your cup of tea later.

However, we all know that not all cups of tea are created equal. What about the tea served at a Japanese tea ceremony or at an authentic English afternoon tea? In both cases, the basic ingredient—the tea—although of different quality levels, is essentially the same commodity, as is the hot water. The service, however, is more elaborate and leaves a lasting memory, so much so that we like to tell people about it and we readily pay more for this offering (which now, technically, is no longer a service, but an experience). Because of the fact that people pay more for experiences, it is worth researching the phenomenon. What exactly is it that people pay so much more for, and how can we replicate and maximize it economically?

In the late 1990s, several books on this "new" economic value were published, including The Experience Economy *(1999, by Gilmore & Pine),* Experiential Marketing *(1999), and* Customer Experience Management *(2003, both by Bernd H. Schmitt). These books addressed the fact that the phenomenon of "service" and its many hybrids deserved a closer look, and from this closer look, a fourth economic value emerged: the experience. Let us go back to the tea example to clarify: loose leaf tea sold by the pound is a commodity, tea bags (readily packaged for faster preparation) are products, and selling a tea bag with hot water in a consumption environment is considered a service, which is interchangeable with all other providers of tea bags and hot water. Therefore, the tea bag and water are measured by their tangibility and the service is measured by its intangibility (putting tea and hot water together). So how, then, do we measure an experience? Gilmore and Pine define an experience as* memorable *by the customer. So, if the customer sees a distinct* value above the tangible and intangible components of the cup of tea, some-thing he or she remembers and (in the best case) cannot wait to share with others, we have a distinctly separate economic value called experience that tops service. Consumers readily pay more for an experience because it meets their emotional needs (the emotional spaces discussed above). Those consumers then tell others about the experience (the best avenue of spa marketing), not to mention the fact that the press loves to write about experiences, giving a busi-ness wonderful, free PR, or marketing through experiences.

There is an additional economic value above experiences called "transfor-mation". A transformation is the ultimate economic offering. It happens when the experience helps people change themselves and they sustain that change: higher financial stability, better health, a longer life, weight loss, more strength, greater ability to deal with stress, and the list goes on. This is particularly im-portant in the spa industry, because some spa goers simply want to escape life and are looking for indulgence (true experiences), but are not looking for a better, healthier life, like many of the core customers.

Now, let's look at these economic values again, and how their value esca-lates, in particular when dealing with Ayurvedic elements.

Ayurveda—commodities: making your own Ayurvedic products from scratch.

Ayurveda—products: purchasing ready-made Ayurvedic products. (Cus-tomers pay for something tangible, $).

Ayurveda—services: get a basic massage with Ayurvedic products. (Cus-tomers pay for something intangible, $$).

Ayurveda—experiences: learn about and be immersed in unique experi-ences of Ayurvedic techniques and products, in an esthetically authentic Ayurvedic environment (architecture, design, props) and stimulation of senses. This is an experience worthy of sharing with others. (Customers pay for something memorable, $$$).

Ayurveda—transformations: authentic Ayurvedic personal assessment, personalized authentic Ayurvedic treatment plan and subsequent sustained and measurable health and wellness transformation. (Customers pay for sustained transformation of themselves, $$$$).

As you can see, the economic value increases with the complexity of the offer-ing. A product alone is worth less than the product in connection with a service. A product connected with an experience is worth more than a product with a service, and a product in connection with a transformation is worth more than a product in combination with an experience. Also see this economic escala-tion on the graph below.

Let's look at one very simple example to clarify. Imagine a high-quality essential oil bath product on a drug store shelf. The $4 price tag seems adequate, for it is a product described on its package. Imagine that same product in a bath someone has drawn for you—all you have to do is slide into the tub, close your eyes and enjoy. The value of this bath is higher than that of the bath oil, and you probably would not mind spending $15 for it. Now, imagine you are in a spa, and a gorgeous, oversized tub has been filled with water, there is soft music, a glass of herbal tea, incredible views of a snow-covered landscape, and your therapist educates you about the therapeutic benefits of this same bath, which is ceremoniously poured into the water. You have a distinct memory of this time, you can tell others about this beautiful bath and the experiences— and you are perfectly willing to pay $45 for the experience. If the experience was particularly good, you may be motivated to purchase this bath product afterwards, and you may even look for products with similar benefits to extend the effect for home use.

Lastly, you have signed up for a 10-session de-stress program at a spa. The expert staff assesses your personal stress levels and educates you about lifestyle changes that will help you deal with and eliminate stress in a completely personalized program. Parts of this program are relaxation baths with the very same bath product. The product has become part of a greater personal transformation process, but it's all about you now, not about the product. However, since you have now learned about all the benefits and essential herbs, and are feeling the positive effects, you are now an expert shopper and can purchase an array of products from teas to supplements to baths and music, which will help you achieve your personal goals. Here you are perfectly willing to spend $150 per session at the spa.

Below is an overview of the above value and the value escalation for the customer.

Value Escalation

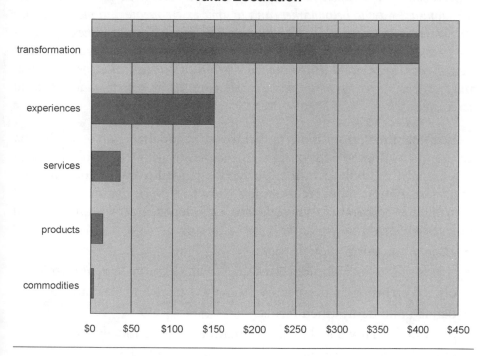

Of course, not every customer is looking for a transformative experience. Most just seek a quick escape, which is located on the experience level. The "core" customer group discussed earlier believes in the transformational value of a spa, however. They have made spa-going an integral part of their life and are willing to spend the money. Most spa customers visit spas for the purpose of indulgence, escape and working on their body. While indulgence and escape are purely experiential values (both are emotional values), working on their body is a pure service (not emotional), an intangible value that can be performed by any provider.

Spas rely heavily on product retail, but often times this happens: The client had a wonderful, escapist, indulging facial and massage in the spa, only to be pulled back into retail reality by being presented a list of "recommended" products to buy. Not only is this offensive to a spa-goer who has just spent a few hours and a few hundred dollars on getting away from it all, it cruelly pulls her back into a world she has spent time and money to escape and destroys the emotional value you have spent hours creating for her. Instead, if a spa created a meaningful experience—that is, including all of the elements we have mentioned above, but above all, authenticity, entertainment and education—the customer will, on her own, be in the mood and frame of mind to purchase products to extend the wonderful memory you have helped create.

In summary, this experiential marketing chapter has given you new and perhaps unusual ways to help market (and to some extent create and manage) your spa. We felt it necessary to give you this angle, because of the uniqueness of a spa's highly emotional offering as well as a new consumer whose demands the spa must meet. Again, understand the consumer, fill their emotional voids, be authentic, and create your offerings on the value escalation scale we have provided. You will never look back.

Learning much from the Uta Birkmayer's model and vision of the spa industry, we adopted a lot of these principles as we were thinking about how to put this book together. Our goal changed from just offering the basic information about treatments to how to support each step needed in making a memorable Ayurvedic spa experience, start to finish and on all levels. To that end we have

- offered you our personal story.
- shared our personal understanding of what Ayurveda is and isn't.
- offered an historical perspective from the Indian and Tibetan cultures.
- defined and demystified terms.
- described what we feel makes a treatment authentically Ayurvedic.
- offered ways to work with the physical and emotional environment in the spa.
- described various ways of understanding body-mind types of clients and staff.
- offered details so treatments can be understood and learned well.
- given home care advice including diet, exercise, meditation and "spa" treatments.
- included testimonials telling of clients' experiences.
- listed resources for finding products, training, places to have treatments, people to help with all aspects of spa set up.

We have shared everything we think is key for an authenticcally Ayurvedic approach. Again, we have never once suggested that you make your spa look like little India and have your staff in Indian dress. Not because that would be wrong but because it would be wrong for us. We have been involved with Indian and Tibetan teachers for thirty years and in all that time we have been more interested in the teachings than the cultural wrapping. Our interest really lies in bringing Ayurveda to the west by authentically sharing the treatments and knowledge. That is our personal choice and your way maybe different for perfectly appropriate reasons. Finding where your heart is, what your core beliefs are, and then perfecting skills to put your dreams into action and finally form is the point we are making here. If you can do that then you will create a spa experience that touches your clients' bodies, minds, and spirits, and sales and repeat business will flow naturally. We wish you blessings on the journey. If it is authentic, it will be nothing but deeply rewarding even when it is hard and be so memorable to your clients they well talk about it forever.

Let us imagine that you have managed to create a top quality, authentic Ayurvedic spa

Experience and business and sales are going well. How can we customize every sales experience? This not so as to be contrived or manipulative, but to more easily

and genuinely connect with clients in a way that feels natural and appropriate to them.

Dosha Guided Sales

It is generally estimated that the average spa makes 60% of their income in product sales. Skin care professionals are more aware of this than the average massage therapist, and their education usually includes some sort of skills in product sales. They are usually comfortable with making suggestions for home care and it is a normal part of their service. The massage community in our experience is less comfortable with the notion of making sales of either their services or of products.

The dictionary tells us that marketing is "an aggregate of functions involved with moving goods or services from provider to customer". Like many things in our modern world, these functions are varied and highly sophisticated. The increased volume of things in the market have only added to the pressure and so it is easy to feel that marketing is about pushing product for profit alone. Ethical marketing is no such thing, however. It is the skill of connecting the individual with a product or service that will improve the quality of their life and be in harmony with their means and values. In a spa setting it is guiding clients to services that meet their needs and products that will provide them with the means to take part of that positive experience home and continue to feel the benefits.

In our experience, the dominant dosha of a particular client can provide us with valuable insights as to how to make this connection in a way that is enjoyable and satisfying to everyone involved.

The more *vata* energy the client has, the more they are sensitive to and influenced by sound and touch. This can even be an indicator to let us know which dosha is out of balance. Do you notice how much louder and more aggravating even the pleasant sound of children playing can be when you are stressed? How can a gentle caress be so pleasurable when you are relaxed and the same type of touch make your hair stand on end and even hurt when you are uptight? Stress increases vata so everything we hear and touch influences our mood more. How can use this in a positive way? When marketing to a client whose vata is high:

- talk enthusiastically and with feeling.
- share stories about the experiences of other clients- naming no names of course.
- describe the sensations and body feeling of a service or product.
- use testers an allow the client to put it on their skin or offer a brief sample treatment.
- cross-marketing works well; put small pieces of one treatment as an add-on in another to kindle interest in something new or different.
- emphasize the mystical and subtle nature of Ayurveda.
- book a series of treatments if possible, as vata clients have the hardest time coming back even if their experience has been stellar.
- call with appointment reminders—high vata makes us all forgetful.
- accept credit cards, as impulse buying is a vata thing.
- sell large sizes of product. Never give samples; the vata client has drawrs full that they never use.
- teach simple regimens.
- offer a variety of services and try to keep up with the new and different or have interesting seasonal variations.

The more *pitta* energy we accumulate, the more we become sensitive to the way things look and how they taste. Have you ever noticed when you clean house or just cannot stop yourself from making that picture perfectly straight? Does the sun or fluorescent lighting bother you more sometimes than other? How is it that some days you obsess about your appearance and other times you couldn't care less? Do you know people that may not have much but you would describe what they have as tasteful? There is pitta on parade. When marketing to a client whose pitta is high:

- make sure your displays and counters are clean and well organized.
- check that testers are fresh.
- have prices marked clearly and be upfront about special offers; confusion about money is not appreciated.
- know the products and services very well; be ready for detailed questions about results, time frames and benefits.
- have beautiful brochures or neatly printed literature to share.

- books sell well; the pitta in us feeds on information.
- simple but elegant packaging is more appealing than fancy extras; they would rather have quality product than expensive packaging.
- emphasize quality, research, and results.
- have important instruction written out clearly in point form.
- never talk about major purchases if the client is hungry or thirsty.

The more *kapha* we carry the more we are sensitive to smell and taste. Imagine the comfort of smelling home-baked bread or the delight of an exotic new treat food on your tongue. Say hello to your kapha! We all have some, some people more than others. Clients with more kapha are often quieter. They hang back from the counter but it doesn't mean they are not interested; they are waiting to be invited in as your special guest. How do we motivate our kapha friends?

- have pretty displays with clever little extras and nonsense items.
- offer a variety of aromas; favorite smells are so individual.
- especially at holidays, make gift baskets with cards and ribbons.
- give out samples; they will be treasured.
- remember a client's birthday or a special day in their lives; you will be a forever friend.
- emphasize tradition and luxury; the kapha in us loves to be treated like a king or queen now and then.
- have gift certificates; they will be given to friends in place of verbal recommendations.
- have special services or deals for regular customers; client appreciation is priceless.
- offer tea and a treat food after services on a pretty tray.

Section
Four

Taking It Home With You

Whatever you can do or dream, begin it.
Boldness has genius,
Power and magic in it.
GOETHE

What follows are suggestions, exercises, and rituals for everyone who wishes to integrate Ayurvedic principles into their daily living. Therapists can use these to improve their own health and wellbeing. Clients can us them as a way of bringing home the Ayurvedic Spa and making it a part of their daily life.

General Principles Regarding Ayurvedic Diet

*I*n the four levels of Ayurvedic medicine and healing as laid out in the Tibetan medical Tantras, we discussed how approximately ninety-five percent of the aches pains and problems most of us contend with or complain about would resolve themselves if we lived a lifestyle that is in keeping with our body constitution and the condition we are in based on age, level of activity, climate and other environmental and seasonal factors, and the way we respond to these conditions.

Of all of the lifestyle factors discussed, diet is the most essential. The reason is that more than any other lifestyle factor, we engage in eating frequently—at least daily—*and*—for the most part—can make a choice as to what it is that we put in our mouths. Other lifestyle factors such as sleep, hygiene, exercise, and relaxation time all contribute to the rate and degree to which our tissues and organs age. However, if our diet is poor, we don't sleep well, we need more products to keep ourselves clean as our body builds up an increased level of toxins, our muscles and connective tissue, starved of proper nutrients, are subject to injury and rapid deterioration, and we remain in a state of nervous tension or exhaustion. Thus, diet contributes to the quality of each of the other lifestyle factors.

If we eat a diet that is healthy for us, the tone, elasticity, and vibrancy of our body endures over time. We age like fine wine rather than sour vinegar. And if we want to recapture our youth in any degree, to re-vitalize and rejuvenate, diet again will be a primary factor. For your clients who seek such in their lives, providing them with useful information on diet will ensure that whatever you do to make them feel better will be enhanced dramatically by what they put on their plates at home or while dining out. As a therapist, the same will be true for you. But more importantly, if you eat a diet that supports your body and mind

appropriately, the work that you love to do, helping and providing healing touch and energy to others, will not fail you. You will find that your
vitality will be more consistent and the likelihood of repetitive injury and
burnout dramatically reduced. Other factors such as exercise and relaxation are also important. But diet is essential.

Melanie and I want to emphasize this latter point simply because we
see hundreds of therapists working wither on their own or in spas by not
giving themselves adequate nutrition during the day to compensate for
the amount of energy they give to their clients. This results in weight
problems (both under and excessive), exhaustion, low back pain, and
carpal tunnel syndrome to name just a few problems. Ayurveda teaches
that this is the direct result of diet, the efficiency of our digestion and
the health of our digestive organs. Basically, there are four steps in this
process.

One of the most common dilemmas we have seen with Ayurvedic
doctors coming from the east who want to introduce an Ayurvedic diet
to their Western clients is that they assume that, like their own culture,
we are a grain-based diet. We are not. Grain used to be the staple of the
American diet, but since the early 1900's, with the erosion of the small
farm, the growth of industry and agri-business, our diet has shifted away
from this sensibility. We have become more urban than rural-based and
our activity has increased. We are on the move. We travel, move vast
distances from our birth places, settle into climates and environments
that more than likely bear little resemblance to the homeland of our
genetic predecessors. As such, we are not settled like an agrarian society. We are more like hunter-gatherers, "cruising for burgers". Even our
food travels great distances. We can eat a tropical fruit in Alaska and
hamburgers in Key West. The reality of transcontinental shipping has
rendered the concept of regional cooking and eating an anachronism.
We can eat whatever we want wherever and whenever we want, 24/7.
And so, if we read a general book on Ayurveda or consult with an
Ayurvedic physician, much of what is recommended seems foreign, either from the standpoint of the food itself, or from the sensibility that
Ayurveda encourages us to have.

It is a common misnomer to assume that if you are going to eat
Ayurvedically, you should get used to curry, dahl, and chapattis, and that
if you go out to eat, you should be going to Indian restaurants! To be
quite frank, the food generally served at Indian restaurants is as Ayurvedic
as McDonalds is an example of healthy American cuisine. More than
anything, Ayurveda teaches principles. Ayurveda's dietary principles can
be applied wherever we are to transform whatever foods are available to

us to provide the greatest delight and benefit for our body and mind. I am reminded of a Japanese chef who walked into a macrobiotic restaurant kitchen to give a cooking class. The two main ingredients he brought with him were a beef steak and white flour. He told the class that he was going to them how to prepare these macrobiotically.

With this example in mind, please understand that an Ayurvedic diet is also not about becoming vegetarian or vegan. There certainly advantages to eating this way. However, some people's bodies can accommodate this and others cannot. A good example of this is His Holiness the Dalai Lama who became extremely ill trying to become vegetarian. In the high plateau of Tibet where there is barley and meat, and very few other vegetables and fruits, generation upon generation has been genetically conditioned to be more animal food/meat based in their eating habits. Thus, we have to accept some of the limitations genetics places upon us. At the same time, we can learn principles that will help us to select, prepare, eat, enjoy, and effectively digest what it is that we do eat, whether it be a fruit salad or shrimp gumbo.

For the most part, the guidelines that we shall discuss are ones that are commonly agreed upon by all of those healing systems that embrace diet as a key factor in health. Some of these will not be new to you. Some will be. All will be discussed in the context of Ayurveda.

Four Basic Principles

Before we go to the Guidelines, there are four principles that need to be addressed with respect to quality eating. These need to be clearly understood with respect to healthy eating and achieving and maintaining health from eating.

FIRST, our diet needs to contain sufficient nutrients that will maintain health and well-being generally. What does that mean? At present, the marketplace is flooded with endless recommendations of what the "right" or "correct" way of eating is. Also, bio-medical research is able to isolate what particular nutrients are beneficial for each and every part of our bodies, including the skin. While Ayurveda, the oldest living healing science on the planet does have very specific dietary regimens to address every imaginable health condition, the general rule is to be on a diet that suits our body, our level of activity, and our environment. Each of our previous books, *Ayurvedic Beauty Care* and *Tibetan Ayurveda: Health Secrets from The Roof of The World*, contain lists of foods based on an understanding of the doshas. Knowing your constitution, you can refer to these lists in order to sort out what are the best, occasional, and least suitable foods for your particular body-mind type. As you get more

familiar with the general guidelines as set out further along, looking at
these food lists will prove useful. However, if you start there and develop
a "Thou shalt" and "Thou shalt not " list of foods, then more than likely
you will feel strangled by limitation. As the Buddhist nun, Pema
Chodron, encourages, "let's start from where we are".

SECOND, our bodies need to have a sufficient ability to be able to
break down the foods we eat into usable nutrients. This ability has to do
with our metabolism—what in Ayurveda is known as agni or "digestive
fire". This will be elaborated on.

THIRD, our bodies must have the capability to absorb, hold onto,
and utilize the nutrients made available to us by our digestive fire. We
are speaking of developing and maintaining healthy digestion, which
leads to the final point.

FOURTH, we need to efficiently eliminate undigested foods and
wastes created by the body. In order to do this the four primary organs of
elimination (the colon, bladder, lungs and the skin) need to be strong.

All four of these processes need to work well to maintain health, well-
being, and beauty. They are all inter-dependent. If we eat inappropriate
or "junk" foods (which, broadly speaking, can be anything our body is
going to turn into junk because it cannot digest it properly, hence creating what in Ayurveda is called *amma* or toxins) our digestive fire or
metabolic heat (Sanskrit *agni*) will become challenged. It may rage too
high to compensate in an attempt to burn up the foods that are not
good for us. The result may be that agni diminishes over time. Or we
can eat things that are like putting water on our inner fires. In either
case, our metabolism is compromised and thus what is passed along for
our digestive organs to assimilate and eliminate creates stress for them
as well. For some, the digestive distress created may be obvious from
the outset; gas, bloating, constipation, diarrhea. For others, perhaps all
of the organs are strong and function well so that an occasional dietary
infraction is just handled with the minimum of discomfort. However, if
such culinary sins are repeated or are the mainstay, eventually, even the
most iron-stomached individual will succumb to gastric distress and the
wear and tear on the body and mind will become apparent.

The Guidelines

The first few guidelines have to do with the context and manner in which
we eat. The eating process, as well as the food preparation process, are
integral parts of Ayurvedic nutrition. For what we are actually talking
about with respect to diet is better defined as nutrition. Nutrition is a
process of nurturing. Each of our five gross senses (hearing, seeing,

smelling, touching, tasting) nurtures our body-mind. Taste and the process of putting physical matter into our body is the material that creates the physical being that supports our mind. But like any one of our senses, the quality of what comes in as nutrition is influenced by environment, our mental state, the quantity of what we are putting in and so on.

Time and Place

Guideline **NUMBER ONE** is to eat in a settled and quiet atmosphere. Do not work, read, or watch TV during meals. Always sit to eat. Eat at roughly the same times each day. Avoid talking while you are chewing. Let's examine each one of these caveats.

- From a general perspective, trying to do a variety of tasks all at once or sitting in a very bustling environment aggravates Vata dosha. If you move around while you eat, your wind or Vata energy is circulating to accommodate your movements. It does not settle into eating and assimilating. Thus excess Vata builds up in the form of gas and bloating.

- Reading or watching TV—basically using one other sense very intently while you eat—also aggravates Vata, but it also challenges Pitta. Eyes and seeing are most associated with Pitta dosha. Pitta is the fire that is also behind digestive fire, or agni. Consequently, if you focus intently on watching something, your digestive fire drops. Have you ever noticed that if you go out to eat, then immediately go to a movie, at the end of the movie, you still feel full from dinner? Similarly, have you ever noticed how drowsy and full you still feel before you go to bed if you sat in front of the TV while eating? A couch potato is what you will become!

- Eating at roughly the same time every day helps to tame or balance Vata. It helps the body to align its digestive process so that you get into a recognizable rhythm. The result is that your body is more prepared.

- Chewing is an important function in eating and will be discussed further later on. However, talking while in the midst of chewing aggravates Vata dosha. Rather than getting into the mechanical, predictable pattern of chewing and swallowing, we get into articulation, moving the mouth in a variety of ways, and taking air in through our mouths rather than our noses. All of these provide more information and stimulation than settled chewing. Bloating, belching, and feeling more spaced out or distracted will be the results.

    Obviously, we do not live in a bubble. We do eat at restaurants, with friends, at social occasions, and so on. Be aware that each of these has their own rewards, but they will still aggravate Vata dosha and create some unintended or unwanted results. Thus if you are needing to get grounded, settle your Vata, and work with your health and sense of stability, try to work at settling down to eat as much as you can. Don't rely on grabbing a snack here or there to or eating on the run, a problem that we especially see with therapists as they scurry from one client to the next. Make a priority of taking some quiet time to nurture yourself so that you can continue to nurture others. Otherwise, you are running on empty.

- Avoid eating late at night or just before bed. Although we have mentioned earlier that you should eat at the same times of day, to have a habit of eating late at night or just before bed is worth breaking. Food eaten at this time cannot be properly digested, disturbs digestive rhythms, and promotes the build-up of toxins. As your body is not resting, but rather actively digesting, you will wake up tired from this habit. And it is a guaranteed way of putting on weight. The great sumo wrestlers of Japan eat vast quantities of food and then go sleep because it ensures that the weight stays with them and does not get worn off from movement.

   If you must have something to eat at this time, have something light, like soup, warm spiced milk, or some tea and fruit—basically something that is very easy to digest. More will be spoken about with respect to times of eating shortly.

Ambience

Guideline **NUMBER TWO** is to dine either alone or with people you genuinely like. Negative emotions, whether yours, theirs, the cook's, or that of other people around you can have harmful effects on your ability to enjoy and/or digest your food (the same is true for business lunches where there can be a lot of apprehension, worry, or uncertainty). Of course, in a family or in any variety of other situations, there will be tensions that may be there at the dining table. Some of this is just unavoidable and will, whether you want them to or not, compromise your digestion.

Beyond any other negative emotion, however, it is best not to eat when you are angry. The emotion of anger can sour the best of meals. It is far better to not eat at all when angry. Take some time to calm your mind or do something that is pleasant. If you get angry while at the dinner table, excuse yourself. Go for a walk and come back to your food. Alternatively, take your food and go eat somewhere peacefully.

Guideline **NUMBER THREE** follows in the same vein. Take a few minutes to sit quietly after eating before returning to or starting a new activity. Abrupt changes from one activity to another aggravate Vata dosha. The result can be the increase of more wind, hence gas, bloating, and a slowing down of the digestive process as other body systems are engaged to do other digestively unrelated work. The most extreme example of this is when you were young and were told not to go swimming until at least 30 minutes after a meal.

Whatever activity you have to go into after eating, do it slowly if possible, at least trying to maintain a slow, rhythmic pace to your breathing. In that regard, some people *do* benefit from a post-meal constitution; taking in some fresh air in a gentle way.

How to Eat

Guideline **NUMBER FOUR** is to chew your food well; the more the better (especially when you feel tired or run down). Chewing aids digestion, providing needed enzymes to aid digestive fire (agni in Sanskrit, pho thut in Tibetan). Chewing is also good for the brain as it allows the temporal lobes to expand and contract. It also aids in tension and stress relief as the jaw is worked and cerebro-spinal fluid is encouraged to move more freely.

A friend and colleague of mine, Lino Stancich, wrote a book called *The Power Eating Program*. In it, he tells the story of his father's experience being in a Nazi prisoner of war camp. There he was only given a small amount of bread and coffee daily. Every day, he chewed each morsel of bread a couple hundred times and swished the coffee back and forth inside his mouth countless times as well. Some prisoners thought he was nuts, while others decided to follow his example as he looked in better shape than most. In the end, only his father and his chewing friends survived the camp.

Grains and other complex carbohydrates need more chewing than fruits or animal proteins. Nevertheless, rather than decide on this basis, thinking of chewing each mouthful 35 to 50 times. And, as was said earlier, if you are unwell, consider chewing each mouthful 100 to 200 times. Not only will your food be more digestible, but because you have maximized the vitality you get out of each mouthful from good enzyme action, you will probably eat less as a result.

Guideline **NUMBER FIVE** follows logically from NUMBER FOUR: Eat at a moderate pace; not too quick and not too slow. If you are chewing your food well, you have no choice but to do this. This guideline also suggests to avoid feeling stuffed after the meal; leave 1/4 to 1/3 of your stomach empty. Start with a portion/plateful that would approximately fill your two cupped hands. Again, if you are chewing your food well, more energy is released from what you are eating. Consequently, you may even find that, naturally, you feel satisfied more quickly. Think of the French way of dining all evening. Their gastric habits yield more delight and little obesity.

If you are still hungry after eating this amount, wait five minutes before taking more. You may be just experiencing the memory of hunger. Breathe for while. If you then still feel the need, take a little more. Leave the meal feeling satisfied.

Another point that goes along with this is that you should not eat in a totally ravenous state. Pitta body-mind types are more prone to this than others. If they are hungry and held back from getting food into their stomachs, expect them to get irritable. But generally speaking, on this point, if you are extremely hungry when you sit down to a meal, start your meal slowly and breathe evenly as you chew. Another Ayurvedic solution is to take a bite of dessert or something sweet to start with. This will create a certain level of satisfaction that will slow you down so you can begin your meal in a more reasonable mental and physical state of being.

Guideline **NUMBER SIX** is to avoid taking another meal until the previous one has been digested (approx. 3 to 6 hours). The only exceptions are those who are hypoglycemic who may need to snack or have small meals more frequently. Our digestive juices and the chemistry of digestion changes as our food is metabolized. Thus, if we start the digestive process all over again by unnecessary or habitual snacking, the mix of new food with more digested food can slow up and spoil the entire digestive process.

Much of the snacking that we as westerners do has to do with the fact that our food sources are depleted of nutrients and/or are so imbalanced and dead that our body seeks more, even when our bellies may be full. Diets full of refined carbohydrates (sugar, refined flour, etc.) will actually leach the body of minerals, thus creating a cycle of craving and dissatisfaction that leads to another sugar binge, on and on. In Ayurvedic terms, these products make our energy spike up, then plunge down, leaving us feeling heavier. Kapha dosha is aggravated and amma, more toxins, are created. As we seek more energy, we go for more sweets and the cycle is perpetuated and the only thing that begins to spike is our weight and sense of depression. One of the solutions to this cycle is to eliminate such products altogether for a minimum of three weeks and increase more complex carbohydrates (whole grains, fruits, and vegetables) and well as other mineral-rich foods. If you have been eating this way for a long time, it may even be useful to take a mineral supplement.

Similar to refined carbohydrates are the effects of eating overly processed or "junk" foods. Such devitalized foods may provide calories, but little benefit for the various systems of the body. Amma is created and a hunger of the body and mind to finally be given something that does satisfy. As these foods have tastes that initially deceive the body into thinking that it is being nutrified, we eat more and more and once again, a cycle that leads to lethargy, weight gain, and negative states of mind is the sad outcome.

Especially for spa therapists, these cycles will wear you down. Beyond all the other recommendations given so far, grabbing a sweet or non-nutritious snack between clients doesn't work. If you have little time to eat a meal, snack on something that is nutritious and easy to digest: a piece of fruit, maybe some lightly steamed or raw vegetables chewed very well.

The last of the guidelines around environment and conditions of eating, **NUMBER SEVEN,** has to do with the optimal times to eat. Under ideal circumstances, those with a dominant VATA constitution or condition should have a rich, warming breakfast, a nutritious lunch, and a warming but light evening meal. PITTA types and those with PITTA conditions should have a light breakfast, a rich and nutritious midday meal, and a slightly smaller but full evening meal. Breakfast can be optional for Kapha-types. Their mid-day meal should be a light, protein-rich meal, with evening meals being similar to the midday meal, albeit a bit smaller.

Such guidelines are great if you are on your own and/or don't have to cook for anyone else, have to go out to work, etc. Thus, in general, try to take your largest meal at lunch, when your digestion (and your agni) is the strongest. If you cannot do this, start your day with a reasonable, but nutritious breakfast, following body-mind type recommendations. However, in our fast-paced urban living, the evening meal is often the one we get to sit down to, eat with friends, etc. As this is our "main" meal, try to observe the following guidelines. These are guidelines that are generally true for all meals, but should certainly be heeded for our main meal.

Food and Beverage Basics

Guideline **NUMBER EIGHT** is to avoid ice water or cold beverages during the meal. It doesn't matter what you chose to eat, be it nutritious or not. If you wash it down with iced beverages, even large quantities of water, you will inhibit digestion. Cool or room temperature juice before meals may be good for Pitta types, but not for Kapha or Vata. Chewing food well during a meal can provide digestive juices to food to alleviate much thirst during the meal. If you must have something to drink during the meal, take some room temperature or warm water or mild tea.

Regarding specific drinks, there are some alcoholic beverages that are good to arouse appetite and others that will aid digestion towards the end of the meal. Few alcoholic beverages are helpful during meals, save for very dry wines. The reason has to do with the fact that such beverages are super-carbohydrate/sugar drinks and will inhibit the release of useful digestive enzymes.

Soft drinks are generally a nice thing to have on their own for fun, but other than that, they are useless. I would rate soft drinks as one of the major contributors to weight gain in western culture. If you cut them out during meals, you will digest your food. If you cut them out altogether, that is best. And absolutely cut out all that contain nutra-sweet and other such artificial sweeteners. Go for a sugar-based Pepsi or Coke if you must.

Drink milk alone (or 20 minutes after a meal) or with sweet foods. We'll discuss more about dairy products in general later.

An excellent practice is to take a cup of hot water 10 minutes after the meal (if you want, add a slice of lemon). The story on the origins of Ayurveda claims that the first medicine was hot water and was used to cure the first illness—indigestion. Hot water actually is quite thirst quenching, will aid digestive fire, and will help curb your desire for dessert! And, if you have dessert, it will be digested that much better.

Although this may sound strange in the melting-pot consciousness of the west, guideline **NUMBER NINE** is to learn about the dietary practices of your heritage. Beyond your dosha-dominance, there are a host of genetic factors we carry from our families of origin. Even certain blood types have their dominance in certain cultures. Often, these foods will work well for you, although they may need to be varied because of availability of regional foods, herbs, and spices, as well as seasonal and climatic changes that are not in keeping with how your ancestors lived. For example, we have seen the devastating effects when Indians from a tropic climate try to eat their indigenous, tropical diet while living in the Thames Valley in England. Interestingly enough, the health of the Chinese population seems to be better because they came from a more temperate climate to start with. At the same time, many of us have mixed heritages, in which case we may need to see what works best in one season or climate for us.

In keeping with this, try to think of your own family history. Tibetan doctors say that if you eat what you were raised on at an early age, these specific foods will not be the cause for any great or serious illness. Certainly, they may not be the most nutritious or give you all of the vitality you would like from your diet. However, they will not cause undo harm. Our recommendation for people who did not have nutritious diets when they were growing up is to find foods that are a better quality, but of the same kind as what you ate when you were younger. Interestingly enough, the natural foods market is leaning in this direction anyway with a wide variety of prepared or typical culturally enjoyed foods of organic quality, although they may need to be modified to suit the climate and seasons you are now in.

Following along with guideline eight, guideline **NUMBER TEN** suggests that we should eat fresh food suitable to the season and your geographical area. The best possible foods for the body are fruits, vegetables, and animal products grown in your area (or similar climate zone). These foods have thrived in the same climatic conditions that you grow in. Thus, when looking at traditional and our historical diets, we should modify them to accommodate where we currently are.

Other than the anecdotal comments made in number eight, I am reminded of a story I read about Alaskan Eskimos who were introduced to orange juice. Researchers thought that some of the health problems of the Eskimos had to do with too little Vitamin C in their diets. And so they shipped up large quantities of orange juice from Georgia. The result? The Eskimos got sicker with new diseases they had previously not encountered. The orange juice was discontinued and they returned to normal. And then researchers began to pay attention to the fact that Eskimos ate lichen, which had a small quantity of Vitamin C. The fact is that in hot, humid climates, Vitamin C helps to keep the body cool and improves immunity against the kinds of viruses, etc. found in such climates. This is not what Alaska is like. So only a little Vitamin C is necessary. Instead, Eskimos need fat-soluble vitamins in their diet, like A and E as found in whale blubber, seal, salmon, etc.

Eating in keeping with our geographical area is problematic because of the transcontinental shipping of foods. So we suggest that if you live in a temperate climate, choose to eat foods that come from other temperate climates, and so on, keeping in mind the above example made of the Chinese and Indians in London.

If at all possible, in making such selections, eat *organically*. If this is not possible, chose commercial fruits, grains, and vegetables that have not been genetically modified. The complication with genetic modification is that no one really knows how they effect the body. All traditional medical literature about the benefits of various foods is based on them being in a natural state. Genetic modification is not natural. True, farmers and botanists have played with grafting and various forms of modification over the years. But this has never been done to the degree of what is possible in science today and we could well be creating a can of health-related worms with Franken-foods.

When selecting foods based on the two previous guidelines, **NUMBER ELEVEN** says that when looking at your historical or traditional cuisines, or one that you are interested in, for the diet to be balanced, try to include all six tastes (sour, bitter, sweet, pungent, salty, and astringent). Traditional cuisines (i.e. Italian, Greek, Slavic, and Asian) often include all these tastes.

For the most part, standard western and especially American diet is heavy on salty and sweet, with only minor variations. These two tastes often attract each other if they are eaten in great quantity and intensity. Other tastes will make the diet richer and feel more settling. Besides what our mouths and tastebuds enjoy, Ayurveda talks about it in terms of *rasa* which, translated, means blood. The taste of our foods affects all of our doshas and are constituents of our blood. Consequently, if we have diets that are heavy in just two tastes, the body is robbed of stimulation. Salty taste is the combination of the Fire and Water elements. So, if in excess, we shall see effects on the organs most associated with Fire and Water, namely our heart, small intestine, glandular and urinary tracts. If we have an excess of sweet in our diet, associated with the Earth and Water elements, we shall see problems with our lymph system, stomach, blood sugar balances, and so on. Clearly, we see a dominance of illness and dis-ease in these organs and systems of the body.

In keeping with a variety of tastes, Ayurveda also says that it is good to create meals of many colors. Colors are pleasing to the eye and also stimulate digestion.

Regardless of where the diet comes from, certain combinations of foods are toxic or do not work well together for any constitution. Guideline **NUMBER TWELVE** is to eliminate and/or be cautious of the following, some of which are quite commonplace and others that you would probably never, ever consider.

These are:
- curds or yogurt mixed with new wine.
- fish cooked in milk products (i.e. British-style poaching, fillet of fish sandwiches topped with cheese, tuna fish casserole, etc.).

- milk cooked with walnuts.
- eggs combined with fish (i.e. tuna salad with mayonnaise).
- mushrooms with mustard.
- chicken cooked with yogurt or curds (although tandoori style with spices is OK).
- fruit juice combined with or followed by milk (i.e. fruit yogurts, fruit based ice creams, etc.).
- honey and oil in equal amounts (more or less of one works fine).
- peaches combined with other fruits.
- food combinations where the food becomes discolored when combined or cooked (i.e. peaches will discolor other fruits as will purple cabbage and beets when cooked with other vegetables).
- heating or cooking with honey (Ayurveda says that eating cooked honey is poisonous, forming a coating in the body that is hard to get rid of; if you have a choice between a cake made with honey or sugar, go for the sugar one every time).
- eating animal and vegetable protein-rich foods together (your body has different enzymes to break down vegetable or meat based proteins. If you eat, let's say, a hamburger and baked beans, or chicken fajitas with a side of refried beans, your body will not know which one to digest. So it will elect not to do very much at all. The result is putrification and gas, which, of course we all blame the beans for).
- eating melon with other fruits or foods (Melons are some of the fastest digesting foods. If you eat them with other foods, your body gets all excited to digest the melon and doesn't tend as well to the other foods. Again, putrification, a buildup of amma, gas, bloating, etc). Melons are best by themselves.

Guideline **NUMBER THIRTEEN** focuses on dairy. Traditionally, Ayurveda has a great deal of reverence for dairy. Fresh milk is considered a panacea, especially for Pitta types. Various grain and vegetable dishes in Indian Ayurvedic cuisine use milk or yogurt. Ghee or clarified butter is used not only for cooking, but also in a number of internal and external medicines. Being a mountainous people, Tibetans, like the Swiss, use cheese. To cope with the dryness and cold, they are known to even put butter in their hair. And in both Indian and Tibetan Ayurveda, fresh, warm milk is sometimes added to medicinal enemas.

The first time I heard of this was when a close friend and Tibetan doctor was working out of our home, giving pancha karma treatments. Toward the end of a week of cleansing massages, steams, and regular herbal enemas, the doctor wanted some patients to take milk enemas. As we were nowhere where we would be able to secure whole, organic milk, I told him that I did not think it was possible. But he thought we could just go down to the local supermarket and pick up milk off the shelf.

I asked him if he had ever heard of homogenization. He had not. I explained how this is a process where the milk is agitated at such a high frequency that the fat molecules of the milk break down and become smaller. The result is increased shelf life, but also ensures that when you drink it, fat goes to where the water portion of the milk would normally go. He was shocked, and decided that such enemas were probably not a good idea.

Beyond homogenization and pasteurization, however, is the enormous amount of antibiotics and hormones that dairy cattle are fed. The end result of this chemical tampering and engineering is that not even baby calves can survive on what the average westerner is told "does a body good".

Our litany against commercial dairy products could take up an entire volume by itself. Instead, we recommend you go to the website of Robert Cohen, www.notmilk.com. Mr. Cohen has done much to expose the travesties of the dairy industry.

Within the context of Ayurveda, our suggestion is that you only purchase organic dairy products. Those of you who are more Pitta will benefit from such products more than others. At the same time, if you are lactose intolerant, which many westerners are, we encourage you to stay away from them altogether or consume them in moderation. Traditional Mediterranean and Indian cooking used spices and herbs to help mollify the mucous-forming effects of these products. Observe the cautions about toxic combinations (fish and dairy, walnuts and milk, etc). And for those prone to tiring dreams or nightmares, yogurt, cheese, cottage cheese or other cultured dairy products should not be eaten at night, especially close to bed time.

Beyond dairy products, see *Tibetan Ayurveda: Health Secrets from The Roof of The World* regarding which body types do best with different kinds of meats. The main suggestion we do have, however, is that you should choose to only eat organic meats whenever possible.

Guideline **NUMBER FOURTEEN** is to minimize your use of raw foods. Raw foods take a tremendous amount of metabolic heat to break down and digest. Pitta-types are much better suited to raw foods, but because our stress levels are higher these days, few of us have the adequate digestive fire to metabolize these properly if we consume them day after day. This may seem to fly in the face of commercial consumer wisdom, but if you have dry skin or hair, have yeast infections or related problems, feel cold frequently, suffer from gas, bloating, or are spacy more frequently than you would like, decreasing your intake of raw foods is recommended.

If you do chose to partake, we advise that you consume them during warm seasons, in warmer climates in general, and/or for a mid-day (rather than evening) meal when your digestive fire is burning higher.

It is also best not to combine raw fruits and vegetables with cooked ones. If you are having raw vegetables at a meal, stick with raw vegetables. If you are eating cooked ones, stick with cooked ones.

Forbidden Foods

In Ayurveda, if you know how to cook well, you can eat almost anything. Ayurvedic cuisine teaches ways of antidoting or balancing even the most sinful of our culinary pleasures. Please see the Bibliography for a list of Ayurvedic cookbooks. Some are western oriented, others more traditionally Indian. The important thing to understand is that Ayurvedic eating is about following principles. If you follow those principles, anything is possible.

That said, guideline **NUMBER FIFTEEN** has to do with the desires and cravings that can arise from modifying or changing the direction of your eating habits. Desires and cravings for specific foods should be examined and at times honored. Sometimes a small amount of a desired 'no-no' food will satisfy some deep physiological or psychological need. On the other hand, if having some makes you only want more and more, then this may be a more destructive habit pattern or craving that comes from detoxifying oneself of the desired food (i.e. coffee, sugar, chocolate, dairy products, etc).

These recommendations and guidelines are intended to improve the quality of how you nurture and nourish your body-mind with food and beverages. They are very general, but at the same time will feel quite revolutionary. Whatever you, do not bend yourself out of shape trying to do everything perfectly. The anxiety and stress alone will make what you eat indigestible, anyway.

At the same time, Ayurveda is a masterful healing science and the dietary recommendations of skilled Ayurvedic doctors and health practitioners can go a long way toward assisting those with serious health concerns. If you are looking for someone to help you beyond the scope of what is discussed here, please refer to the Resource Guide provided at the end of this book.

CHAPTER 12

Exercise and Relaxation

*A*s is evident from our presentation, all human activity and endeavors can be classified Ayurvedically. Exercise, as one aspect of building a healthy lifestyle in the first level of Tibetan Ayurveda, therefore, is given the same scrutiny as other aspects such as diet, spa treatments, etc.

Like the literature on diet, be it from conventional or alternative perspectives, forms of exercise have been elevated to panaceas. When aerobics was first touted as the answer for cardiovascular health in the 1980's, there were those who pushed their bodies to cardiac crisis or chronic fatigue. The cycling and spinning became the answer and an inordinate number of men riding on tiny hard seats developed long-term prostate problems. Of course, over time, research has been done and there are many forms of exercise that are suggested and done with greater discretion and prudence. Had the wisdom of Ayurveda been applied in assessing for whom each form of exercise is good, the learning curve and the damage done would be, in my estimation, much lower.

Thus, the "But for Whom?" question posed by Dr. Vasant Lad regarding diet and Ayurvedic herbs and treatment, is equally valid when it comes to exercise. Thus, first we shall look at the different dosha types and what sports or forms of exercise are most appropriate and, because they are appropriate, they feel better, are more fun, hence giving more lasting benefits. In addition, we shall look at two forms of exercise from the Tibetan tradition, one that is excellent for joint health and particularly useful for therapists, and the other that is a yogic series of exercises that are for rejuvenation. The Tibetan Rejuvenation Exercises as we call them are great for the home and will be an added plus in any day or destination spa where they are taught and practiced.

But before we embark on these discussions, let us first discuss exercise in general. In our post-industrial societies, most of us no longer perform work that is as physically demanding on us as was done in previous times in history. Our sedentary, convenience-based lifestyle means that many of the parameters for eating, resting, exercising, and so on are different than they were for our ancestors. One example I can think of amongst my own circle of acquaintances is a gentleman whose father worked ten hours a day down in coal mines. In the evenings, this man went down to the local bar to be with friends. After sweating all day doing backbreaking work, each of them would consume ten or more pints of beer. And yet they wouldn't get drunk and they all stayed lean. But not my friend, who worked as a chemist and manager of his own company. He had a sedentary life and only did a little exercise on the weekends in his spare time. Yet because of the culture of drinking he was a part of when growing up, he would drink like his father. Unlike his father, he put on weight, his joints suffered, and he felt intoxicated a good many more times than he would have been prepared to admit.

Beyond needing to change our concepts around meals, portions, what is best for us at the dining table, we also need to look at what it takes to keep us mobile and supple in our body so that we can feel more comfortable in our own skin and enjoy our days of activity.

Consequently, whereas for our ancestors, their physical work demanded for them to relax and be more still in their home time, we need to create a post-work lifestyle where the benefits of physical exercise are combined with relaxation. We do not consider this to be a luxury as much as a necessity if we are not to succumb to stress and degenerative illnesses whose origins are over-consumption and ineffectual detoxification.

Exercise should be challenging, yet fun. It should stimulate the body to overcome built up stress and tension and facilitate the elimination of toxins that build up, especially in a more sedentary lifestyle. To meet these criteria most effectively, knowing one's constitutional balance of doshas is most useful.

Please bear in mind that the listing of exercises below is not exhaustive. However, once you get the common sense that is being applied for each of the body-mind types, you can then apply the same criteria to other forms of exercise you may be considering.

For Vata Body-Mind Types

Vata-types do best when an exercise program is gentle and consistent. And yet, because of the tendency for Vata to unbalanced in times of stress and change, Vata types can be energy and exercise junkies, pushing things too hard and for too long. Many a Vata-type woman has found herself suffering from chronic fatigue after years of high impact aerobics. For in general, these types need to keep their breath smooth and relaxed when they exercise. They also need to be wary of doing any kind of exercise that puts too much strain on their joints—a focal point for the Vata body-mind type.

In any kind of exercise, Vatas should start slow and build up stamina. Types of sport and exercise that best suit Vatas are

- Yoga—especially emphasizing inverted postures as this helps to cleanse and tonify the colon, the seat of Vata (the use of inversion machines can also be of benefit for Vata types for the same reasons).

- Tai Chi—as breath and movement are evenly coordinated and there is an appreciation of the flow of energy that is most appealing for Vatas.

- Qi Quong (Chi Kung)—for the same reasons as Tai Chi.

- Swimming—as it stretches out the joints. But Vata types also need to be wary of the harsh effects of such chemicals as chlorine as this dries out the skin and will aggravate Vata. The same is true of salt water. Rubbing the body with sesame oil after swimming is recommended to counter this effect.

- Stretching Programs—working the joints is excellent for Vata types. To enhance results, oil all the joints before exercise.

- Road biking—being on smooth and even surfaces (as opposed to off-road mountain-bike conditions) is best. Oiling of the hips and knees is recommended, as is stopping before one gets winded. Spinning under the guidance of someone who monitors breath and heart rate is an excellent alternative.

- Weight training—oil the joints with sesame oil and go for less weight and a slow, progressive buildup of repetitions.

- Walking—better than running. Good-fitting, supportive shoes are essential.

- Water exercise and aerobics—especially useful for those with joint problems and/or injuries and elders in their Vata stage of life.

- Generally, any exercise that is gentle on the joints, keeps the breathing even, and focuses on slow, long-term benefits.

- PRECAUTIONS: If one does like to engage in sports where there is impact on the joints (running, mountain biking, tennis, etc.), oiling of the most used joints is essential).

Beyond the recommendations and precautions listed above, Vata body-mind types do best to **AVOID** those sports where breathing is strained (**high impact aerobics, mountain climbing, scuba diving, or generally just over-doing it**), joints are strained or there is strong impact on them (**mountain biking, volleyball, handball, intense contact sports such as rugby, football, kickboxing, boxing, etc**), or where there is a high degree of unpredictability (**extreme, dare-devil sports, combat games like paintball,** etc).

For Pitta Body-Mind Types

These are the more athletically inclined of all of us. Good stamina and well-balanced proportions give Pittas the edge in most sports. However, because of their competitive nature, they sometimes find enjoying exercise a challenge and can put as much zeal and intensity into their exercise as they do for work. The result is stress in exercise that diminishes cardiovascular and other benefits. Pushing themselves to the max and beyond, Pittas can suffer from sudden exhaustion, burn-out, and even more physically debilitating events as heart attacks in the activities they consider "fun". Thus although you will probably not get the Pitta person to abandon competing with themselves or others altogether, a mantra they should keep in the back of their mind when exercising or engaging in sport is "fun and relaxation".

Although we shall discuss relaxation in greater length later on, it is important to emphasize that cool down and time for relaxation processes as part of exercise are a must for the Pitta body-mind types. This not only balances their intensity, but also entrains their body to be more prepared when exercise is done in the future. Besides these caveats and suggestions, one other major **PRECAUTION** is to **not exercise to a profuse sweat.**

In general, Ayurveda suggests that one only exercise up to the point where a small amount of perspiration is felt on the surface of the body. **Breaking into full sweating is considered to be injurious to the heart.** And the buildup of internal heat and then its dissipation in profuse perspiration is particularly harmful for the Pitta types.

All this being said, let's look art the various recommended sports and exercises for Pitta types:

- Yoga—best if it is a dynamic form, such as Iyengar style, etc. Pitta types like the martial approach, but also respect the tradition and will more than likely comply with the relaxation that is recommended in such forms. At the same time, Anusara-style yoga with its playfulness is also good. Postures emphasizing compression in the torso and twisting are excellent for Pittas. **Bikram or hot-style yogas are not recommended for the reasons given above.**

- Tai Ch'i—This may be considered almost adjunctive to more physical and intense forms of exercise. Will be appreciated more later on in life when the heat is dissipating and Vata is on the rise.
- Qi Quong (Chi Kung)—for the same reasons as Tai Ch'i.
- Swimming—mainly because of its watery, cooling nature. But Pittas are very sensitive to chemicals and this may cause breakouts and skin rashes. The same is true with salt water. What Pittas need to do is be sure that they rinse thoroughly after swimming to get off the residues that may cause these problems.
- Mountain Biking—because it is unpredictable and they can test themselves, sharpen their focus, and let go. Still, road biking is also fine, but they should be sure to get a soft, gel-like seat as the pressure on their reproductive organs can cause problems later on. This is generally true, but especially true for Pittas who have a great focus of energy in their glandular system.
- Weight training—oil the joints with sesame oil and go for less weight and a slow, progressive build up of repetitions.
- Running or Walking—Just keep cool and don't do it in the mid-day sun. You might even combine running with walking to give yourself permission for a good cool-down.
- Generally, almost all other forms of sports and exercise are fine, provided that the Pitta types stay cool, don't build up to a fighting frenzy, and do quality relaxation afterwards. Also, it is best if they **AVOID iced or very cold drinks at the end of exercise as this rapid cool-down can deplete their heat too quickly.**

For Kapha Body-Mind Types

Kapha body-mind types do not particularly go for exercise. They like to watch sports, sit on a park bench and ponder why people will run around knocking themselves out on fitness. Yet the truth of it is, they are the body-mind type that benefits most from daily exercise and will see the greatest benefits from it.

Motivating the Kapha person to exercise needs to come both from an inner intention and possibly some outside coaxing. As they put weight on easily, they can get discouraged by not losing weight and becoming as svelte as their leggy Vata or Pitta athletic friends. If their motivation overcomes their lethargy, they will discover that they have more stamina, strength, and resilience that them all. As they become more alert and feel the benefits, this will convince them to stick with it.

For this to happen, exercise and sport need to be interesting. Looking at the lists from the Vata and Pitta types and modifying them for our Kapha friends:

- Yoga—especially emphasizing inverted postures as this helps to backwash their lymph system, which can get congested, forward and backward bending postures to increase spinal flexibility (along these lines, they can derive much benefit from small personal trampolines, i.e. rebounding, as well as the use of inversion machines). Twisting postures are also helpful. Like Pittas, the forms of yoga can be more dynamic, but can also include such styles as Bikram.

- Tai Bo—taking the principles of martial arts, boxing, dance and Tai Ch'i, originator Billy Banks has created a form that keeps the Kapha up and interested.

- Qi Quong (Chi Kung)—helping to re-oxygenate their bodies, hence overcome lethargy.

- Aerobics—better equipped physically to take the impact. However, few Kaphas may gravitate towards this to start with. They need to be pushed into a class. After a few times, they will see the benefits and really get into it.

- Biking—road and mountain.

- Weight training—oil the joints with sesame oil and go for less weight and a slow, progressive buildup of repetitions.

- Running—Cross-country style, giving them interesting terrain to look at. If done around a track, they should intersperse sprints with long distance. If the Kapha person is not inclined to start with this, walking may be an alternative. If this is what is chosen over running, encourage them to consider speed walking.

- Generally, all sports are fine, but they will find sports that have unpredictable movements more fun and beneficial; i.e. **basketball** (many pro basketball players are big Kapha guys), **racket games such as tennis, squash, handball** (They have enough thickness in their skin and lubrication around their joints to handle the impact), **contact sports such as boxing and forms of martial arts.**

Of all the body types, as they get conditioned, they are the ones who can allow themselves to work up a sweat. However, this sweat usually has a strong discharge with it. Traditionally, Kapha types are encouraged to get oil on their bodies, work up a sweat, and then cover their bodies in red lentil flour to pull the toxins out. At home or with a trainer in a spa, such a practice will help the Kapha person experience even greater benefits from their exercise. The alternative, but not as effective, is to be sure to take a good shower before this sweaty layer dries.

Age and Seasonal Considerations for Exercise

Regardless of our constitutional mix of doshas, age factors will contribute their doshic signature on the age phases we pass through over the course of our lives. When we are born and for the first eight years of life, we are more Kapha in the expression of our constitution; we're rounder, softer, mucousy, and bounce better when we fall or are dropped. From eight until our mid-forties, we go through our Pitta phases; the rising and settling of our hormonal intensity that gives us our lust for life and the dramas that go with it. Coming through a menopausal tunnel— something that both women and men do—we are drier, both within and without, and go through the Vata phase of life.

What this means is that your needs for exercise change from your twenties to your forties. It is not just a matter of running out of steam. It also has to do with the manner in which the body needs to be treated for it to derive the benefits it requires for the new stage of life. In other words, you may have done aerobics when you were in your early thirties. But now that you are in your fifties, you should not lament, nor become dejected because aerobics doesn't feel right, makes you feel weaker than stronger. At fifty, in the more Vata phase of life, aerobics just doesn't work. And if there is strong wish to do it, the considerations for Vata need to be observed; oiling the joints before exercise, watching that the breath stays more regular, and so on.

Beyond applying this common sense to ourselves, this wisdom from Ayurveda is invaluable for fitness educators and trainers in spas. Not only does it hone fitness programs to best benefit the client, it will also reduce the risk that a spa member is injured or worse at your facility.

There is also the fact that the seasons have their influence on how we should exercise. In the changeable seasons of spring and fall, our Vata will tend to become more naturally aggravated. This will be especially true for those with a dominance of Vata in their constitution. Keeping to a fuller schedule of exercise rather than really intensely working out one week and then nothing for a few weeks is recommended. If doing aerobics, shifting to more low impact forms and focusing more on warm downs and relaxation is advisable. In the summer, with the heat up, Pitta can be aggravated. Thus Pittas need to be especially mindful of not overdoing it, sweating profusely, jogging in the mid-day sun. Cool down times and relaxation, doing exercise early in the morning or towards sunset are best. In the cool of winter, Vata and Kapha can become aggravated. If it is a cold, damp climate, this aggravates Kapha. If cold and dry, this aggravates Vata. With this awareness, exercise should be done to build up heat and energy, but not get to the point of dissipating heat by breaking a sweat.

Another factor consider that is similar to seasonal changes is the fact that most of us have a dominance of two doshas; Vata-Pitta, Vata-Kapha, Pitta-Kapha. Thus, depending on environmental, seasonal, and lifestyle factors, it may just be that there are times when we elect to do one form of exercise over another. The important point here is to be mindful and flexible. There are no panaceas. Ayurveda insists that in all aspect of our lives we are mindful and make choices that are appropriate for today.

Deepening the Benefits: Breathing and Mudras

One way of ensuring that you breathe properly with maximum results from both exercise and sports is to use what in the tradition of yoga is called *Ujjayi Pranayama*. Pranayama is the science of breath. *Prana* is the subtle life force that is the most refined aspect of Vata. In the Chinese tradition it is called Chi, in Tibetan it is Lung, and in the Japanese it is Ki. Pranayama relies upon regulating the breath in a variety of way to effect physical, emotional, and spiritual growth.

Ujjayi Pranayama is a particular form of breathing, where you rest your tongue behind your top front teeth (as spoken of in the section on the preliminaries for offering treatment rituals), close your mouth, and breathe both in and out exclusively through your nose. The breath comes in naturally and on the breath out, you contract the throat slightly, so that the out breath sounds hollow, like Darth Vader in "Star Wars". In the practice of Pranayama, this becomes refined until you are breathing very deeply, both in and out. However, in the case of exercise and sport, just regulating the breath like this improves the quality of your workout. **It is also excellent for therapists to keep to this style of breathing throughout a treatment.**

In an interview with Melanie, Ayurvedic chiropractor and master, Dr. John Douillard says of Ujjayi breathing:

We find that when people breathe like this while they exercise, they feel in the zone. They feel blissful. They enjoy their workout. They are not stiff or uncomfortable the next day . . . there have been proven chemical changes that happen naturally in the body just from changing the way we breathe, changes that involve nitric oxide . . . Nitric oxide, which is more available when we do this 'Darth Vader' breath, regulates blood pressure, boosts the immune system; kills cancer cells, bacteria and viruses; increases blood supply to the cells; aids muscle control, balance and coordination.

(Page 97, Les Nouvelles Esthetique, April 2004)

What is also nice about this form of breathing is that it will help you regulate becoming out of breath. When you are building up your workout or in the middle of a sport, when you can no longer hold the breath in and out in the above manner and you start panting with your mouth open, you are out "of the zone" and the benefits of your exercise will begin to diminish. At the same time, if you stop then, regain your composure and get your breath back into control, over time you will find that you are able to keep your breath like this longer and your stamina, strength, and endurance will grow exponentially.

Besides Ujjayi-style breathing, there is a *mudra* which we find particularly useful for exercise, especially for walking, running, and any floor exercise, be it low or high impact aerobics.

A *mudra* (pronounced moo-drah) is a seal, the creating of a circuit. In virtually all spiritual traditions, mudras are used. The Angele (hands held together, palm to palm) is a mudra common to both eastern and western spiritual traditions. Tibetan Buddhists use a wide range of mudras in some of their meditations to create the movement of specific energies in the body and mind. The martial arts tradition also uses such mudras as the hopjang positioning of the hands, again to elicit and channel concentration and force of the subtle life force (prana or chi).

The mudra that we suggest for the styles of exercise mentioned above is one where the tip of the thumbs are placed at the base or root of the fourth finger, with the remaining fingers wrapped around the thumb.

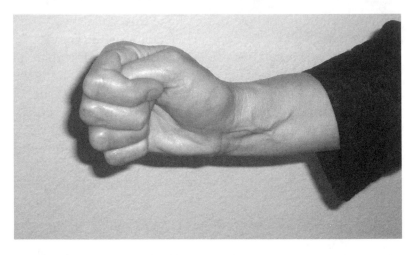

   In the Buddhist tradition, this is the mudra of the Bodhisattva, the Enlightened ones who walk amongst us helping us to awaken to our full potentials. This mudra is intended to awaken compassion. This is its higher purpose and it is an excellent mudra to use when sitting in meditation. In this case the hand position is palms facing downwards resting on the knees as opposed to upwards the way many people think of positioning their hands.

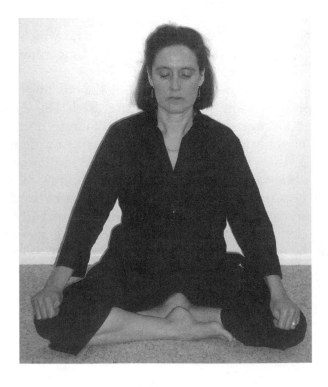

At the same time, this position creates a seal or circuit between specific energies in the body. From the Ayurvedic point of view, the thumb represents the Ether or Space element and is associated with the brain. The fourth finger represents the Water element and is associated with the kidneys. From this point of view, the brain, which governs our Central Nervous System, and the kidneys, which play an essential role in the functioning of our autonomic nervous system, come together to help our alertness and coordination. As Water nourishes the Ether element, fluidity delivers its energy into an element most associated with Vata, hence movement. If we look at this from the Chinese understanding of the Five Elements, the thumb is associated with lung energy and the fourth finger with metabolic heat, the Triple Warmer. With the two joined, more prana, chi, or—more from a physical standpoint—oxygen is delivered to the fires that must burn strongly in order for us to move dynamically and with precision. The location of these three warmers of the Triple Warmer are in the Svadhisthana or Hara region, just below the navel, the solar plexus, and the throat, the glandular regions whose subtle aspect are the second, third, and fourth chakras, respectively.

When you keep your hands in this mudra and exercise, you feel more balanced and alert, do not tire as easily, and find your second wind to revitalize your efforts. Combined with Ujjayi-style breathing you are making your mind and body work together more efficiently and with greater results.

Quality Relaxation

In the spa or at home, quality relaxation is an important aspect of any wellness and rejuvenation program. That said, most people do not achieve any deep quality of relaxation and because of this, they never get proper rest when they sleep, either.

In the section of the book devoted to treatment rituals, after the Tibetan Blissful Sleep ritual, we made several recommendations to help you and your client to sleep better. Many of the suggestions will certainly help you to relax. However, here we are speaking of learning and conditioning yourself to experience a deeper level of relaxation in your life generally. It seems odd to think that we would need to 'learn' to relax. But in the pace of modern life that often spins seemingly out of control, to re-introduce and learn effective relaxation methods is extremely useful. There are two aspects we will focus on: relaxation in relation to exercise and relaxation as a form of exercise in and of itself.

In both the yogic and martial arts traditions, there are moments of stillness. In yoga, not only is there savasana (the corpse posture) at the end of the session, but there should also be a period of rest in between each posture that is done.

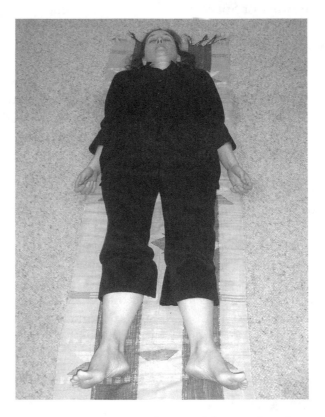

The same is true in moments of inward focus after forms or *katas* or such cycles of exercise as chi quong or tai chi. The purpose of such moments of stillness is integration and entrainment. What this means is that you are giving the body and mind time to come together, to fully experience the benefits of the exercise that you have just completed. As this takes place, a deeper connection between your central nervous system and your body is forged to ensure that the next time you come to do the exercise, your body and mind will be more alerted, prepared, and able to do the exercise with greater efficiency and ease. This is entrainment.

Too often, exercise classes and poorly trained teachers in the martial arts and yoga try to pack the class full with things to do. With no proper space or time for integration and entrainment, students will get more frustrated as they progress more slowly and run the risk of becoming injured. Taking moments to pause during and leaving a sufficient amount of time at the end to allow the person to warm and wind down after a class is an essential ingredient in a quality class. It will make the class more enjoyable and will ensure that people leave the class alert and focused, but relaxed.

This advice also applies to those who work out on their own. For especially at home, one gets to thinking about what needs to be done next when finishing whatever form of exercise you have 'scheduled' into your day. Take the time. Especially in a home environment, the use of relaxation music as a reminder that it is time to slow down is quite useful.

Besides relaxation as a part of exercise, it can also be used as a form of rest and rejuvenation in and of itself. Here we are speaking of what many people know or may have heard of in many forms and by many names: skilled or progressive relaxation, autogenic training, biofeedback, guided imagery, etc. Essentially, the deep relaxation sought by all these forms comes when we are able to pull our senses away from the myriad of distractions in our day, focus more inwardly on such physical aspects as our body sensations or breath, on an imagined image that elicits serenity and peace, or a combination of these three. Music or voice cues, such as relaxation music or guided imagery or instruction can be helpful in encouraging the process of relaxation to unfold. Because Pitta becomes more active when we use our eyes, the use of vision and visual cues generally does not work so well. Some people may claim that they get relaxed by watching T.V. Mostly what this is is distraction and in fact, will leave the person more tired than refreshed. Of course, there are more and more companies creating relaxation videos with wonderful audio tracks. These may be helpful on an airplane or in a waiting room. There are also a number of brainwave light devices that help to trigger the "relaxation response." For home or spa use, such devices can be helpful in entraining people to experience relaxation. However, they will never be as effective only because of the Pitta stimulation that runs counter to deep, quality relaxation. In truth, like the simple yogic asana of the corpse (*savasana*), the deepest results come from just relying on one's own breath and awareness.

In speaking earlier of brainwaves and the "relaxation response," we get to the crux of what one is trying to achieve in doing any one of these exercises. As we pull our attention inwards and come to a less distracted focus, our brainwaves shift from the normal, discursive Beta-wave frequencies, and move towards an increase of relaxing Alpha-wave and imaginal or hypnogogic Theta-wave frequencies. As the amplitude of these particular waves increase and dominate our brainwave activity, there is an increase of oxygen-rich blood that goes to the brain, which in turn balances both the central and autonomic nervous systems. This causes a release of our 'fight-flight' response and greater circulation gets into our organs and muscles. Toxins are cleansed away and the body is left feeling deeply rested.

For such results to occur, most experts of this "relaxation response" suggest a minimum of 20 to 30 minutes to do such an exercise. Obviously, in the case of *savasana*, where much preparation has been done through the poses and pauses done throughout a yoga session, the time to elicit such a response is usually about 10 minutes. Regardless of the method learned, the one suggestion all experts on relaxation make is to **not do these exercises while in bed or wherever you associate with sleep**. The reason is that during and immediately after the exercise you do not want to fall asleep. You may dip in and out a bit during the exercise, but in order for you to receive the replenishing effects from the exercise, you need to get up and move around afterwards. If you do it in the place you are conditioned to think of as your sleep place, you will, by habit, fall asleep. Certainly, the preliminaries to these exercises are great for learning how to get to sleep and rest more effectively. But in order to do the excericse properly, you should find somewhere else that is quiet and comfortable that has few associations with sleep in order to subvert this tendency.

If one has an extremely stressful life or a dis-ease that creates ongoing debility and impairment of your functioning and joy in life, such exercises are invaluable. In such cases, developing a daily routine of relaxation is recommended. And, in the context of the spa environment, to have someone educated and/or qualified to offer skilled relaxation to clients and guests is equally invaluable and a wonderful training that they can then take home and implement into their daily lives.

One may wonder if there are any precautions when doing such exercises. The answer is, not really. However, there can be effects that one would not expect. For example, after experiencing deep relaxation for the first time in years, people may feel a bit disoriented. In this circumstance, it is best to give the client ample time to get up and re-integrate back into the world. Get them something to drink, a piece of fruit, etc. This is not that dissimilar from those who have experienced shirodhara. Another reported effect is that the client says that the day after the relaxation, they felt sore everywhere. This may persist for several days. What is happening here is that the muscles are finally receiving fresh blood and eliminating toxins from the tissue. Thus, like working out for the first time and feeling sore the next day, the person needs to understand that they are detoxifying and that as they persist with daily practice of their relaxation, these symptoms will go away. An Ayurvedic explanation of this is that prana, the life force that is the subtle aspect of Vata, has been unable to enter and encourage *amma* or toxins to leave muscles that are overly contracted due to stress. Where the mind focuses is where the subtle aspect of Vata, prana, will flow. Especially in those forms of relaxation that have you observe regions and muscles in your body, you may be following along a muscle and then come to a place that feels like it is dammed up—usually the places where there is a buildup of tension and toxicity. The suggestion then is usually to spend some time focusing on this area. As stillness, focus, and the breath penetrate into the afflicted area, mobility returns, and the prana helps to hasten the release of what has been built up.

Perhaps the most extreme examples of this you will find will be when you see people that are flaccid everywhere, exhibit little tone in their muscles, and seemingly are hyper-mobile; you can bend and twist them any way you want. And, in fact, that is usually the problem; they have many demands and an inability to set boundaries that would allow them to rest and recuperate. The rest is that the tension lasts for so long that the muscles become starved and as a result, go beyond tense to flaccid. This is an extreme Vata condition where people are adrenally exhausted and depleted in general. In such cases, I have seen the relaxation response elicit massive bruising as the life force floods in and you bring them back through tension into a state of tonification. **NOTE that in spa environments, it is important to watch for such people, for their response to touch therapies is not the norm. With the pain and bruising that may arise, you may need to spend more time explaining their condition, smoothing matters out. It is best to be proactive in such cases. Also, as part of the services that you offer, relaxation therapies are invaluable for two reasons. First, it is most beneficial for them. Secondly, as the pain and bruising comes out, they have no one to point at and say that such and such a therapist was rough with them, etc.** Once they have gone through this phase of their rejuvenation, a re-introduction to soft-contact (not deep tissue) therapies is advised. To replenish the system, the Tibetan Shirodhara as outlined in the treatment rituals is recommended.

Short and Lazy Relaxation Exercises

The tradition of yoga as well as the modern practices of skilled relaxation mentioned earlier can be found in any number of sources on relaxation and biofeedback. Thus I shall not go into these. I strongly encourage everyone to learn one of these methods for daily wellness and rejuvenation.

That said, there are any number of short relaxation methods from the east out of both the yogic and martial arts traditions that help us to dismantle the stress we build up during the day. Though not as therapeutic as the deeper relaxation methods discussed above, they are handy to know if you are feeling the need for a break from stress without the usually culturally chosen toxic excursions into caffeine, nicotine, or alcohol.

One exercise I learned years ago that I feel is worth learning and passing onto clients as it is so easy as to be what I would call, a lazy man's approach. It comes from the Taoist tradition and was past on to me by my dear friend and master shiatsu therapist, Rex Lassalle.

What is most important here is to find a place where you can either sit up well supported or lie down. A chair with arms or a 'lazy boy' is fine as is the ground, a couch, etc. Again, your bed may not be the best place, but this exercise is almost so fool-proof, that you can lie there if you so chose.

1. Place both hands in the mudra that we described earlier (your thumbs touching the base of your fourth fingers and the other fingers wrapped around). Your hands are thus in loose fists with the thumbs wrapped.
2. Lie back and let your head cock forward slightly so your chin almost rests on your chest (if you are lying down, you may need a pillow to do this).
3. Place your right loose fist over the region of your heart.
4. Place the left loose fist over the region just below your navel—again svadhisthana or hara.
5. Close your mouth and allow your tongue to rest behind your top front teeth.
6. Close your eyes.
7. Allow yourself to let go—as if you want to sleep.

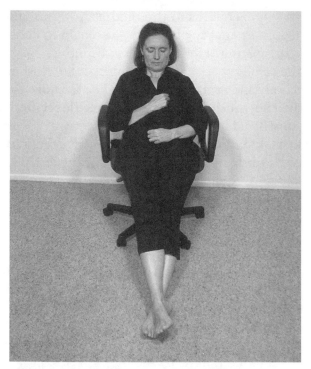

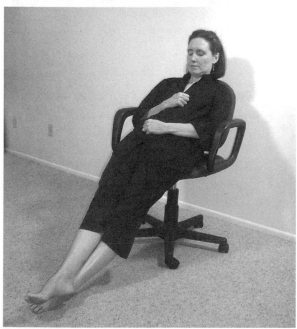

Within ten minutes or less, you will wake up spontaneously, feeling relaxed and refreshed.

The secret of this exercise is in the mudras. Mudras, along with connecting us to a certain quality of energy, also help to keep energy from leaking out or dissipating. Here your hand mudras are being used to settle and, at the same time, charge the area of the heart and the center of our physical body and seat of Vata. (**NOTE: Be sure that you keep your hands in the mudras and positions described during the exercise. If your hands unwind or they fall away from their positions, you *do* risk falling asleep. To avoid this, you can place pillows or props under your arms to guarantee that your hands do not fall away.**) Distraction and anxiety drop away as new energy pours into us as we let go. And when the body feels full up for the time being, we wake up. It is that simple.

Such an exercise can be done at work (unless your afraid of being seen by your boss—although they may want to learn your secret) or at home. If you are a therapist and have a short time between clients, this can help to re-balance you and renew your vigor. I have even used this at rest areas while on the road.

Another exercise that can be done in about the same amount if time is a three-part technique taught to me by Dr. Lobsang Rapgay. Unlike the Lazy relaxation, this exercise is more active in that you do not risk falling asleep. It is also an excellent method of getting yourself to relax before meditating.

1. Begin by sitting on a cushion on the ground. The cushion should be high enough to ensure that your knees are below the level of your navel. Place your hands in your lap, the back of the right hand resting in the palm of the left hand with thumb tips touching. Allow your spine to feel straight, your neck slightly tucked and relaxed. Your tongue rests behind your top front teeth. Your eyes are gently closed. At the same time, you can sit in a chair to do this exercise. If you do so, be sure to have your back slightly away from the back of the chair.

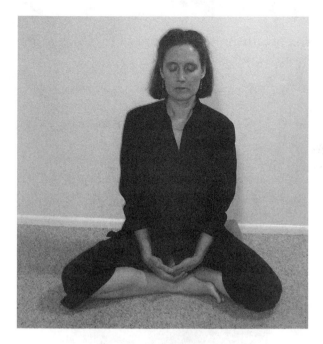

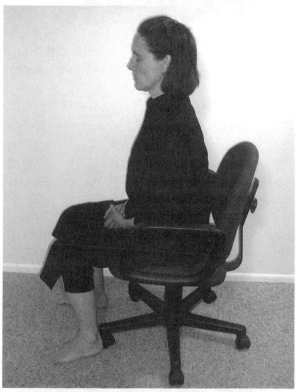

2.

a) As you breathe in to the count of five, slowly draw your shoulders up towards your ears.

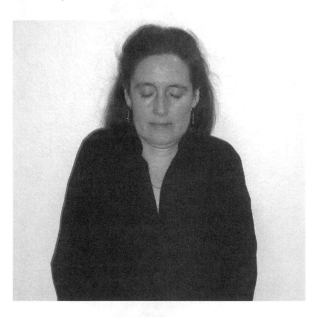

b) Closing your right nostril with your right middle finger, breathe out to the count of five while you lower your shoulders back to their normal position.

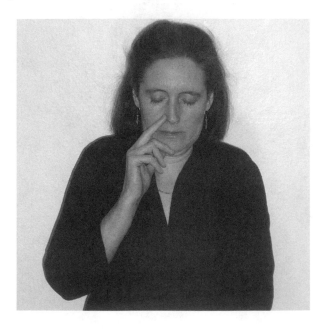

c) Place your right hand back on your left palm, breathe in a repeat steps a and b two more times.

d) Repeat this process three times, blocking the left nostril with the left middle finger.

3.

a) Like in 2a, breathe in to the count of five as you draw your shoulders up towards your ears.

b) As you exhale to the count of five, slowly bend forward so that you bring your forehead lower and lower. If you are on a cushion, try to come down to the ground. Do this without straining.

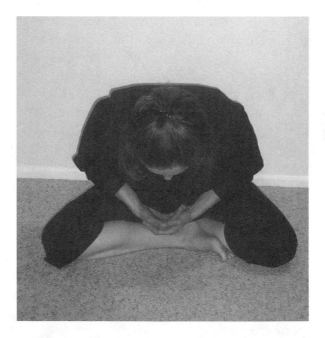

c) As you breathe in to the count of five, slowly bring yourself upright and then breathe out to the count of five.

d) Remaining upright, just breathe in and out to the count of five for one cycle. Then repeat steps a through d two more times.

Tibetan Rejuvenation Exercises

The process of staying in balance and in accordance with our body-mind type constitution requires us to constantly adapt to our circumstances. Thus, although it would be nice to think that our lifestyle would adequately sustain a level of wellbeing that would ensure us aging like fine wine, more often than not, because of our Three Poisons, we don't understand what changes are happening around and, hence, to us, and we get fixated on what has worked in the past and cling to it for dear life, resisting the changes that are necessary. The result is that we find ourselves congested, experience some level of dis-ease, and age more like vinegar. Ayurveda does not judge this as either good or bad. For life just is and we must learn how to embrace whatever it is that we come to experience. That is why, as part of bringing us back and into balance, Ayurveda includes detoxification and rejuvenation processes. As you have learned throughout this book, Ayurveda is very serious about detoxification and rejuvenation. Such methods as pancha karma can be quite extreme with respect to the demands it places on one's time and lifestyle. Yet the rewards often outweigh the inconvenience. At the same time, there are practices one can engage in that may yield slow but increasing benefit if practiced regularly and over time. From the Tibetan Ayurvedic tradition, there is a series of five exercises that slow the aging process and, when coupled with some of the body-mind type lifestyle recommendations suggested at the *first level* of Tibetan Ayurveda, such as proper nutrition, can actually help to reverse the aging process. In both the first and second editions of my book, *Tibetan Ayurveda*, I call these Tibetan Rejuvenation Exercises. A simple form of yoga that was taught in Tibetan monasteries and retreats, serious meditators, monks and nuns, performed them, not because they wanted to look young and beautiful, but because they helped them maintain a suppleness in mind and body that would allow them to engage in their spiritual practices with greater focus and clarity for as long as they were alive.

If practiced in the morning, Tibetan Rejuvenation Exercises will get the body and mind up and ready to face the day. If done at the end of the day, even before bedtime, they help to relax one and smooth out the stresses and strains of the day. They actually improve the quality of your sleep. If done before meditation or prayer, they will facilitate a deepening of your experience.

These exercises are very easy and can be integrated into any spa exercise program. As they are based on very standard yoga postures, they are also an excellent introduction for those who may wish to sample what yoga can do for them. And it is my experience as a yoga instructor that I have never seen series of yogasanas as succinctly deliver as many benefits. What is also nice is that each of the exercises can be modified to suit older and infirmed guests and still create wonderful results.

Exercise #1

We start with spinning, like the whirling Dervish tradition of Sufism. In this context, the spinning activates the chakra/endocrine systems. It also activates our vestibular system, engaging our brain and nervous systems. The physical stimulation and energy activated by the spinning makes all of the other exercises of this series beneficial.

It is natural for a person to feel some level of dizziness from doing the spinning. That is the sign of a healthy vestibular system. Thus, do not be alarmed. Also, as with all of these exercises, start slow. Begin with 7 spins and gradually work up to 21. For those who feel too dizzy or nauseous, before starting to spin, focus on a point in front of you. Make it so that as you complete each spin, your eyes return to the same point. This is what ballerinas and other performers who are required to spin do if need be.

Stand straight and allow your arms to be outstretched with fingers extended, palms downward. Keep your arms at shoulder height; not above, not below. Rest your tongue on the roof of your mouth, just behind your teeth. At a physical level, this allows for a freer flow of cerebro-spinal fluid to move along your spine. In turn, at a more subtle level, it activates a *marma* or vital energy point, which in Sanskrit is called the Brahma-Randra, the crown point of the skull. This allows more psychic and spiritual energy to enter the body. And where the tongue is touching is an important Taoist point that connects the Brain Governor and Conception Vessel, the two primary meridians of the body, creating a powerful flow throughout the body. **You will keep this tongue position for all of the exercises**.

Spin in a clockwise direction. This means that your right arm drops back as your left arm moves forward. Spin at a comfortable rate.

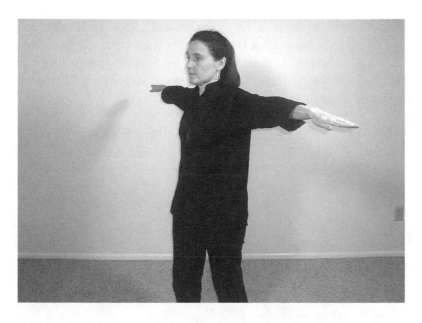

At the end of the number of spins, place your hands on your hips. Breathe in through your nose and out through your mouth 2 to 3 times. Then lie down on the floor (preferably a carpet or cushioned surface or mat) with your arms to your sides, palms down. The palm-down position of the hands seems to lessen the dizzy feeling. Allow your breath to return to a normal, even pace. Observe your body sensations as you rest. As in the performance of any yoga program the rest between exercises is important.

Exercise #2

Lying on your back with your arms to your sides and the palms downward, inhale while simultaneously bringing your head off of the ground so that your chin comes towards your chest and raising your straight legs so that they come perpendicular to the ground. A little beyond perpendicular is fine, but try to keep the legs as straight as possible. Then exhale and lower your head and legs to the ground, again simultaneously. Allow all of your muscles to relax for a moment, then repeat the exercise. Work up to 21 repetitions.

As mentioned earlier, there are modifications you can make to this if you have injuries or weak abdominal muscles. If there are low back problems, tuck your hands, palms down, under the small of your spine. If there is still too much strain, bend the knees to the degree that helps. Over time, through repetition, you may find that your back and abdominal muscles will become strong enough to perform this exercise with straight legs. **At the same time, the tradition of yoga teaches that you should visualize in your mind's eye that you are performing the exercise perfectly. Body follows mind, thus you may find that your back and abdomen become stronger to perform this or any of the other exercises without modifications.** *This advice is applicable to all forms of exercise.*

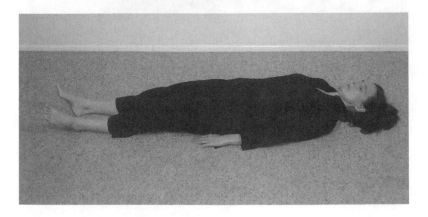

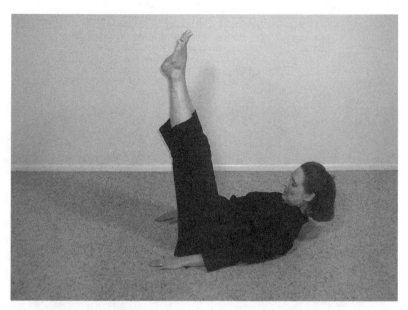

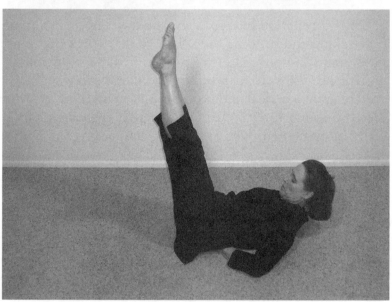

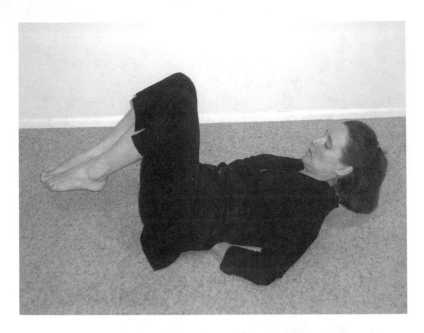

All of the Rejuvenation Exercises that follow the initial spinning emphasize stretching and bending the spine. Yoga teaches that in order to stay youthful and to rejuvenate, we need to maintain flexibility in the spine. In Exercise #2, you are working the sacral and occipital pumps while stretching the cervical and lumbar spine. This allows for more efficient cerebro-spinal fluid movement through the entire spine. This benefits the entire nervous system and encourages proper circulation in all internal organs.

At the completion of however many repetitions that you do, lie quietly, allowing your breath to return to normal, observing your body sensations.

Exercise #3

Position yourself now so that you are in a kneeling position, your knees about one fist distance apart and your toes curled up. Your torso is straight and in line with your upper legs. Allow your hands to clutch just below the buttocks on the back of the thighs, or on the buttocks themselves. Rest your chin on your chest.

As you inhale, lift and draw your head back as far as it will go while you lift your chest and throw open your shoulders so that your upper spine is arched. Then, as you exhale, return the chest and shoulders to a more natural position and allow your chin to once again rest on your chest. Repeat this as many times as you feel comfortable, up to 21. Once you are finished, sit back on your legs or any way in which you feel comfortable. Close your eyes, settle your breath, and observe body sensations.

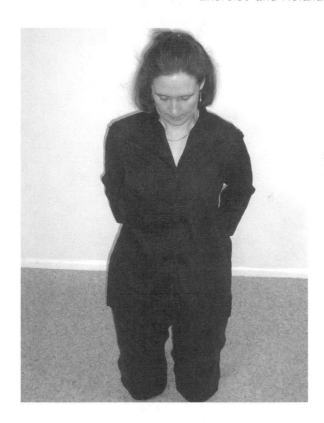

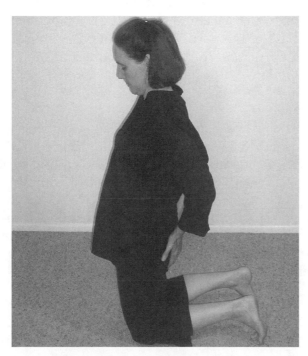

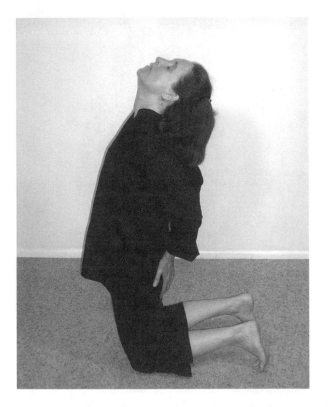

This activates the thyroid, parathyroid, and thymus, the energy vortices/chakras of the neck and chest. It also stimulates the brachial plexus at the base of the neck, strengthening the arms and shoulders, and increasing circulation to the lungs, heart, and the chest region in general.

Exercise #4

Sit so that your legs are before you and outstretched, with your feet about twelve inches to a shoulder width apart. Place your arms to your sides so that your hands are palms down on the ground beside your buttocks, your fingers pointing towards your feet (if your arms are shorter or longer, so they don't feel comfortable directly beside your torso, you may need to adjust your arms so that your hands are resting slightly behind or in front of the line of your torso. As you do the entire exercise, experiment to see where they seem best positioned). Your chin is, once again, touching the top of your sternum, as in Exercise #3.

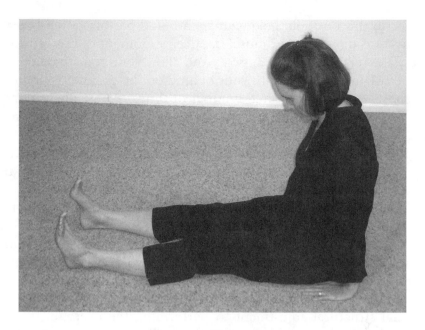

You will now perform what is basically the Table Pose in yoga. As you inhale, lift your buttocks off of the ground and allow your head to drop back. The final position of this movement should be where your legs are bent at a right angle at the knees with your feet on the ground, your abdomen and chest parallel to the ground, your arms straight, and your head tilted back so that you are looking at what is behind you upside down.

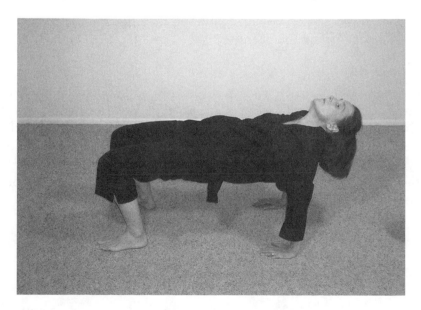

Once in this position, hold your breath and perform a full-body isometric—tensing all of your muscles. After a moment of this tensing, as you exhale, relax all of your muscles and allow your body to come down into the original posture, with your behind on the ground, your chin on your chest. Repeat the desired number of times, eventually working up to 21. Then sit comfortably with your eyes closed, observing body sensations, allowing your breath to return to normal.

This exercise tonifies the abdominal muscles and organs and energizes the region of the solar plexus. Prana is driven deep into the body as a result of isometric tensing.

As this is a strenuous exercise, remember to maintain regular and balanced breathing. Slow down or pause if you become winded. Two other difficulties that people report in doing this exercise are pains in the shoulders and an inability to bring the torso to the parallel position. Regarding the first, unless you have a rotator cuff or other specific shoulder or upper arm complaint, the pain experienced during or after is a beneficial structural adjustment to performing the exercise. If such a pain persists for longer than a week, it is advisable to consult a health professional (massage or physical therapist). Then again, some people with specific shoulder complaints find that a lower number of repetitions of this exercise promotes faster healing. As regards the second difficulty, where one cannot bring oneself up for the torso and legs to be parallel with the ground, this often arises from weak abdominal and lower back muscles. Try to lift yourself up to the best of your ability. And, as mention earlier, visualize yourself moving into the perfect position while performing the exercise.

Exercise #5

This exercise is akin to Upward and Downward Facing Dog, only more dynamic. Place yourself into a push-up type position with both your hands and feet spread about two feet apart. Your toes are be curled (not pointed back) and your back is sagged and you are slightly arched so that you are actually looking forward. You are actually holding your body off the ground with your hands and toes. Not even your knees or any other part of your hips or legs should touch the ground.

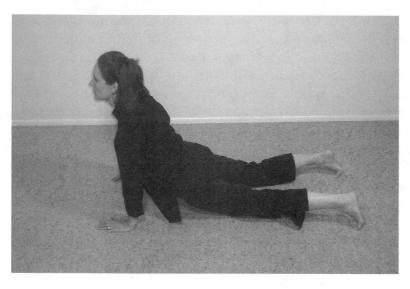

As you inhale, drop your head and shoulders towards the ground and raise your behind so that you are looking between your own legs. Your behind should be higher than any other part of your body. As you exhale, reverse this flow so that you lower yourself down into the original position. Repeat this for a number of times that feels comfortable, working up to 21. At the completion of this exercise, stand erect with your hands on your hips, breathing in through the nose and out through the mouth a few times until your breath returns to normal. Allow your entire body to relax.

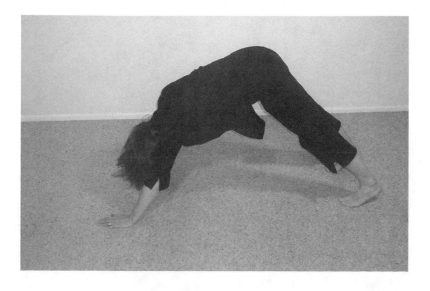

The arching of the entire spine in this exercise rejuvenates the nerves in the spine and improves the functioning of the immune system. Both the arms and legs are also strengthened.

This can be a difficult posture, especially for those who either have weak abdominal muscles or suffer from low back complaints. Of course, this exercise will help such conditions, but it may be necessary to initially modify the exercise to prevent more strain or injury. The following modifications I have found to be useful and still provide positive results. And remember to always visualize doing it perfect anyway.

The first posture is where you *do* allow your knees to rest on the ground. Arch forward as best you can, at least trying to look before you. In what would be the Downward Facing Dog posture where your behind would be up, here, as you inhale, draw yourself back onto your haunches, providing a good stretch to the entire spine and hips. Then, as you exhale, come off your haunches and return to the original modified position.

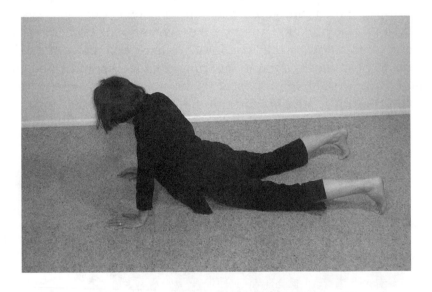

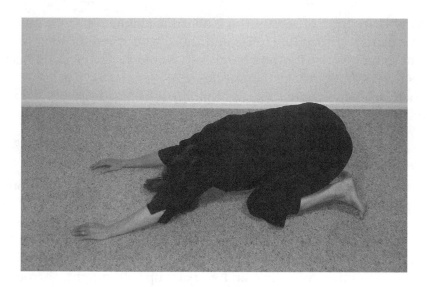

These five are the foundation of Tibetan Rejuvenation Exercises. They are excellent for all Ayurvedic body-mind constitutions. For such a short and simple series, the benefits of their practice are very rewarding, on the physical, psychological, and spiritual levels. Once one becomes proficient in these five, there is an additional, more esoteric practice that one can learn about by referring to *Tibetan Ayurveda*. But even without adding this component, these five will promote greater mental and physical flexibility and openness and you will experience a state of being that is radiant and joyful; a reflection of true rejuvenation. This is the promise of Ayurveda.

Tai Wu

The tradition of Tibetan Tai Ch'i was taught at the Shaolin monastery in China. Kept separate from its Chinese counterpart, students were hand selected to learn this special art. It is said that this form of Tai Chi came from the lineages of the Dalai Lamas. I had the good fortune to train with a man who spent thirteen of his summers at Shaolin before the Japanese invasion during World War II, when Shaolin was overrun. My teacher's name was Liu Siong. He and his wife, Marilyn, ran a school called the Garuda School of Tibetan Tai Chi and Chuan Fa in Albuquerque, New Mexico. Liu Siong passed away several years ago, but his wife, Marilyn continues to teach. What she offers is rare and in danger of passing into the mists of history. I am indebted to both her and Master Liu and offer these exercises in their honor.

Tai Wu is a form of exercise that helps to keep flexibility in the upper and lower body. It is done in preparation for doing the slower, more contemplative form of Tibetan Tai Ch'i. At the same time, it is an excellent series to learn for therapists and those who stand for long periods of time and/or work with their hands—as would be the obvious case for aestheticians and massage therapists.

There are six separate exercises that are a part of Tai Wu. One is devoted to the legs and pelvic girdle, two for the fingers and hands, two for the wrists, and two for the arms and shoulder girdle.

Exercise #1

Either stand behind and hold onto the back of a chair, or hold onto a railing, table, or other surface that keeps you standing upright. With your feet pointing forward, breathe in and laterally lift your entire right leg out to the right side, with the foot parallel to the ground, then, as you exhale, swing the straightened leg in front of you to the left so that your toes are now pointing upwards. Inhale and go back up to the right, then exhale and swing to the left. Do this 25 times. Repeat for the left leg.

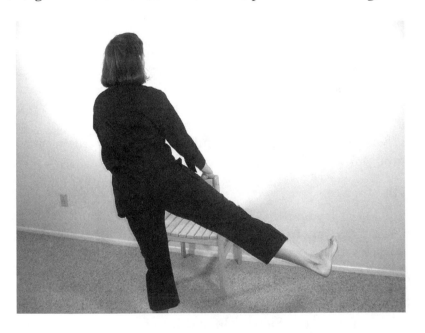

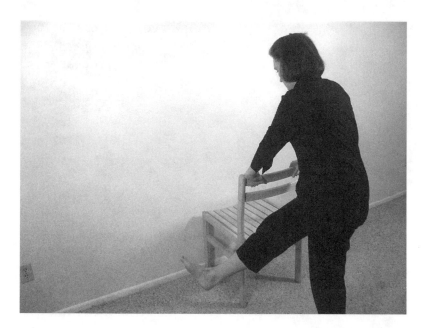

Exercise #2

There are usually variations on how you stand for the finger and wrist exercises. However, for simplicity, we shall stick to one stance only. Stand in what is known as the 'horse riding' position. Your knees are slightly bent, your back straight. Let your tongue rest behind your top front teeth and breathe naturally in and out through your nose. Rest your arms to your sides, but lift your forearms so that they are parallel to the floor and your palms are facing upwards. Starting with your little finger, close your fingers into a fist, one finger at a time until your thumb, which you wrap over the other fingers, then immediately open them up in the opposite order, finishing with your little finger. Do this as rapidly as you can, closing to a fist, then opening fully so that the palm feels stretched and the fingers are straight. Do this 35 to 50 times. While you do this, you may feel some burning in your fingers or wrists. To help with this, imagine that as you breathe out, you are sending your energy out through your fingertips.

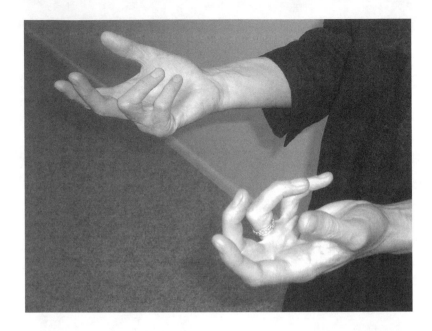

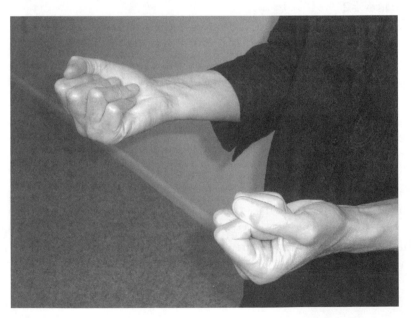

Exercise #3

While in the same stance, keep your arms to your side, but turn your forearms over so that your palms are now facing downwards. You will now flick your fingers, which will help to prevent the normal curving of the fingers that happens with age. Place your thumb on the nail bed of the little finger. Imagine that there is something on your little fingernail that you want to get flicked off. Placing pressure against your thumb, snap your finger so that it straightens. Then go to the fourth finger then repeat all the way through to the index finger, each finger snapping to straight, then go back to the little finger. Repeat this motion 35 to 50 times.

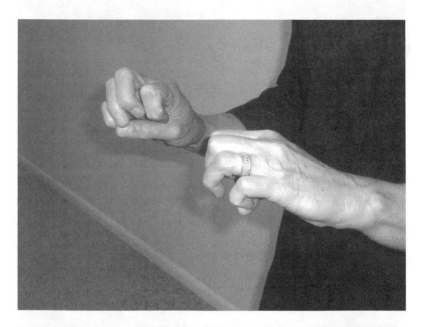

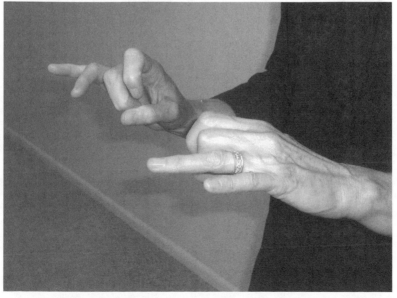

Exercise #4

With your stance, arms, and hands in the same position as #3, flap your wrists up and down vigorously, but not so intensely as to cause discomfort. Do this 35 to 50 times.

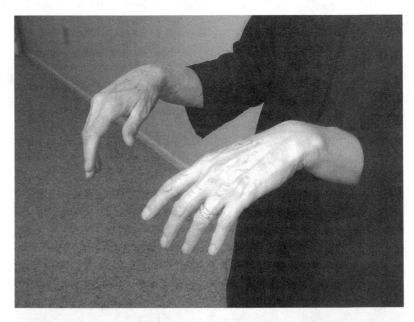

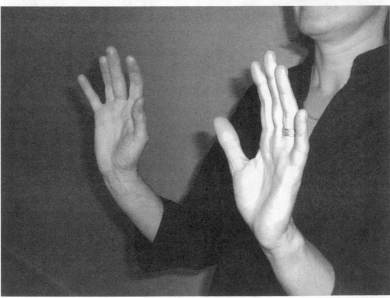

Exercise #5

In the same stance, rotate your forearms so that your palms are facing each other. Now flap your wrists towards and away from each other. Do this 35 to 50 times.

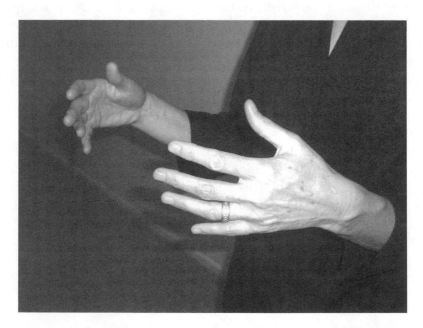

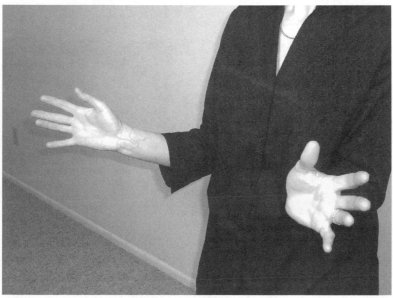

Strengthening and getting energy flowing through the wrists is extremely important for overall wellness. Essentially, the polarity of the meridians running through the arms changes at the wrists, which is why it is such a complex joint. Exercises #4 and #5 help to improve the flow of energy through the wrists and are great preventive exercises against carpel tunnel syndrome, a common repetitive motion injury for aestheticians and massage therapists. Anyone who uses their hands in a similar way as these two professions will find great benefit in this exercise.

Although Tai Wu does not include a similar exercise for the ankles, one will be shown following the Tai Wu exercises.

Exercise #6

This exercise is for the shoulder girdle. It has three phases to it. Stand so that your heels are together and your feet are fanned out at about a 45-degree angle. Stretch your arms out to the sides and allow the wrists to relax so that the fingers kind of droop. Move your thumbs so that they dangle down between the third and fourth fingers.

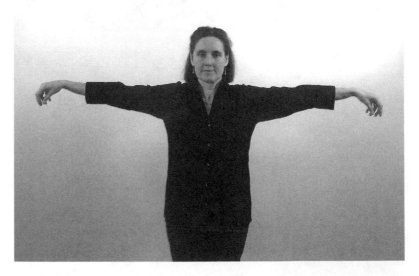

a)   In a simultaneous motion, inhale, turn your head to the right, turn your palm so that it is facing upwards, and bend your elbow so that you are bringing your right hand towards your face. As you exhale, allow the right hand to pass in front of your right shoulder and swing back to its original position.

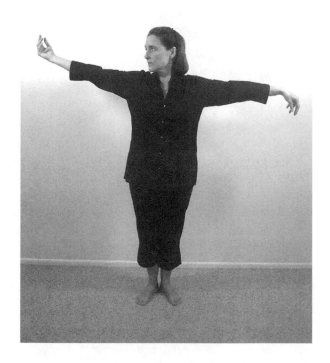

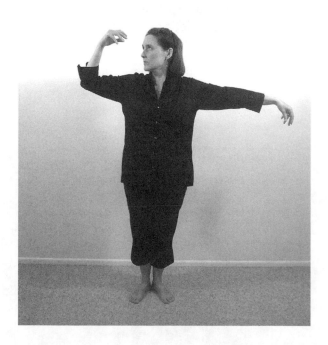

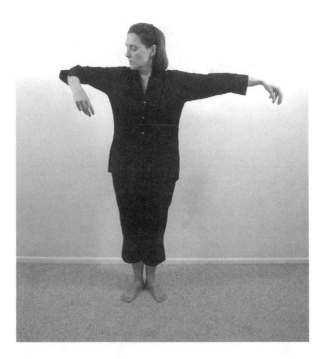

b) Repeat this for the left arm.

c) Looking forward, inhale and bring both arms towards you at the same time, and as you exhale, pass them in front of your shoulders, down, then out to the sides again.

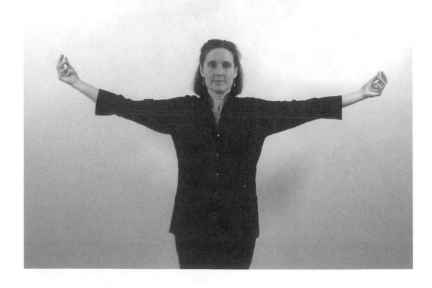

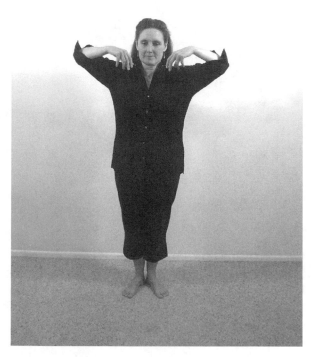

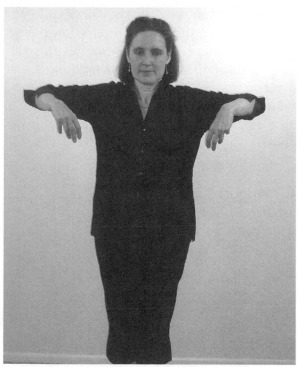

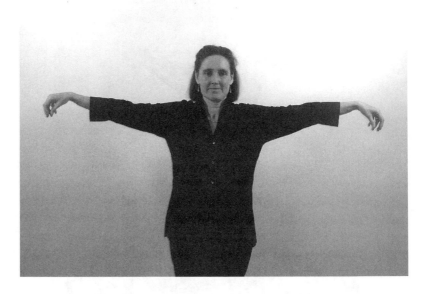

d) Do this cycle of a, b, and c 7 to 10 times. If you cannot do 7, start with a lower number and work up to a larger number of repetitions. Try to work up to 15.

NOTE that during this exercise your shoulders can get tired and you may feel the urge to lower or drop your arms below being parallel to the ground. This is actually more tiring. To counter this tendency and to override some of the discomfort, imagine that there are strings running from your wrists that are tied to the walls on either side of you, supporting your arms. You can also imagine that your arms are like wings. You rotate one wing in and out, then the other, then both together, feeling a sense of openness and expansion as you exhale and fully stretch out both arms.

Exercise #7

Keeping your stance as in #6, your arms are out to the sides, but this time, draw your fingers so that they are pointing upwards with your palms facing away from you.

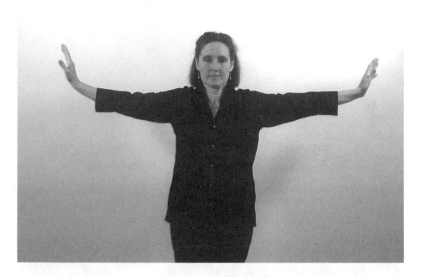

a) Breathe in and out naturally for one cycle.

b) Breathe in, then breathe out vigorously, like huffing your breath out and as you do, keeping your hips straight and looking forward, rotate your upper torso and shoulder girdle so that your right straight arm moves slightly behind and your left straight arm rotates slightly forward.

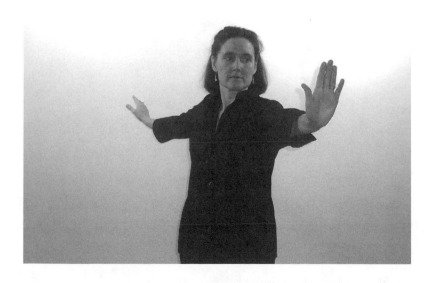

c) Inhale and bring your arms back to their original position.

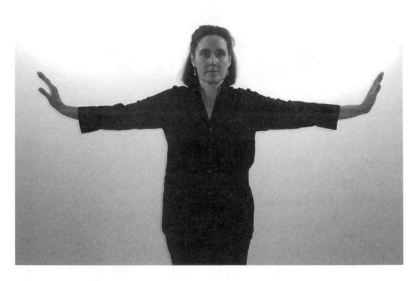

d) Inhale and then exhale out vigorously in a huff and now drop your left arm back with your right arm moving forward.

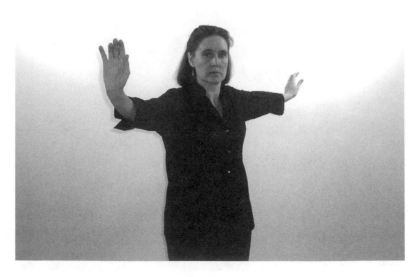

e) Repeat c and then go on to b.

f) Do a cycle of both arms like this for 5 times to start with, gradually working up to 15.

Again, this exercise can be strenuous, but lowering your shoulders will only make it feel worse. Imagine that you have wings when doing this. Alternatively, feel that there is a string from the center of your palms that is connected to a real or imaginary wall on either side, providing support.

Exercises #6 and #7 will help with rotator cuff problems, improve the quality of energy that moves through your arms, and improve posture.

Ankle Excercises

As mentioned earlier, energy changes its polarity at the wrists and ankles. You have learned the Tai Wu exercise for the wrists. And of course, there are a number of yoga poses that work on the flexibility of the ankles. Here is a variation that is simple to do and can be done during the day to ease back tension and improve circulation into your knees and feet.

Sitting on your haunches with your feet underneath you and your toes pointed back in what is known is known as *seiza* in Japanese, inhale and as you do, lift your behind off the backs of your legs and bend the feet so that the toes are curled. Exhale and sit back on your calves, putting some pressure on your arched feet. Then, inhale and come off the back of your legs, straighten your toes, and as you exhale go back to the seiza position. Repeat this 25 times.

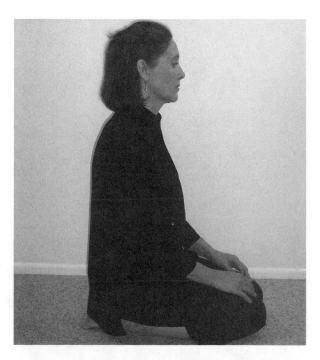

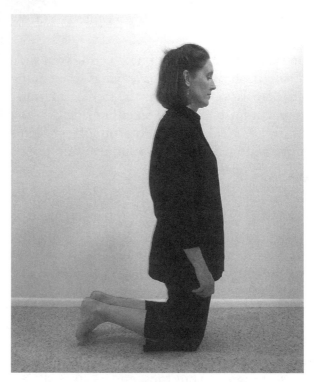

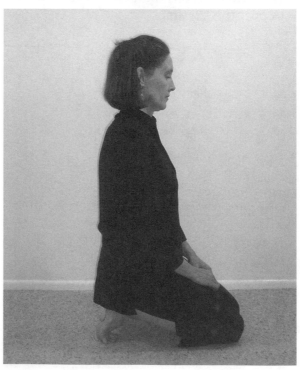

CHAPTER 13

Meditating

*A*s should be clear in what we have presented so far, Ayurveda is more than just a series of treatments. It is a paradigm based on a philosophy of the unity of all things. To experience this unity and live in the light of love and compassion that this unity reflects is the goal of Ayurveda. Ayurveda wants each of us to be happy, healthy, and inspired.

When we wrote earlier of the Four Levels of Tibetan Ayurveda, we discussed how diet and exercise were crucial aspects of the first level and massage and other body therapies were important parts of the second level. These aspects have been what we have focused on for the greater portion of this book.

Of course, it is always nice to find someone who can give us a great massage, tell us what is best for us to eat, and what exercise regimen will work well for our body-mind type. But all too often, we put off going to the spa or getting a massage, can't find the time or inclination to exercise, and slide into comfort foods and convenient eating rather than making our daily nutrition a priority. We see the benefits of all of these things, even know them to some extent. But habits that create tension and dis-ease can be so hard to break. In the Buddhist tradition, habits—especially unhelpful ones—are caused by what are known as the Three Poisons of ignorance, attachment, and aggression. Simply put, we are confused and do not understand the world around us and what is ultimately useful for us. As a result, we get distracted, then fixated by what attracts us based on our desires rooted in that confusion, and get moody and irritated with anyone that points out to us that maybe what we are doing isn't the best thing after all. We act from these Three Poisons in every aspect of our life; from not seeing the correlation between our back pain and the six espressos we have each day, getting caught in confusing and problematic relationships again and again, and so on. This is where meditation comes in.

Of course, meditation can be defined and looked at in religious terms. But here we want to concentrate on the pragmatic benefits of including meditation in our life. Here we are focusing on the broadest notion of what is spiritual; that we are—in the words of Teilhard de Chardin—"spiritual beings having a human experience."

If we can sit quiet and relaxed and free ourselves from distraction, clarity and calm will naturally arise. With this sense of space, we are able to look more closely at ourselves and what is around us. We can then see how distraction, confusion, and our moodiness often fuel poor choices in daily habits and are the real culprits in the tangled webs that we weave. As we become accustomed to just being—here and now—our identification with our turmoil and confusion is disrupted. We can then become more active in making choices that are not just knee-jerk reactions. We also come to understand how easy it is to get sidetracked, lured by one emotion or another. Thus, our compassion for others grows naturally as we come to understand how easy it is for others, too, to be trapped in realities that they may not even want but don't know how to get out of.

Being more specific, as a therapist interested in benefiting your client with whatever you offer them, having a daily meditation practice will keep you centered, more in tune with the energetics of your client, and will allow you to be more creative and flexible with your treatment delivery. **Especially in treatments that deal with subtle body energies, acupressure points, marma points and chakras, a more meditative state of mind is a necessity to be effective.** We also feel that beginning a spa staff meeting with even a short meditation is a great way to help people stay focused and more open with each other. There are endless numbers of studies that confirm the benefits of meditation for team building and problem solving. And then there are your clients, who would like help in learning how to decompress from the pace of their lives and stick with the positive lifestyle suggestions you and others may offer them. It is not surprising, therefore, to see classes in relaxation, meditation, and meditative exercises on spa menus or included in destination spa services. Especially for the client that is interested in Ayurveda and similar energetically-based spa experiences, it behooves therapists to learn to teach or suggest such classes.

The practices offered here are meditative exercises based on Buddhist tradition or are, in themselves, traditional meditations. All of them are suitable for everyone, regardless of faith or orientation.

How to Begin and Stick with a Meditation Practice

When we add something new to our life, such as finding time to meditate on top of all the other things we need or would like to do, other parts of our life get shoved around. Most of us already feel pressed for time. Without some kind of tangible reward, we may place meditation as something lower down on the list of daily priorities. But this is not understanding meditation. And it turns an activity that yields the potential of creating more joy and ease in doing everything else seem one more burden. This is no way to approach meditation.

In his "Instructions on Meditation", the great Tibetan master, Dudjom Rinpoche, wrote

> Allow yourself to relax and feel some spaciousness, letting
> mind settle naturally. Your body should be still, speech
> silent and breathing as it is, freely flowing. Here there is a
> sense of letting go, unfolding, letting be.
> What does this state of relaxation feel like? You should
> be like someone after a really hard day's work, exhausted
> and peacefully satisfied, mind content to rest. Something
> settles at the gut level, and feeling it resting in your gut, you
> begin to experience a lightness. It is as if you're melting.
> (Dudjom Rinpoche, care of Vajrayana Foundation, Hawaii)

Settle down to meditation in this way. It is a time to feel nourished, to feel replenished. Enjoy it! If it becomes stiff, habitual, and an enforced discipline, meditation will provide you little benefit and you'll probably start finding a million and one excuses not to do it. For sure, in the beginning, there will be some amount of awkwardness. To get over these speed bumps, a little serious push is necessary.

Start with small increments of time and work up to a time frame that feels comfortable and doesn't make you feel like you are being squeezed in other aspects of your life. Over time, as meditating becomes a part of your daily life, it will feel more and more natural and your sense of joy and commitment to the process will grow. Then, if there is an opportunity to do more- say, on a weekend—or a retreat, go for it!

Clarifying Intentions

It is always good to first ponder why you want to meditate. To overcome stress, fine. To become healthier and be more focused on developing a more positive lifestyle, great. But even better, consider that when you are less stressed, when your mind is not crowded with the Three Poisons running the show, you are actually a nicer person and can be a better spouse, parent, worker, and citizen. Altruism, thinking of others when you meditate, actually strengthens and deepens the benefits of meditation. In that way, taking some time to yourself is not being selfish. It is an act of kindness, both to yourself and others. With such an attitude, you will notice that when you come away from your meditation time, you can listen and communicate more easily with everyone around you. And a deeper calm will begin to enrich your life.

Breathing Exercise to Transform the Three Poisons

This exercise was taught to me by Dr. Lobsang Rapgay, a Tibetan doctor and former monk who is now a well established clinical psychologist in California. The purpose behind this exercise is to help us loosen the grip of the Three Poisons on our consciousness. This is done through focusing on the movement of breath and working with our subtle energy body. It is a great exercise to begin your day with. It is also a simple technique to share with clients as well as a great technique to do together with co-workers before a meeting.

Many in the west are familiar with the term *chakras* or energy vortices that are mentioned in these eastern traditions. Besides those who study oriental medicine, spirituality, and philosophy, mention of them happens frequently in yoga classes everywhere. Along with these chakras are the channels that they are made up of; two that run from about 3 finger-widths from below the navel and finish at the edge of each nostril and a central or main spiritual channel (Shushumna) that begins in the same area below the navel and goes up to the crown of the head, then drops down around the middle of the forehead, turning inward towards the center of the brain. In theory and practice, the two side channels wrap around the central channel and it is where they wrap and constrict around that central channel that you find the chakras. Meditations are done to focus on the various chakras, loosen the constriction of the two side channels and allow for the movement of spiritual energy to ascend through the central channel. According to Tibetan tradition, the "opening" of the chakras can only be done through the strong blessing of a master or through the individual doing intense and effective meditation practice. Contrary to popular belief, no one else, like a massage therapist or healer placing special stones or toning over your chakras, can open them for you. However, both in Indian and Tibetan Ayurveda, there are forms of bodywork that can awaken a person's sensitivity to the chakras. A form of Tibetan Chakra Massage actually follows in accordance with the exercise that is described below, using pressure and stones associated with each chakra.

The visualization for this particular exercise does not have the side channels wrapping around the main channel. For this exercise, the right smaller channel should be viewed as transparent RED in color and is representative of the female (wisdom) energy. It is hollow and its thickness is about that of your little finger. It starts three finger widths below the navel and moves at a distance of one "tsun" (about ½ an inch) from the right side of the spine (neither to the front or back, but deep within). It passes through the neck, over the brain, but underneath the skull bones, drops down from the right side of the central fontanel, ending at the outside tip of the right nostril. To the left, also hollow and of a similar thickness is a transparent WHITE channel, representative of male energy (skillful means) which mirrors the RED channel pathway on the left side. The Central or 'spiritual' channel is visualized as a straight tube that is two little finger widths in diameter. We see this channel as a transparent DEEP BLUE tube that starts 4 finger widths below the navel and goes up through the body anteriorly to the spine. It goes through the neck and head to the central fontanel point where it makes a tight turn downwards to the area of the "third eye" and hooks inwards (or posteriorly) towards the pineal gland.

The Practice:

You can sit cross legged to do this exercise or be in a chair, so long as your spine is upright and your back is not pressing against the back of the chair. You do not want your lungs or diaphragm to feel constricted in any way. This means that if you are sitting cross-legged on the ground, you should sit up on a cushion so that your knees are below the level of your navel.

1. To cleanse the right RED tube, visualize that the beginning of the WHITE channel or tube is slightly smaller and inserts into the beginning of the RED channel below the navel (the RED tube opening is seen as larger and capable of accepting the smaller WHITE tube end).

2. With your right thumb resting at the base of your fourth finger, wrap your other fingers around the thumb, with the exception of

your index finger. Have this finger extended. Block your right nostril with your right index finger and inhale through your left open nostril. Imagine that the air you are breathing in through your left nostril is clean and fresh and that it is being carried down through the WHITE channel to where the WHITE channel is inserted into the RED channel below the navel.

3. At the point where you are visualizing that the clean, fresh air is at the beginning of the RED channel just below the navel, release the right nostril and with your left hand in a similar arrangement as your right one, with your left index finger, block the left nostril. As you exhale, visualize that the clean, fresh air is pushing out what is unclean, contaminated, and polluted out of the right RED channel. Especially see that as you breathe out you are releasing the defilement or poison of ATTACHMENT or clinging. These negativities are seen as smoke or soot leaving the right nostril.

4. Repeat this two more times. After this, breathe through both nostrils and visualize the right, RED, channel as being luminous and purified of all negativities. Breathe in and out naturally three times, seeing this right channel as radiant as a ruby.

5. Now repeat a through d for the cleansing of the WHITE channel. See the RED channel end fitting inside the end of the WHITE tube end. Start with blocking the left nostril. As the clean air goes from the RED channel and then into the WHITE channel, imagine that you are breathing out the impurities and the defilement of AGGRESSION, again in the forms of smoke and soot. Do this three times and then breathe in and out normally three times, seeing the WHITE channel now as luminous and pure, like a diamond.

6. Now visualize Shushumna, the Central, spiritual channel. It is BLUE and the thickness of 2 small finger widths. Visualize that both the lower ends of the WHITE and RED channels are inserted into the base of the Central Channel. Once you see this in your mind's eye, place your hands in your lap. Allow the back of the right hand to rest in the palm of the upturned left hand. The thumbs then touch to form a triangle. With your hands in this configuration, place them around your navel so that they form a triangle around your navel.

7. Breathe in through both nostrils so that the pure, fresh air goes up through the nostrils, down through to the openings of the RED and WHITE channels fitted into the bottom entrance to the Central Channel.

8. As you exhale, feel this pure air moving up and cleansing the Central Channel and with it the defilement of IGNORANCE. Visualize that IGNORANCE and all of the impurities are pouring out of the region of your third eye, like smoke.

9. Repeat this two more times. Then lower the hands into the lap and breath normally three times, experiencing the Central Channel as luminously blue, supple, and purified. It is radiant like a deep blue sapphire.

Energetically, this simple visualization practice acts like a more advanced practice of counting to ten when emotions are running high.

Three Sounds and Three Lights Meditation

The following meditation is a combination of a relaxation exercise as taught to us by Dr. Lobsang Rapgay and the traditional Three Light Meditation as taught by Danish Buddhist Lama Ole Nydahl. Combined, they form a very wonderful relaxing and deep meditation that is wonderful to do on ones own or in a group.

Step One:

Let us first begin by focusing on posture. Sit in a comfortable manner. If it feels comfortable or natural to sit cross-legged on the ground, sit so that you maintain the natural curve of your lower back. You may need to sit on a few cushions to achieve this. Generally, it is best for your behind to be somewhere between four to six inches off the ground with your knees below the level of your navel. If you know various yogic or meditative sitting poses, feel free to choose one of those. Allow your hands to rest, palms down, on or just above your knees. You can also try a simple meditation *mudra*. Place your thumbs at the base of your fourth fingers and wrap the other fingers over the thumbs. This is the hand posture is said to help us to connect with our compassionate heart.

If you need to sit on a chair, sit with your back away from the back of the chair so that your chest can expand fully. Your feet are placed squarely and firmly on the ground, about shoulder width apart.

Step Two:

Allow your neck to relax with your chin slightly tucked and your throat soft. You should not feel as if your head is craned back or tilted forward. Moisten your lips with your tongue and then place your tongue just on the top palate behind your top teeth. If you are sitting on the ground, your eyes should have a slightly downward gaze, resting approximately eighteen inches to two feet in front of you. If you are on a chair, aim your gaze between your knees, letting it go a bit farther. In either case, it is generally considered best to have your eyes just slightly open. This helps to keep you grounded, oriented in the space that you are in, and relaxed. If you find the room or space too distracting, then close your eyes. However, if what you get when you close your eyes is a great movie, keep your eyes partially open as originally instructed.

Step Three:

Take a deep breath in, draw up your pelvic muscles, tense your buttocks and abdomen, straighten your arms so that your palms or hands are pushing down on your knees, and lift your spine. Hold the tension for a moment, then slowly exhale and as you do so, let all the tension leave with the breath out. You want to feel really settled onto your cushion or seat. Allow your diaphragm to become soft and your breath natural as it rises and sinks from deep within.

Step Four:

We first start with sound. The sounds we are going to focus on are what in Tibetan are called "seed syllables". These sounds or syllables have no particular meaning per se, but are the root sounds of many mantras and help to open what are called the Three Gates of body, speech, and mind. These sounds are:

OM   AH   HUNG

OM is one of the most universal sounds. It is actually a combination of the sounds AH+OO+MM, but pronounced so that it almost sounds "home" without the letter 'h'. AH sounds like you would expect. HUNG is more like HOONG. This is the Tibetan pronunciation. In traditional Sanskrit it is HUM or HOOM. You can use whichever you prefer.

First focus on saying these sounds mentally to yourself coordinated with your breathing. You are not trying to do yogic breathing or regulate your breath in any way here. All you are doing is naturally breathing and out, using the syllables with the rhythm of the breath. To get a full and natural breath, as you breath in, feel the air passing in through the nostrils and moving down along through your abdomen to a point about three finger widths (about one-and-a-half inches) below your navel. As you breathe out, the abdomen contracts slightly as the air moves upwards and passes out of the nostrils. In combination with the sound, the purpose of this is to help you to relax at all levels of your being: body, speech, and mind.

a) As you breathe in, hear in your mind the sound **OM**.

b) Hold your breath just briefly and in that breathing cycle pause, hear in your mind the sound **AH.**

c) Then, as you naturally exhale, hear in your mind the sound HUNG.

d) Repeat a through c a total of 5 times.

Step Four:

We now go to saying the sounds out loud, but coordinating it with our breathing and specific colored lights. The colors of the lights are

WHITE   RED   BLUE

a) Imagine in your mind's eye that just above the level of the horizon of a beautifully turquoise blue sky there arises a radiant WHITE disk of light. As you breath in, feel that the white light is shining into your forehead through to your brain, enlivening your nervous system and from there, your entire body. As you breathe out, continue to feel this radiance shining into your forehead as you sing out loud the sound OM. Do this 3 times. Then breathe in and out normally a few moments as you sit in the presence of this experience.

b) Now imagine that the WHITE disk goes further up into the sky and just below it, again on the horizon, there appears a warm, shimmering RED disk of light. As you breathe in, feel that this red light is shining into the area of the region of your neck, throat, and upper body, giving warmth, joy, and passion to your speech and all modes of expressiveness. As you breathe out, feel this light continue to shine into this area as you sing out loud the sound of AH. Do this a total of 3 times. Again, follow this with sitting in the presence of this experience.

c) The WHITE and RED disks now go further up into the sky and below them on the horizon, imagine the arising of a deep sapphire BLUE disk of light. As you breathe in, feel that this deep blue light penetrates into your heart, giving you clarity, peace, and a glimpse of the true nature of your mind. As you breathe out, feel this light continue to shine into your heart as you sing out loud the sound of HUNG. Do this a total of 3 times, then rest in the presence of this experience.

d) Now, in your minds eye, see all three disks of light, one above the other in the sky above the horizon; blue at the horizon, red above that, and white above the other two. As you breathe in, feel that all three lights are shining down on you all at once; the white light fill-ing your head, the red light blazing into your throat, the blue light pouring into your heart. As you breathe out, still feeling the lights shining into you, sing out OM AH HUNG. Breathe in again and repeat this for two more cycles. Then rest in the presence of the experience.

e) Now imagine that the white disk comes closer, then enters into your body through the crown of your head, filling your head with white light. This light strengthens your entire body and makes you feel more alive. The red disk now comes closer, enters through the crown of your head, dissolves in the area of your throat, and you are filled with a sense of warmth and joy. Finally, the blue disk draws near, enters into you through the crown, moves down to the heart where it dissolves, and you are filled with a sense of space and possibility. Rest in this full experience for another few minutes.

Step Five:

Enjoying how these sounds and lights have enriched you at all levels of your being, imagine you that you are filled to the brim with these lights and sounds vibrating inside you. As you breathe in and out naturally, feel as if these qualities are radiating from you, filling space in all direc-tions, and touching everyone around you, whether you know them or not, regardless of whether they are friend, foe, or unknown to you one way or the other. Sit in this state of peace, equanimity and compassion for another few moments.

Step Six:

Finally, bring your attention, once more, to your breath and hearing the sounds within as you breath in and out. OM as you breathe in, AH in the pause between the in breath and out breath, then HUNG as you breathe out. Do this a total of five times. On the fifth time, as you breathe in to the sound of OM, you are preparing yourself to move out of the meditation. With AH, you pause in preparation, feeling yourself full of all the strength, joy, and clarity of the meditation. Then, with HUNG, you bring your eyes into a natural focus and begin to move once again into your daily activities.

CHAPTER 14

Home Care Rituals

Ayurvedic Face Rejuvenation Home Care Ritual

Touch these points when you do your regular skin care routine, when cleansing, or when applying oils or lotions. If you want to do the whole technique for yourself, you might try it lying down so you can support your upper arms and relax your shoulders. Men love this experience so it is great to try with your partner.

We have found that one of the best ways to unwind from a long day, especially one in front of the computer screen or a classroom of students—where you are "on view", is to massage your face with oil and then do a steam. Jojoba oil works for all skin types, even those prone to congestion. Essential oils can be added. Check the appendices to see which ones we suggest for each skin type. For a home face steam, bring an inch and a half of water to the boil in a wide pan, turn off the heat add fresh herbs such as lavender, rosemary, mint, and rose petals or a few drops of essential oil. Set the pot on a table securely on a trivet. Sit comfortably leaning forward a little, rest your elbows on the table, and support your head with your hands. Leaning over like this encourages greater circulation to the lymph and blood vessels in the face which deeply refreshes the complexion. Drape a large towel over your head and shoulders to make a steam tent.

Breathe deeply for 5–10 minutes. Pat dry with a towel. Use ubtan or a light clay mask afterwards to remove the extra oil on your skin. A little oil mixed with essential oil of nutmeg on the back of the neck eases tense shoulders. This is wonderfully relaxing and replenishing in the evening, or a wonderful start to full body massage.

Self-Massage Ritual
Massage of the Scalp

Originally in the face rejuvenation treatment, the scalp was worked using a fair amount of oil. Hair oil and head massage is very popular in India, but we find that skin care clients in the west were not enthusiastic about going home with that greasy hair look. Oiling the scalp is a marvelous way to relax and renew, so you might try it at home. Wrap your head in an old towel and leave the oil on as long as you can, overnight is best. You can use a plastic shower cap underneath the towel during the day, but I find that at night, this makes your head sweaty. In the morning, the most effective way to get the oil out is to put shampoo on first before you get your hair wet. Using the three points on the midline and oiling the feet will help with restful sleep.

Massage of the Head

Pour oil on the point that is on a central hair parting eight finger-widths above your eyebrows. Massage the oil down both sides of the scalp towards the ears as if shampooing. Next, pour oil on the crown point and again massage the oil into the scalp towards the ears. Tilting the head forward, pour oil onto the point on the back of the head and rub towards the ears. Finally, apply oil at the back of the head at the hairline and rub the oil along the sides of the scalp towards the back of the ears. The whole scalp should now be oily. Use both fists to gently tap the head all over. This stimulates the circulation and awakens the nervous system. Next, take a hold of locks of hair all over your head and give them a gentle wiggle and pull from the roots. This helps relieve muscle tension that keeps the head feeling tight. In particular, be sure to pull the hair over the three points where you initially poured the oil.

Quick Massage of the Face

Keeping the fingertips well oiled, do massage strokes from the central portion of the forehead (above and between the eyebrows) outward toward the hairline on both sides of the face. Continue to stroke over every contour of the face, from the midline of the face outward and upward, over the forehead, above and below each eye, along the cheeks from the nose, above and below the lips, and be sure to include underneath the chin and up under the jaw. Tap under the chin and pinch along the jawline. Press and release three times on each of the marmas that are on both sides of the face that you can touch together. You can touch particular problem areas such as points for eyestrain or insomnia. If any of the points are tender, touch in gentle clockwise circles. Working with marma points will bring light and vitality to your face that cannot be achieved by products alone.

Self-Abhyanga Home Care Ritual

Abhyanga can be as complicated or as simple as you want to make it. It is an oily process and has the potential to be messy at home, but it is worth the effort. Nothing balances my energy and brightens my mood faster or better than a good self massage—except a great spa treatment. No matter how tired I am to start with, am I so filled up at the end that the few minutes' cleanup is a breeze. We have two approaches. One is for the distinctly cold types and one for the more robust amongst us. But first warm the oil. You will need 2–4 ozs depending on your size. You can warm it in a pan on the stove, a food warmer, a baby bottle warmer, or put the bottle of oil in boiling water for 5 minutes. It should feel good and warm to your hand.

The Tub Approach

Run a tub of hot water deep enough to completely cover your body. Sit on the side and massage your legs and up to your waist. Carefully get into the bath. Massage your feet, then massage all other parts. When you are covered, submerge your whole body and soak for 10–20 minutes. Mix one cup of ubtan powder with an equal volume of warm water so that it makes a creamy consistency. You can do the same with Ayurvedic mud. Put it on the top half of your body while sitting, then stand and do your legs. Take a few minutes to rub gently all over. Your skin will be soft and polished looking. Dip down in the bath and rinse. Finish with a cool shower. This works in a hotel, and their shampoo does a good job of cleaning up the oily ring so your room service doesn't have extra work. It is a great way to overcome jet lag and get a good night's sleep. Mud works better than ubtan for jet lag or deeper tiredness.

The Sheet Approach

Find a space in the house large enough to spread out a single sheet. When you are massaging with oil it does tend to flick about if you are not careful. Get naked and stand in the middle of the sheet and go through the massage as suggested below. The sheet will catch the dry ubtan and make clean up easy.

Home Abhyanga Sequence

What follows is a simple sequence that you can use with beneficial re
sults. You will be focusing on delivering the oil evenly over your entire
body, giving an extra focus to large muscle areas, joints, and special energy points (or *marmas*).

What You Will Need:
- dosha-balancing massage oil
- Tibetan Lotion for stiff muscles (Nutmeg) or sore joints (Ginger)
  (optional)
- pomegranate or shatavari ghee if you are doing breast self-massage
- ubtan powder, bowl, and pot of warm water to mix it into a paste
- 2 sheets; one for the ground and one for covering you that can both
  get oily
- a couple towels that you don't mind getting oily

Procedure:

Remove all your clothes and any jewelry that will get in the way. If you
have some particularly sore areas, use the appropriate Tibetan Lotion or
other product and rub into the affected joints or muscles. Leaving this
on through the remainder of the massage allows the lotions to penetrate
more effectively.

Using the dosha-appropriate oil, follow the following sequence:

Scalp—Spread the oil through your scalp and then use your fingertips
and scrub back and forth vigorously. Afterwards, following the direction of the subtle energy, stroke your hands over your head, starting
at your forehead and moving back over the skull. Then find 3 marma
points, one at the crown, one at the anterior fontanel, one at the posterior fontanel. Lightly press and massage with clockwise circular
strokes each point in the above sequence.

Side Face

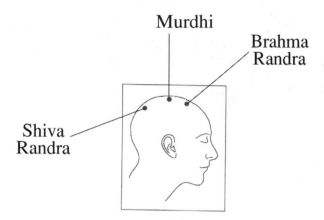

Marmas on the Bottoms of the Feet

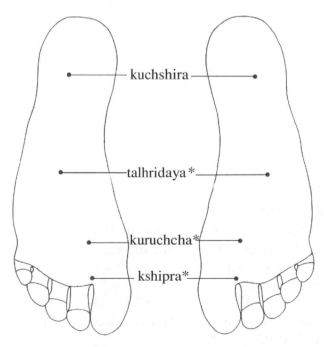

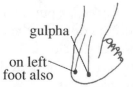

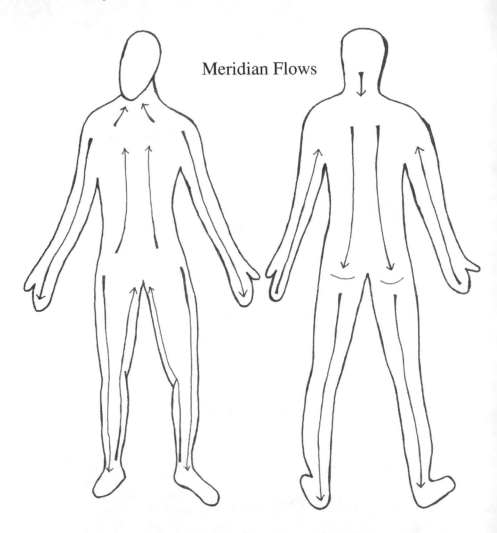

Meridian Flows

Ears—Massage along the outer edge (pinna) of your ears, from top to bottom. Pull on your earlobes, then rub the ears back and forth.

Face—Starting at your chin, spread the oil up over your entire face. Then rub the cheeks vigorously, especially along your jaw joint. Then rub back and forth across your forehead. Place your three middle fingers on each temple, another marma area. Close your eyes and just for a moment, think of a beautiful place that makes you think of peace and relaxation.

Neck—With long strokes, let your fingertips put oil on either side of your throat. Stroke from below your chin down to the top of your sternum. Do this several times. This improves the circulation to your complexion. Then stroke along the side and back of your neck, from the top down.

Shoulders—Starting with the right shoulder, rub down from the neck, then vigorously over the shoulder joint (where the shoulder meets the arm). Repeat on the left side.

Chest—from the base of the ribs and sternum, bring oil up along the right side of the sternum, over the breast and then down the right side. Do this 5 to 7 times, in a continuous circle. Repeat this on the left side. Find the marma in the center of the sternum (*hridayam*), and do light clockwise circles on this point (you can finish like this or do the Breast Self-Massage).

Abdomen—Lie on your back with your knees drawn up. Apply the oil in clockwise circles around the abdomen. Using both hands, alternate going lightly and deeply around and around the entire abdomen, from below the rib cage to the top of the pubis. Do this for a minimum of 3 minutes. Then, placing both of your hands on the area just below the navel, breathe in and out deeply for at least a minute. With each breath in, feel your belly rise and with each breath out, feel like your back is just sinking and settling and becoming more relaxed onto the ground.

Arms—Starting with the right arm, massage each finger joint with oil. Rub along the back of the hand, then smooth out the thick pads on the palm. With your left hand's fingers, make a band around your right wrist and rotate your right arm so that you are getting a good rubbing (like an old-fashioned Indian rope burn) around the wrist. Then rub oil up along the forearm. Rub vigorously around the elbow joint. Squeeze up along the muscles of the biceps and triceps. Do meridian stroking of the arms (see diagram) at least 7 times. Finally, place your left thumb in the deepest part of your right armpit. Press gently in and massage the marma point with clockwise rotating motions. Do this for a few moments. Rest a moment. Then repeat on left side.

Legs—Sitting with your legs in front of you, start with the right foot. Massage and rotate each toe, starting with the big toe. Rub between the bones on the top of the foot. Rub the bottom of the foot back and forth. Rub all over the ankle joint and slowly move up the calf to the knee. Squeeze up along the calf muscles. Rub vigorously all around the knee. Then work your hands up over the upper leg muscles to the hip joint. Apply light meridian strokes up the inside and front of the leg, then down the outside and back of the leg. Repeat this on the left leg.

Buttocks and Genital Region—Much stress and tension is carried in this area. At first you may feel uncomfortable touching yourself in these areas. But with time, you will see the benefits of ease in movement and improved libido and sexual performance. **FOR MEN**: Oil the space between the back of your scrotum and the front of your anus. Rub back and forth in this crease between your legs. Apply thumb pressure up into this space to benefit the prostate. Holding onto your right testicle, gently pull down, then release. Do this 25 times. Do the same for the left testicle. Apply oil (You can use Ashwagandha ghee to do this) onto the penis and pull from the base, allowing your hand to slide up over the shaft and come off the tip. Do this 25 times. **FOR WOMEN**: Oil the area between the back of the vagina and the front of the anus. Press up and massage into this area. With some additional oil (You can use Shatavari Ghee to do this) you can gently take hold of the labia and massage the lips with the oil. Stretch the tissue to improve elasticity. **FOR BOTH:** With regular dosha-appropriate oil, apply deep, clockwise circular motions with your fists or the palms of your hands to your buttocks. As these have large, strong muscles, apply this motion 25 to 35 times.

BACK—Apply oil to the lower back as high up as you can get. Do the same from the back of the shoulders down. Rub up and down along both sides of the spine as best you can. To get additional stimulation to the rest of the spine, lie on your back with your legs curled up. Rock back and forth on your spine 25 to 35 times.

Cover your body with a sheet and rest quietly for about 3 to 5 minutes. If you are more Vata in your body-mind type, you may want to put a blanket over the sheet. Allow the oil to penetrate for a few more moments as you rest.

Take about 1 cup of ubtan powder and mix it with warm water. You can also use Ayurvedic mud or even a mixture of mud and ubtan. Starting at your head, put a light coating of this paste all over your body. You can also take the ubtan powder and sprinkle it on dry. Make sure you are entirely covered, from head to toe. Wrap yourself up again and rest for another 2 to 3 minutes.

Get up, drink a glass of room-temperature water, and then shower.

This self-abhyanga ritual can be done early in the morning, in which case you will feel light and relaxed all day. It can also be done in the early evening, in which case it will prepare you for a quiet, blissful night of sleep.

Home Breast Massage Ritual

STROKING THE SIDES OF THE NECK—With the head turned slightly to the left, place the fingertips of your left hand just behind your right earlobe where you feel a small bony bump. Just behind this bump is *karna marma*. Rub this area gently, moving in 5 little clockwise circles. You might feel tension in your jaw release. Then stroke down the side of the neck, following the large muscle down to *arshak marma* which is on the top surface of the right collar bone where it joins the breast bone. Rub this area using 5 clockwise rotations. Now turn the head to the right and repeat the same procedure on the left side of your neck using your right hand. Repeat this process 15 times, alternating between the right and left side.

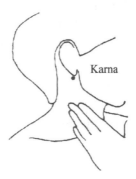

PRESSING ON THE COLLAR BONE—With your head turned slightly to the left, use your left thumb or fingers to press down upon the top surface of your right collar bone from the breast bone out to the tip of your right shoulder. Turn your head to the right and repeat the same on the left side.

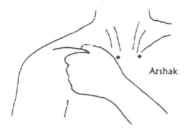

RUBBING BEHIND THE COLLAR BONE—With the same alternating method as in the last step, using clockwise rotational pressure, touch in the hollow space behind your collar bone, starting again from the breast bone and moving up along the tops of the shoulders. This helps your body relax and does a great job of combating fatigue.

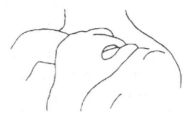

PRESSING UNDER THE ARM—Starting under your right arm, press gently into the deep hollow of the armpit and apply clockwise rotational pressure into *apalapa* marma. Do this 3, 5, or 7 times. Repeat on your left side. This point activates the lymph system in the upper torso and releases tension around your shoulders and arms.

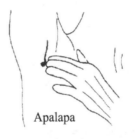

Apalapa

TOUCHING YOUR JOY POINT—Touch the point four fingerwidths below the top of your breastbone, approximately a half-inch below the sternal angle. Press and release this point (upper *hridayam marma*) in a gentle, pumping action 3, 5, or 7 times. This point allows you to more joyfully connect with your body and the world around you.

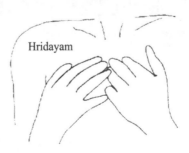

Hridayam

TOUCH YOUR HAPPY POINT—In the same way you touched the upper *Hridayam*, find the point that is approximately 4 centimeters below and to the right of *hridayam*. This point, known as *apastambha marma,* balances energy in your lungs and helps your body let go of grief and sadness.

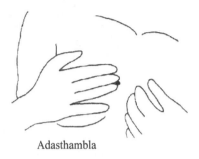

Adasthambla

TOUCH YOUR HEART POINT—Locate a point that is in the middle of the sternum, roughly at the level of the nipples. Apply gentle clockwise rotational pressure to this marma, also known as *hridayam,* and then proceed down the remainder of the sternum with circular massage strokes. This helps to alleviate depression.

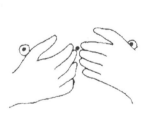

OVER THE TOP AND UNDERNEATH—With your left hand on your right breast, stroke over the topside of the breast with the flat of your hand, moving from the breastbone towards the armpit, using the pressure you would use to pet a cat. Use the right hand and repeat this movement over the left breast. Then, with your left hand, stroke the underside of the breast, starting at the breastbone and moving towards the armpit. Repeat with your right hand on the left breast. Do these strokes in an alternating fashion; left hand over right breast, right hand over left breast. Be sure to touch every part of the breast. *Pay particular attention to the outer upper quadrant of each breast, as this is the most common area for problems to arise.* Remember to end each stroke at the armpit.

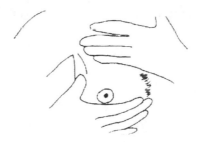

AROUND AND AROUND—Do 100 circular strokes on both breasts simultaneously, keeping the shoulders relaxed and projecting positive thoughts towards yourself and your breasts. The circles should cover the outer portion of the breast and the tissues just slightly above, below, and to the side of each breast, allowing the circles to get gradually smaller, working towards the nipples. Massage to the area directly below breasts stimulates blood circulation. Massage to the portion of the breast below the nipple increases sensuousness and a sense of self-confidence. All in all, this step helps maintain a pleasant shape to the breasts.

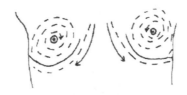

FOR ALL THE FINE CAPPILARIES—Pull the nipples, using gentle pressure between the thumb and index fingers. Nipple stimulation excites the finest capillaries and lymph tissue in this area of he breast.

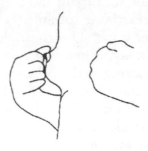

BACK TO THE ARMPIT—Repeat the massage of *apalapa* marmas.

Home Steam Box

Portable steam boxes are now readily available in the United States. They are easy to set up and safe for the whole family. After doing home self-abhyanga or treating each other to a massage, we often finish the ritual with 10 minutes in the steam box.

Remember that is best to use **purified water** when steaming. You can make the steam even more effective for yourself by putting the tri-doshic blend of essential oils (bay, eucalyptus, and ginger) in the steam unit. Also, for those who are more Pitta in nature or condition, wrap a cool, moist cloth around your forehead.

A source for these units is mentioned in the Resource Guide.

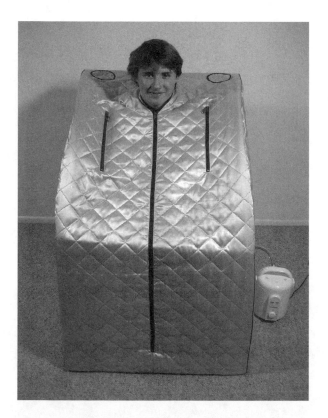

Tibetan Eye Rejuvenation Home Care Ritual

Remove your shoes and socks. If you are in trousers, roll up the cuffs. If you have a microwave, place two stones (flat river rocks or the "Body and Sole" stones) in your microwave for 2 minutes. Alternatively, put them in your oven on the lowest temperature setting for about 15 minutes to 20 minutes.

Sitting comfortably in a chair, with a warm cloth wipe your feet thoroughly, then pat dry. Using the Tibetan anise butter lotion or anise lotion, massage each foot for five minutes, starting with the right foot. If you know reflexology, pay particular attention to eye, liver, spleen, and kidney reflexes. According to oriental tradition, the liver governs the sight in the left eye and the spleen, the right. The actual structure of the eye itself is governed by the kidneys.

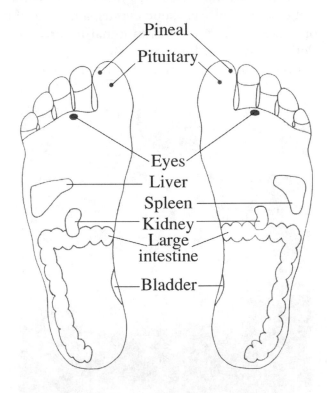

Pineal
Pituitary
Eyes
Liver
Spleen
Kidney
Large intestine
Bladder

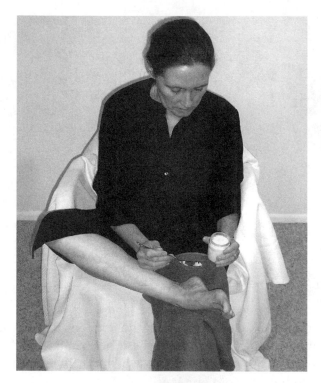

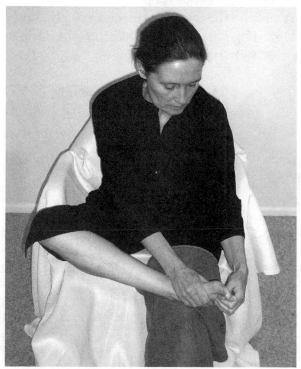

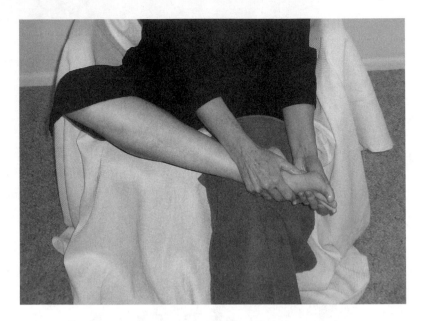

After the right foot, cover it and do the left foot in the same manner. Cover the left foot as well and leave the lotion on an additional 5 minutes. Breathe in and out and just relax as you let the anise lotion penetrate deeper into the bottoms of your feet.

Remove the cover on the feet and rub chickpea (besan) flour or ubtan into each foot, starting with the right. Cover, then allow the ubtan to rest on the feet for about five minutes.

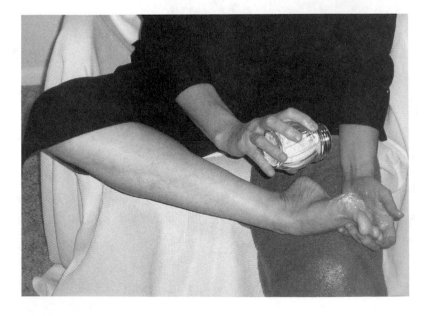

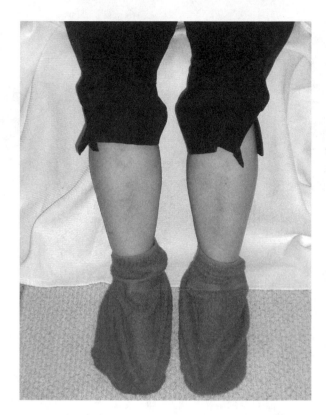

Wipe the powder with a dry cloth and then a warm, moist cloth. Pat the feet dry, right foot, then left. Take the warmed 'Body and Sole' stones (or other set of stones of equal size—traditionally round river rocks) that have been heated up and place them on a towel on the floor near your feet. Then rest your feet on the stones so that they are under the ball of each foot, just behind the toes. If you use the "Body and Sole" stones, the little bumps can be positioned directly under the eye reflexes, found on the under side between the base of the fourth and fifth toes. **Remember to hold these stones in your hands a few moments to check their temperature.** If they feel too hot, place a thin towel or dry washcloth between the feet and the stones. Again, the therapeutic action comes from the earthen quality and consistent deep heat that the stones radiate. Wrap a towel over the feet while the stones are in place (**resist the temptation to step down hard onto the stones, unless you want to feel more warmth**). Allow your eyes to stay closed and just notice and enjoy the warmth on your feet. The heating benefits of the lotion and the stones reduce Vata which can take the form of stress and tension exhibited in the face. This treatment literally draws this stress and tension away from the eyes and face and out of the body via the feet.

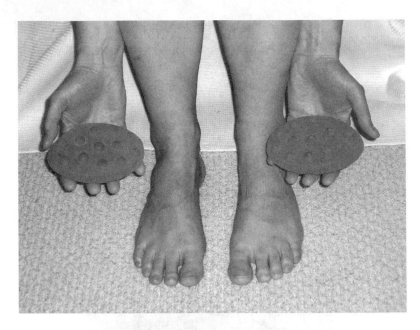

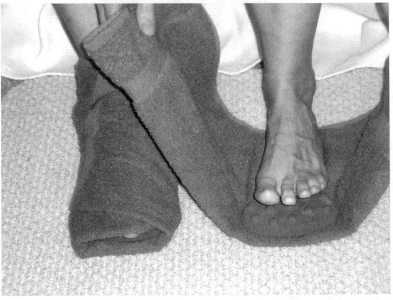

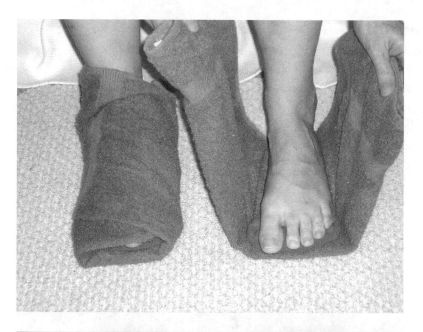

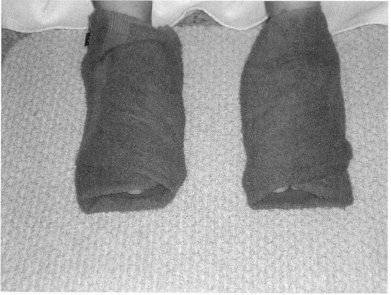

After 7 to 10 minutes, lift your feet and remove the stones, right foot, then left foot.

Shirodhara Home Care Ritual

Shirodhara is a difficult treatment to give to yourself. However, there is a way to derive some of the benefits of shirodhara through the following technique.

1. Start by taking a small amount of warm oil (sesame is best, but sunflower or almond will do) and rub it lightly through your hair to the scalp.

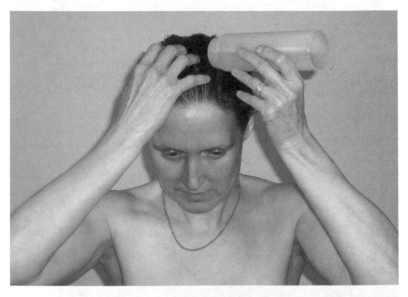

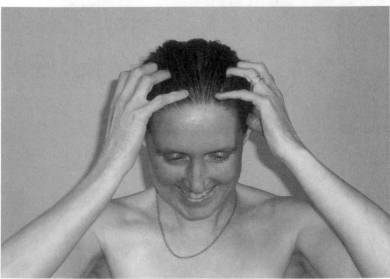

2. Lightly massage in clockwise rotational circles over the following
   marma points on the head.
   a) Murdhi
   b) Brahma Randra
   c) Shiva Randra
   d) Shankar

   Do these points in sequence 3 times.

Side Face

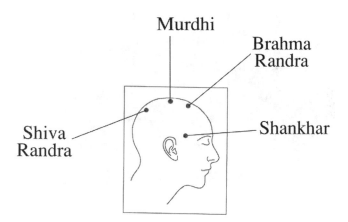

3. Along with the marma point in the middle of the forehead, there are
   several other marmas all along the forehead, from above the eyebrows to the hairline. Take a washcloth or an absorbent terrycloth
   towel and fold it so that it is the width of the space between your
   eyebrows and your (original) hairline. Then saturate it in warmed,
   unrefined (but *not* toasted) sesame oil. This can be purchased from
   any natural food store. The oil in the cloth need not be dripping, but
   it should feel well saturated (do not warm the oil in a microwave.
   Use a pot on the stove. It should only take 10 to 15 seconds to get
   the amount of oil you need warmed sufficiently).

   Place a towel beneath your head and lie back comfortably, perhaps after doing some exercise or yoga. Place the cloth over your
   forehead, close your eyes, and relax. Allow the oil-saturated cloth to
   stay on your forehead for about 10 minutes.

The sesame oil that lies on your forehead's vital energy (marma) points will penetrate and begin to relax your entire scalp and calm your mind.

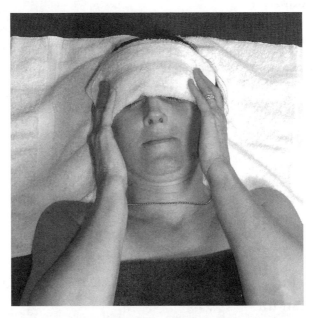

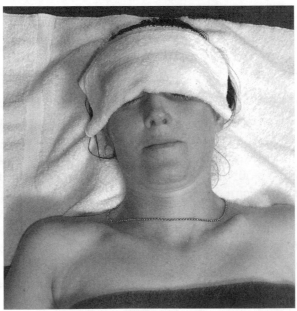

As a stress management technique, this procedure can be done daily.

Three Marma and Mud Magic Home Care Rituals

Home Foot Soak

Fill a small bucket or basin with 1.5 gallons of comfortably warm water. Then take 2 tablespoons of the Tridoshic Bath Salts mixture and stir it in. Place your feet in the water, sit back and relax. For a bit more stimulation, sprinkle some marbles or glass beads (easily available at hobby stores) into the bottom of the soaking basin and rub the bottoms of your feet along them. Rinse your feet with tepid or cool water afterwards.

This is a wonderful treat at the end of a busy day.

You can also place 1 cup of the bath salts into a tub and soak your whole body for 15 to 20 minutes to shed the tensions of the day. Remember to rinse off afterwards.

Home Kansa Vataki Treatment

Place a towel over your lap and bring your right foot up and rest it on the towel. Coat your foot with either the clarified butter (ghee) or the Anise Tibetan Lotion. Then, holding your three-metal bowl by the handle or clutched around the edge, massage your foot with the following steps.

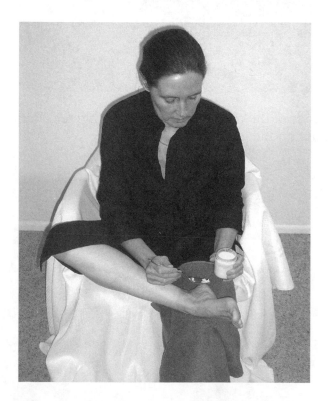

1. Start with the bottom—rub back and forth along the entire length of the foot at least 21 times.

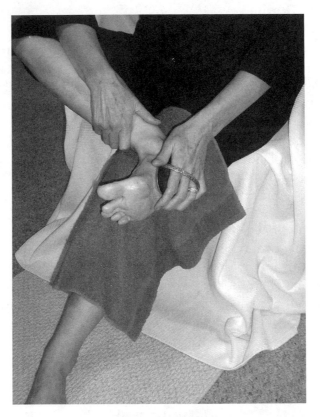

2. Do the ends of the toes, starting with the big toe. Perform 7 clockwise circles on the very tips.

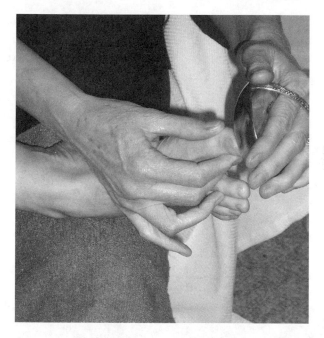

3. Starting at the edge of the big toes, make small clockwise circular strokes along the inner side and arch of the foot, around the back of the heel, and finally up along the enter outer edge of the foot up to the toes. Go around like this 3 times.

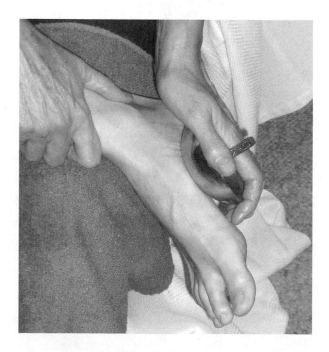

4. Do the top of foot. As the area is bonier with less dense tissue, use lighter pressure. Go as high up and over both medial and lateral aspects of the ankle joint as is comfortable. Do strokes back and forth along the metatarsal lines.

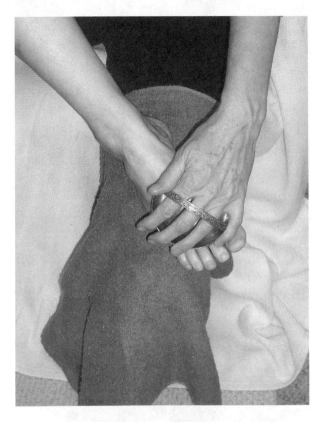

5. Go back to bottom again, this time doing clockwise circular motions, followed by figure eights over the entire bottom, then deep rotations into the arch.

6. Do 3 spins on the tips of the toes, starting with the big toe. The motion is that of trying to untwist a lid off of a can.

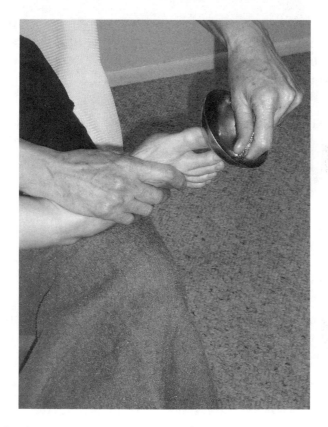

7. Wrap the foot in a warm towel and repeat steps 1–6 on the left foot.
8. Sit and relax for a few minutes.
9. Then unwrap your feet and sprinkle them with ubtan powder. Massage the powder into the right, then left, foot and re-cover. Allow your feet to rest with the powder on them for a few minutes.
10. Unwrap your feet, rinse in warm water, and pat dry.

Home "Herbomineral" Mud Treatment

You can use this warm mud on your arms and legs (fingertips to elbows and toes to knees) as was done at the spa *or* you can apply over your entire body. Just doing it on your arms and legs can be almost as relaxing and beneficial as doing the entire body. But we'll leave that up to you.

If you are preparing mud for your arms and legs, you will need about ½ cup of the dry mud. If you are doing your entire body, use a cup of the dry mud. To either amount, add enough warm water to create a slightly runny paste. Apply the mud in a place where you don't have to worry about it splashing.

If you are doing just your arms and legs, do the right arm, then the left arm, then the right leg, and finally the left **(note: For a more restful sleep, you can just do your legs a half-hour before bedtime. The manufacturer of this product has other home-help suggestions. See our Resource Guide).**

If you are doing your entire body, put the mud on in the following order:
- face
- neck and shoulders
- chest
- belly
- right arm, then left
- right leg, then left
- genitals
- back

Try to keep the mud moist. If it begins to dry, have a spray bottle around with some water and spray a mist onto the mud. Allow it to be on the body a minimum of ten minutes. Then rinse off and pat dry.

Blissful Sleep Home Care Rituals, Exercises, and Recommendations for Insomnia

The following three exercises can be done while you are lying in bed.

Abdominal Massage

1. Lie on your back and have your legs drawn up so that the bottoms of your feet rest on the mattress and your knees are drawn up.
2. With your fingertips, rub firmly down from the top of the sternum (breast bone) continuing down the middle of your abdomen (belly) until you get to about 1 ½ inches below the navel. As you get into the soft part of your belly below the rib cage and chest, press deeper. Do this 4 to 5 times.

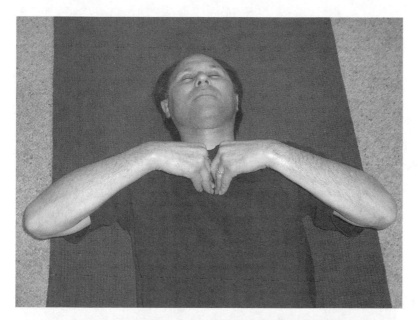

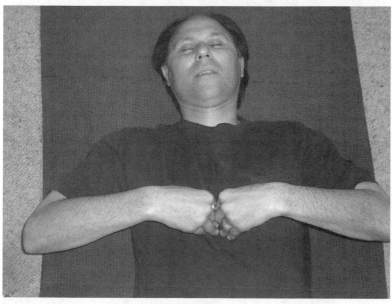

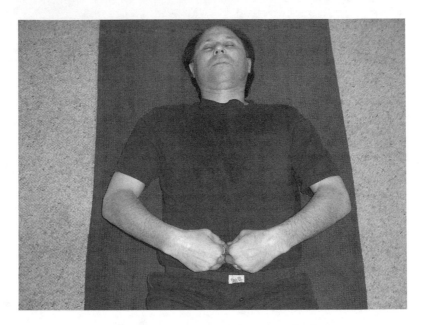

3. Starting below the navel, press down on points around the abdomen as if each point was a number on a clock. Go in a clockwise direction. Repeat 3 times, pressing in as you breathe out and releasing as you let your breath in again.

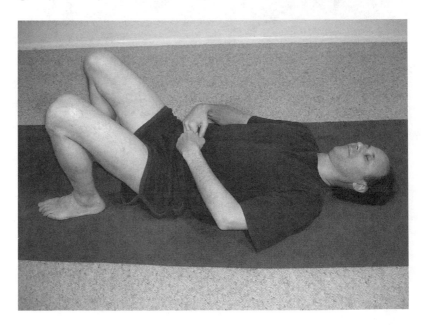

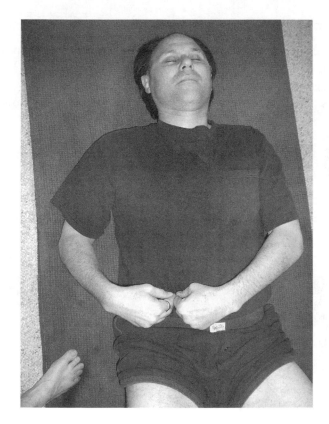

4. Use both your palms to rub your belly in a clockwise motion for about a minute.

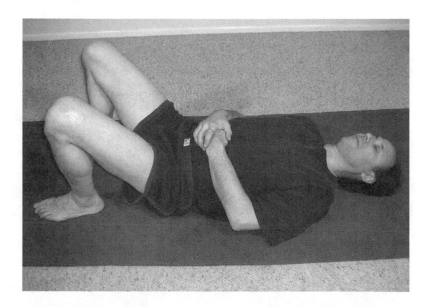

Leg Tensing

1. Still lying on your back, have your legs flat on the mattress. Breathe in, tense your right leg and press the back of your right heel into the mattress while holding your breath, then relax your leg and breathe out. Do this 5 times. Repeat this with the left leg.

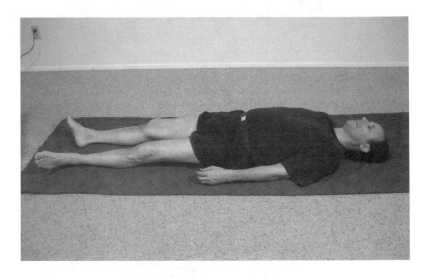

Upper Back and Neck Tensing

1. Still on your back, rest your elbows on the mattress with your arms beside your body. As you breathe in, arch your upper back and your neck so that the top of your head is on the pillow. Then breathe out and relax your back and neck. Repeat this 5 times.

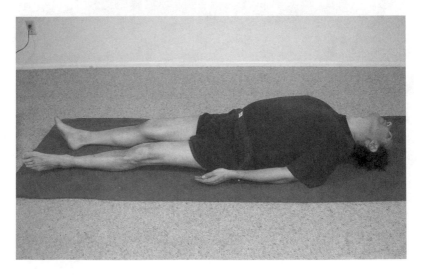

After these 3 exercises, place your hands so that your fingers rest just below your navel. Observe your breathing, allowing your belly to rise and sink with each breath. With each breath out, imagine that you are allowing yourself to sink deeper into the mattress.

To Relax the Spine

Sit cross-legged on the floor next to your bed and hold onto your feet. Allow yourself to roll back gently on your spine as far as you can go and then roll back into a sitting position. Do this for about 2 minutes.

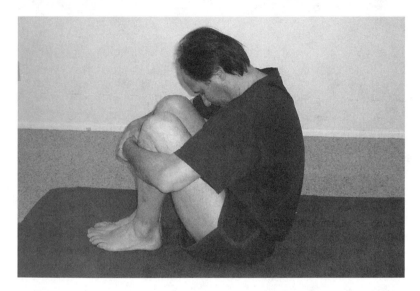

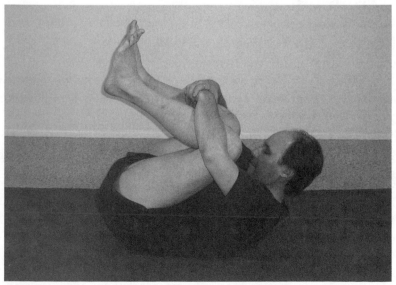

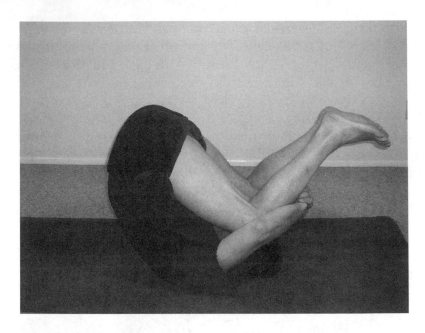

Other Helpful Hints

Even following just 5 or 6 of the following recommendations will dramatically improve the quality of your sleep. Some we have asterisked (*) to indicate their effectiveness.

- Exercise between 4pm and 8pm. This can help clear the body of adrenaline.
- Do some yoga, especially cobra, shoulder stand, mountain, and corpse poses.
- Avoid caffeine after midday*.
- Take a warm bath with baking soda and essential oils or herbs, or at least wash your hands and feet and clean your teeth. A hot bath may be too stimulating. If you shower, keep your head dry and allow warm water to flow on your shoulders and back (this will pull circulation away from your head).
- Oil your feet with "Calm and Clear" or another Vata-balancing oil. Also, put a little of the same oil in your ears and on the three special marma spots on your head*.

Side Face

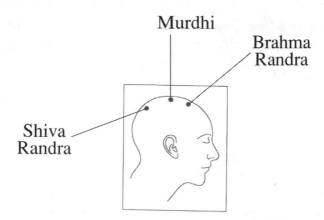

Murdhi

Brahma
Randra

Shiva
Randra

- Herbs such as hops and chamomile contain calcium, help alleviate cramps, and promote cell regeneration. Passion flower relieves pain and nervous irritability, especially around hormonal change times. Valerian and Ayurveda's Jatamamsi ease muscle tension, slow the heart, and help concentration.
- Learn an effective form of skilled relaxation. Many recordings of relaxation methods are available. These will entrain you to let go more when you go to sleep.
- Learn to meditate as a way of loosening your fixation on thoughts that keep your mind churning*.
- Many herb pillows are available, or you can make one with the essential oils or actual flowers of linden, lavender, violet and myrrh.
- Avoid being in a space where cooking smells linger. These can keep your brain active*.
- Have your physician or health care practitioner check your calcium, potassium, and B vitamin levels.
- Place your bed so that your head is in the south. This works with the polarity of the earth. Better still is to imagine that your head is resting in the lap of someone you admire or love.
- Rest on your right side. It helps to cut off attachments and fixations.

- Keep the temperature of your bedroom cool—60 degrees Farenheit if possible. Keep a window open, again if possible*.
- Spend money on a good bed. Remember, you spend a third of your life there*!
- Don't have a bed directly on the floor. This does not allow for there to be a circulation of energy around your body while you sleep.
- Use natural bedding. Synthetic sheets, blankets, and foam pillows all hold electromagnetic charges which can keep you more churned up. Cotton and wool give the body energy. This also applies to what you wear to bed*.
- Keep electrical appliances away from the bed, such as electric alarm clocks, computers, etc. If you have an electric blanket, *turn it off and unplug it once the bed is warm*. We have seen people who wake up every twenty minutes because that is when the thermostat on their blanket turns the blanket back on*.
- Sleep in the dark. Use an eye mask or hat if necessary. Have whatever covers your eyes also cover the middle of your forehead as light hitting there can stimulate the pineal gland and keep you awake*.
- Be aware of your emotions, especially negative ones. If it is possible to resolve a matter with a loved one before you go to bed, do it.
- Eat light at night—sleep does not stop digestion but digestion does interfere with sleep. Breakfast is supposed to be about "breaking" "fast". If you have been metabolizing a late-night pizza throughout the night, chances are you will awake feeling sluggish. In that respect, **especially avoid fermented dairy products such as yogurt, sour cream, or cheese late at night.** These will give you intense, sometimes violent dreams. If you must, drink something hot or cool (but not cold), or eat something light, like a piece of fruit, some apple sauce, etc—generally something that is light and easy to digest*.
- Use a negative ion generator or one of the many energy enhancing and air filtering systems currently on the market.
- Don't read or watch something very engaging just before bedtime.
- If you have a TV in your bedroom, turn it off at least 20 minutes before you go to bed. TV's produce many positive ions, which can keep the room feeling electric. This also applies to computers*.
- Stick to a routine. Routine in your life will help to calm Vata.
- If you are moreVata in nature, be aware that you sometimes forget to rest. Try to simplify what you do, at least close to bedtime. Waking in

the early hours and not sleeping again until morning is a sign of high Vata. If this is also what you are experiencing, naps are useful, but try to keep them to 20 minutes.

- If you are more Pitta in nature, you generally will do fine with 6–8 hours of rest but your sleep will be lighter than either Vata or Kapha types. Be particularly mindful of anxiety and getting too caught up with goals and a driven achievement orientation. Avoid daytime sleep unless you are elderly, sick, or tired from sex, overwork, or emotional distress. If you exercise during the day, also learn to have a cooling down or relaxation period after the exercise.

Nadi Swedana Home Care Follow-up

A gentle oiling with the dosha-appropriate oil blend, plus a warm face cloth soaked in one of the essential oils mentioned above can accelerate the easing of discomfort if any remains. At the same time, if such areas are chronic, it is a great home preventive health care practice to encourage. Of course, always tell people to consult with their health care practitioner if any pain persists.

Nasya Home Care Ritual

A short form of pacifying or *Shamana* Nasya can be taught to clients for them to do at home. One of the best oils to recommend is a standard formula called *Vacha* or *Sidda Soma* oil, although plain organic sesame oil or warmed ghee can also be used.

The procedure for your client is simple:

1. Warm a small portion of the chosen oil by standing a small bottle of it in a cup of boiling water for a few minutes.
2. Take a warm washcloth and apply it to the forehead and cheeks to increase the circulation into the cheeks.

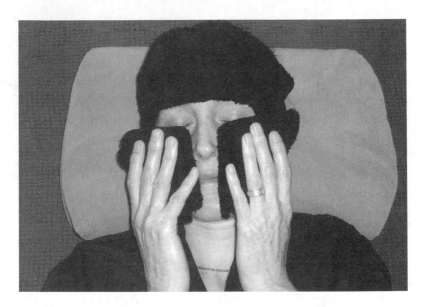

3. Lying on your back with a supportive pillow under your neck, block the left nostril first. Administer three to five drops of oil into the right nostril. As the oil goes down, breathe normally and massage along the side of the right nostril for deeper penetration.

4. Then block the right nostril and repeat step 3 on the left side.

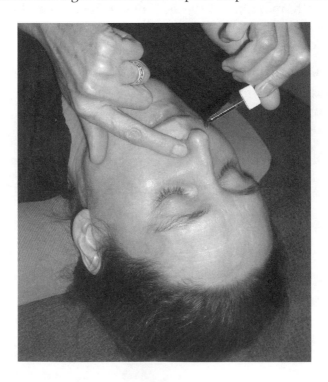

Besides the above home protocol, you can also encourage your clients to invest in a *neti pot*. If you are involved in practicing yoga, perhaps you have heard of neti pots. A neti pot is something like a small teapot that is filled with a mild saline solution or herbs to wash out the sinuses. Such pots are now on the market from a number of distributors, all of which provide instructions.

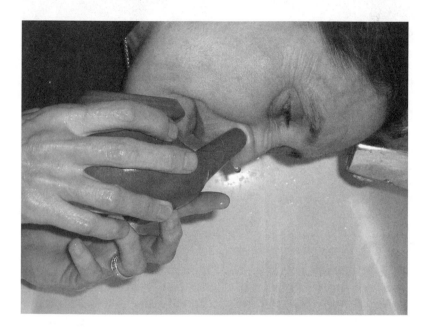

For other people, especially those suffering from stress, anxiety, or depression, there are several Tibetan incenses that are available and can be found using our Resource Guide at the end of the book. Several Indian and Japanese incenses are also excellent, although the authors are unfamiliar with their particular uses.

And for those more adventurous, one can direct them to Indian grocers who carry a number of medicated snuffs that can be used periodically for sinus conditions, etc.

Netra Basti Home Care Ritual

Netra Basti can actually be done at home, but for shorter periods of time. What you will need to do this is ghee, a cheap set of swim goggles that has the thick foam on the edge that presses against your head, a tower, some tissues, and a rolled-up towel that you can put under your neck.

To start with, remove all eye make-up, then take a tissue to wipe around your eye so that the skin around your eyes is as dry as possible.

First start with a simple massage of the following points around the eyes. Start with pressing the points closest to the nose first, seven times. Then go farther along to the points under the eyes and then the points towards the outer edge, pressing each seven times. Then pinch along the eyebrows, starting from the center and moving outwards.

Eye Massage Points

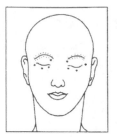

Warm the ghee so that it becomes liquid and just slightly warm. Wag your finger back and forth in the ghee to make sure it is not too warm. Then pour a small amount into the cups of the swim goggles, so that they are about ¾ of the way filled. Make sure you don't get any ghee on the foam edge. If you do, wipe it off.

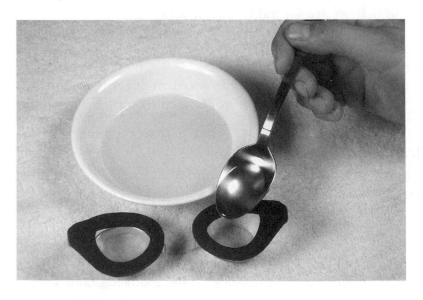

Now put the goggles up to your eyes and press them firmly up around your eye sockets. Then lie back so that the rolled towel is under your neck.

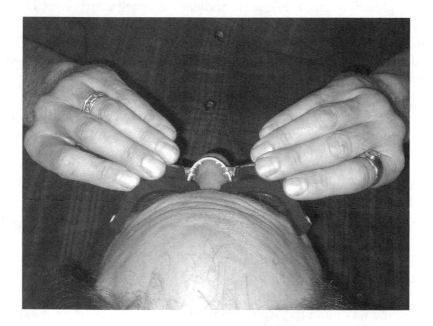

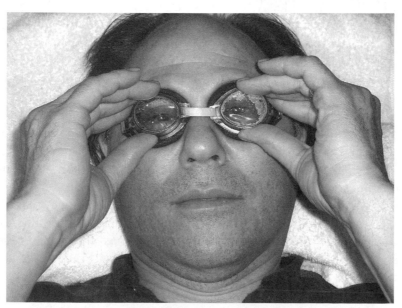

This takes a bit of coordination to start with, so don't wear anything that you may be concerned about getting oil on. Initially, the pressure may be uneven and you may spring some leaks. If so, simply adjust the pressure.

Even though this may all seem a bit complicated to start with, the rewards for doing this at home periodically are well worth it. **It is especially good for those who work around computer screens or have a lot of redness or feelings of strain in their eyes.** REMEMBER: the ghee may make your eyes sting a bit to start with. Just breathe and relax. Allow about 5 to 7 minutes for the entire treatment.

When you are done, turn over. Lower the goggles onto the towel. Then take a tissue to wipe the excess oil out of your eyes and out from around them. Expect your eyes to be a bit bleary for about 20 to 30 minutes.

Karna Purana Home Care, Exercises, and Recommendations

Here are a number of simple suggestions for ear hygiene and a number of conditions.

For cleansing your ears, periodically take a small amount of hydrogen peroxide and put it in your ears. Lie on your left side first and pour a few drops into your right ear. It will gurgle and crackle as it dissolves some wax buildup. After about 3 to 5 minutes, drain that side and repeat on the other side. Afterwards, let each ear dry out for about 10 minutes, then put in a few drops of almond or sesame oil (almond, garlic, or mullein oil are especially good for earaches).

When you travel, especially by air, place a few drops of sesame oil into each of your ears. This will help with jet lag, make you more relaxed, and ease the hissing sounds that often persist from the white noise of the planes. Generally, it helps to calm Vata dosha.

If you have tinnitus or ringing in the ears, before you go to bed, take a small amount of Nutmeg Tibetan Lotion and massage it into both *karna* marma points behind and slightly below each ear. This can be done nightly for relief.

If you suffer from jaw tension, for daily maintenance, place a few (3) drops of sesame or almond oil in your ear canals. Then take a bit of this same oil and massage the following marmas and stress relieving points: 1. *krikatika* marma, 2. *karna* marma, 3. Jaw Point, and 4. point of "old tears".

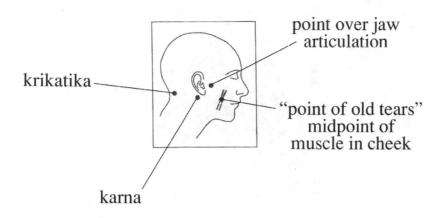

krikatika

karna

point over jaw articulation

"point of old tears" midpoint of muscle in cheek

To help with jaw tension and TMJ Syndrome, try the following exercises that were taught to us by a dear friend and master dentist, Dr. Ballard Morgan. They are called the "Six by Sixes".

1. Say the word "CLUCK" six times. Note how your tongue goes to the front of the roof of your mouth.
2. Keeping the tip of the tongue behind your top front teeth, open your mouth as wide as you can and then close it. Do this six times.
3. With your fingers clasped or interlocked, place your hands over the nape of your neck and rock your head back and forward, pressing the back of your head against your clasped hands, then forward to bring your chin to your chest. Do this six times.

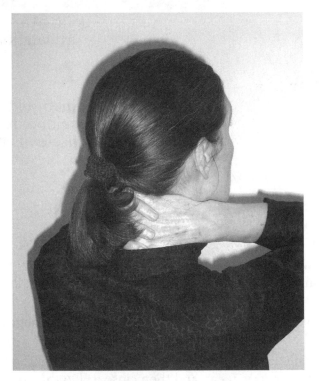

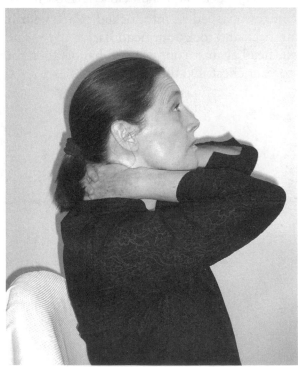

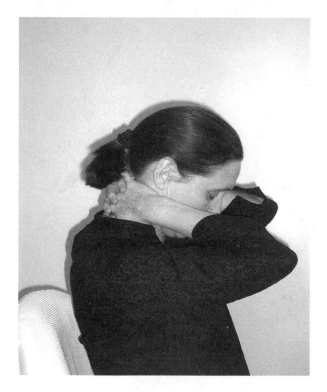

4. Repeat this entire series 3 times a day.

Section Five

Last Minute Essentials

Shirodhara Information and Advice Form

Please read and sign prior to your treatment—thank you.

The shirodhara treatment can evoke an extremely deep relaxing state and have a profound effect on the psyche. It is not uncommon for some clients to experience dreamlike states, lights, colors, and/or strong emotions. Others simply experience lightness, clarity, and sense of open awareness that is both freeing and somewhat magical.

Experiences like these in our mental state can often leave us feeling more open, but sometimes a little more vulnerable. For this reason **we strongly recommend** that you do not drive, return directly to work, or go into any circumstance that you deem to be stressful immediately after your shirodhara treatment. Allow at least 30 minutes after your treatment to dress slowly and be our guest for tea and a snack. Then return to a place that is quiet and supportive for a few hours.

You get the greatest benefit if you leave the oil in your hair for a minimum of an hour, but overnight is best. Oil is best removed by applying shampoo before you get your hair wet.

Please help us help you to fully honor your shirodhara experience and get the most out of your treatment.

I_____ have read and understood the above information.

Client's signature_____

Therapist's signature_____

Date_____

Some General Skin Care Treatment Suggestions

*I*f your client checks predominantly **Vata** qualities, then you should use products that are warming, grounding and calming, nourishing, hydrating, toning, warming, focusing, clarifying, energy giving, are emotionally balancing.

Some of the base and essential oils we have found useful separately and in combination for Vata skin conditions include:

- Avocado—hydrates and nourishes, high in protein, vitamins A, E, and C and potassium, the "youth mineral"
- Jojoba—repairs/protects
- Hazelnut—warms, strengthens and nourishes
- Vitamin E—repairs/rejuvenates
- Rosewood—regenerative, relaxes wrinkles, warming, steadying, uplifting when stressed
- Rose Geranium—warming, relaxes and eases pain, healing, reduces anxiety and nervousness
- Rose—hydrating, rejuvenating, relaxing, sensual, balances mood swings
- Palma rose—regenerative, toning for mature skin, nourishing, relieves nervous exhaustion
- Neroli—stimulates new growth, moisturizes, reduces anxiety before stressful events, improves depth of rest and level of self confidence
- Carrot Seed—improves tone and elasticity, nourishes dry and mature skin

If your client checks predominantly **Pitta** qualities, then you should use products that are fresh, clean, spacious, cooling, calming and soothing, and increase patience, sensitivity and self love.

Some of the base and essential oils we have found useful separately and in combination for Pitta skin conditions include:

- Apricot—activating, cooling, toning
- Sunflower—cooling
- Vitamin E—repairs/rejuvenates
- Lemon—balances sebum, acidity, discoloration, antiseptic, clears and tones, cools head, helps focus
- Bergamot—balances sebum, soothes inflamed breakouts, lifts spirits but still relaxing
- Frankincense—preserves youth, helps get more in touch with reality
- Vertiver—cooling, refreshing, helps resist temptation, "oil of tranquility", helps with being more "in your body" than "in your head"
- Jasmine—"king of oils" reduces heat and sensitivity, warms and lightens the heart, helps open to new ideas
- Spearmint—cooling and refreshing

If your client checks predominantly **Kapha** qualities, then you should use products that are warming, rich, luxurious, comforting, clearing and gently stimulating, energizing, uplifting, and inspiring.

Some of the base and essential oils we have found useful separately and in combination for Kapha skin conditions include:

- Jojoba—repairs, protects and helps ease congestion
- Vitamin E—repairs, rejuvenates
- Orange—stimulates flow of lymph and circulation, uplifting
- Bergamot—balances sebum, reduces perspiration, curbs appetite, lifts the spirits, helps you feel constructive
- Rosemary—antiseptic, stimulating to nervous system, reduces cellulite, cleansing, gives clarity, and strengthens will
- Juniper Berry—reduces congestion, stimulates circulation, helps with letting go and breaking limitations.

Rave Reviews:
Testimonials of Happy Clients

*R*ather than fill the book randomly with quotes from students and clients who have experience the beauty of Ayurvedic treatments, we thought we would place them as an Appendix and allow you to choose which of them you would like to use to spice up your spa menus or as wall quotes in your spa. If you are already reading this book, chances are you are already convinced by Ayurveda and know that it is here to stay. So with the exception of a few quotes which mention our teaching and the classes some have taken in other schools, most of these quotes will inspire your clients.

(Regarding Ayurvedic Face Rejuvenation)

"After the Ayurvedic Face Rejuvenation treatment I slept better than in a long time. I normally don't have difficulty sleeping but this was a different kind of sleep, really deep. I felt that there was a lot of good energy flowing, I felt I was unblocked in different places. In a half-asleep state, I was thinking "wow" this is really good, this is really deep."
—AYURVEDA LIVING'S CLIENT, CA

"This form of massage (marma point) will change my life and my business. I'm very excited about this change and I look forward to the journey."
—SANDRA B.

"Giving the movements felt sacred to me. I feel it is what has been missing in the approach to beauty care."
—COLLEEN

"It's by far the most wonderful treatment I've given and received. The whole treatment was quite enjoyable and truly mesmerizing."
—SUSAN

(After a training the Face Rejuvenation with Melanie)
"I was able to put into practice the Marmassage right away with some very pleasing results. Life is a little more interesting now because I look at people and try to determine what their Dosha is. It also helps me to understand them a little more."   —CONNIE F.

(Regarding Shirodhara)

"I experienced a deep and profound sense of relaxation and wellbeing I have not been in touch with for several years. I also saw several comforting and inspirational images."   —SHARRON M.

"I felt like I was floating in a safe, warm place totally at peace."
—GLORIA H.

"I'm teaching Shirodhara this weekend at the AHG meeting in New Hampshire. I've pulled two or three people out of a deep psychosis with daily shirodhara treatments and other things."
—MICHAEL TIERRA OF PLANETARY FORMULAS

"Shirodhara is SOOOO wonderful! If psychiatrists knew what it can do, with or without some other Ayurvedic support, they might be short on business. After moving across the country dealing with heartbreak, breast cancer, and financially on a total leap of faith, I signed up for one every two weeks for about 4 sessions. It gave me a feeling of groundedness, wholeness, ease, and wisdom in my awareness and body, and renewed simplicity about restoring my health and strength—and my career! It served me better than massage or any other treatment I can think of."   —ISHA, AGE 55, FROM RIVERSIDE DAY SPA
AND WELLNESS

"The lines in my face seem to soften, my eyes got brighter and colors seem more vivid after I experienced one of Karyn's shirodhara therapy sessions."
—HALLIE BROTHERS FROM RHODE ISLAND
(FROM THE ISHA CREATIONS CENTER FOR
HOLISTIC EDUCATION AND THERAPY)

"During the shirodhara treatment I experienced my body opening and it felt like the oil was lubricating the opening of my 3rd eye. The oil felt like it facilitated the release and opening of past-old "stuff" that can now be shed. It felt like my eyes were open even though my lids felt shut. It felt like lots of spirits came into the room and it even felt crowded with them, but they all came to help."

"After the treatment I felt more fluid and the pain in my hip which was bothering me before the treatment was completely gone. I felt very relaxed and calm, happy and sad at the same time."

"My clients love it. A lot of what I've been hearing from my clients is that they feel reborn. They also include stories about traveling "somewhere" during the procedure. My lady on Tuesday said that she felt like she was in China and that she had experienced something very spiritual. This lady comes to me because her Vata is extreme. So extreme that her own immune system is attacking her hair follicles. I have also had clients tell me they felt" silent". It is truly a deep spiritual procedure . . . . Thank you so much for teaching it to me!"
—MELANIE O.

(Regarding Nasya)

"We had a client who had sinusitis and was recommended for Nasya (series of 5). From the second day onwards, she started feeling better and by the end of the series she was totally free from congestion and was happy and energized. "This is an amazing treatment for anyone suffering from congestion and sinusitis and it works. I'll be back for more," she concluded."
—SHYMALA AYURVEDA, LONDON

(Regarding Netra Basti)

"After the Netra Basti my peripheral vision was immediately affected. One and a half days later I had a splitting headache from my eyeglasses being too strong. Now I am having to be more sparing in my use of them. Hopefully this will last . . ." —CAMBRA C.

"On the way to (the class), I was in a pretty bad state of mind—tired, depressed, overwhelmed, very negative . . . I felt like I would be in that state for a while—at least several days.

Once the treatment began, however, I was able to let go—my eyes relaxed so much, the rest of me followed. When leaving after the treatment, I felt like I 'saw the world through different eyes'. I no longer felt down or distressed. Instead I felt renewed and I remained that way.

The following nights, for perhaps a week, I slept very well . . ."
—JILL

(Regarding Tibetan Marma Sequences)

Just to let you know the Tibetan Treatments I learned last year with Robert are amazing. I can't really explain what is happening to my ladies! Most of the ladies I get for this treatment are practitioners themselves.

One particular lady asked me to contact you and tell you that during her treatment she went into all those unfinished past lives and cleared them all up!!! That is a bit spooky for me, but she insisted you knew."

—SALLY M.

(Regarding Abhyanga And Ayurvedic Massage In General)

"A client came in with severe shoulder pain. He could not lift his hands as it was too painful. After recommending pindsweda and marma massage for two days, the client was able to lift his hands and even some weights. " I am feeling 100 % better now. I tried all kinds of medicines but that didn't work. I am really surprised and happy about the treatments I received and I am interested in learning more about Ayurveda."

—SHYMALA AYURVEDA, LONDON

"I noticed after the first day . . . how my arthritis in my ankles and knees did not bother me and when I awoke in the morning, I feel as if my joints were more lubricated and not as painful as they usually are."

—KRISTY H.

"I felt this treatment addresses the full body, therefore I completely relaxed compared to when only parts of my body are worked on. Working on marmas to balance the full body certainly has a long term, lasting effect. Thank-you Bob and Melanie. You're the best."

—SYLVIA G.

"Himalayan Mountain Abhyanga has had a deeply relaxing effect on my entire body. I saw some colors during the time when certain marma points were being stimulated. I felt my skin and face looked fresher and more vibrant. The techniques were easy to pick up and I feel will work well in our spa at the St. Regis Monarch Beach.   —TRISH L.

"I hadn't given Ayurveda much consideration as a modality. Now, the energetic, common-sense bodywork approach has made me re-evaluate my entire approach with clients. Robert and Melanie work together to create a complete environment from yin and yang, east and west approach. They compliment one another from academic and practical aspects. I am extremely satisfied with the skills and knowledge I gained from the Abhyanga class and feel confident practicing this knowledge with my spa clients."

—GWEN F.

"The Himalayan Mountain Abhyanga left me feeling energized, clear and very calm, relaxed. One has a complete nurturing feeling that one has been touched deeply. I loved the feel and smell of the oils and the dry brushing at the end. I think my face was brighter and clearer after the treatment."
—MARY S.

"Robert and Melanie have shared their massage technique and I shall be happy to share all the fantastic info at my spa.

The Abhyanga massage has a huge benefit in terms of energy being re-vitalized and feeling refreshed at the end of the 90 minutes. The abdominal massage technique will be shared with our therapists also..."
—LEIGH H.

"I feel that when giving (the Abhyanga) massage I was not as tired and worn out as from traditional massage, which makes me happy because of the tremendous effect it has on a deep level without using as much energy."
—KRISTY H.

"I traveled to Portland from Alberta, Canada in order to experience 5 days of Panchakarma. It was totally awesome! I was pampered from the moment I arrived to the moment I reluctantly left. Richard and his well-trained staff did everything to make my Panchakarma experience blissful. And blissful is was. Comfortable lodgings and delicious Ayurvedic meals were provided for me. The most wonderful experiences were the daily, time-honored Ayurvedic treatments. Abhyanga, Nasya, Swedana, shirodhara and Pizichili massage: all were done with loving care while I experienced a blissful state of well-being. When my week was over, I virtually floated back home, wishing I could stay indefinitely. Thank you, Richard, Nick, Theresa and Mary-Jo for giving me one of the best and most profound experiences of my life!"
—ANN SCHUSTER

"I felt so pampered and special after I received one of your hot oil (abhyanga) massages 6 years ago! I have traveled all over the world since, trying different types of massages, but still, this form of Ayurvedic massage makes me feel deeply healed, grounded and renewed. I just love it."
—GRETA FROM HOLLAND (PROVIDED BY
SACRED STONE CENTER FOR HOLISTIC
EDUCATION AND THERAPY)

"After graduation from CCA, I started my Ayurvedic medicine and Pancha Karma practice, first in San Francisco and now in Idaho. I'm amazed how my education prepared me to help people in basic ways that make a real difference in their health and happiness."

> —C.S. APRIL, 1999 CLASS, CALIFORNIA SCHOOL
> OF AYURVEDA

"Recently a client was preparing for her wedding. This client was a very strong Vata personality and shared with me how nervous she was becoming. My wedding gift to this client would be an Ayurvedic treatment. On the day of her wedding she came for her treatment. At the conclusion of this treatment she stated she just wanted to stay and sleep for awhile. Her first visit after her marriage, I asked her how she handled the remainder of her day and she responded, 'I can't believe that I was so calm even into the next day.'"

Resource Guide

Ayurvedic Schools and Training

American University of Complimentary Medicine
11543 Olympic Blvd.
Los Angeles, Calif. 90064
Phone: 310-914-4116
Fax: 319-479-3376

www.aucm.org

Ayurveda Institute of America
561 Pilgrim Dr. Ste B
Foster City, CA 94404
(650) 341-8400
www.ayurvedainstitute.com
jayapte@ayurvedainstitute.com

Ayurvedic Institute
11311 Menaul Blvd. N.E.
Albuquerque, NM 87192
505-291-9698
www.ayurveda.com

Ayurveda-Yoga Institute
Trainings in the Ancient Ayurveda system
New York City and New Jersey
212-631-4283
201-440-3106
www.ayurvedayogainstitute.com
gandharva@earthlink.net

The Balanced Approach
1025 Maxwell Ave, #2
Boulder, CO 80304
(303) 447-9484
www.thebalancedapproach.com
info@thebalancedapproach.com

California College of Ayurveda
1117A East Main St. Grass Valley, CA 95945
530-274-9100
www.ayurvedacollege.com
info@ayurvedacollege.com

Diamond Way Ayurveda
P.O. Box 13753
San Luis Obispo, CA 93406
805-543-9291, toll free 866-303-3321
www.DiamondWayAyurveda.com
ayurveda8@earthlink.net

Affiliated Regional Diamond Way Trainers:
EAST COAST
Dawn Tardif (Ayurvedic Face Rejuvenation, Tibetan Shirodhara)
Phone: 978-977-9966
dawn.tardif@verizon.net
MIDWEST:
Jon Alan Vice (PediKarma™)
Phone: 317-414-6821
jonalanatelier@sbcglobal.net
SOUTH:
Tracy Adele Henson (All Diamond Way Ayurveda treatments)
Phone: 772-334-6362
tracy@alohahenson.com

Dr. John Douillard's LifeSpa School of Ayurveda
6662 Gunpark Drive
Suite 102
Boulder CO 80301
Phone: 303-516-4848 / 866-227-9843
www.LifeSpa.com
School@LifeSpa.com

Florida Vedic College
4926 Buchanan Place
Sarasota, FL 34231
941-929-0999
www.ayurvediccollege.com

John Holmstrom III, Ayurvedic Teacher
Shivalchemy Transmutational Ayurveda Educational Corporation
President: John Holmstrom
15332 Antioch Street, Suite 507
Pacific Palisades, CA 90272-3603
www.SuryaSpa.com
Email: Shivalchemy@mindspring.com
(research and training, non-profit for Ayurvedic Acupuncture, herbs, and all modalities and styles of Ayurveda)

Institute for Wholistic Education
Dept. AS
3425 Patzke Lane
Racine, WI 53405
Ph: 262-619-1798
Website: www.wholisticinstitute.org

London Centre of Indian Champissage International
136 Holloway Road
London N7 8DD
ENGLAND
Phone: +44 (0) 20-7609-3590
          20-7607-3331
FAX: +44 (0) 20-7607-4228
www.indianchampissage.com
www.faceliftmassage.com
kundan@faceliftmassage.com
indianchampissage@yahoo.com

Mahindra Institut
Forsthausstrasse 6
63633 Birstein-Obersotzbach
GERMANY
Phone: +49 060 54-91 31-0
Fax: +49 60 54-91 31 36
www.mahindra-institut.de
info@mahindra-institut.de

Michael Tierra' East West Herb course
PO Box 533
Soquel, CA 95073
(800) 606-6226
www.planetherbs.com

Sacred Stone Center For Holistic Education & Therapy
554 East Main Road
Middletown, RI 02842
toll free: 877-832-1372 or 401-846-6380
www.sacredstonehealing.com
k@sacredstonehealing.com

Sparsha Trainings for Ayurveda and Spa Therapies
Toll Free and Fax 888-522-6860
(India) +91 80 2528-8630 or 2525-4654
www.SparshaTrainings.com
SparshaTrainings@yahoo.com

SWA MA CHI—Sacred Window Ayurveda for Mothers & Children
Postpartum Kayakalpa and Basic AyurDoula Care, Correspondence/ Intensive
    Training,
PO Box 2276 Alachua, Florida 32616
352-378-3660
WEBSITE www.sacredwindow.com
(Discussion site) www.groups.yahoo.com/mygroups
    "Perinatalayurveda"
AyurDoulas@sacredwindow.com

Centre TAPOVAN
Adi Shankti
9 rue Gutenberg
75015
Paris
France
Phone: +33(0)1 45 77 90 59
www.tapovan.com.fr

Tara Spa Therapy, Inc.
26384 Carmel Rancho Lane
Suite 203
Carmel, CA 93923
831-624-9570 or 800-552-0779
www.taraspa.com
customerservice@taraspa.com

Ayurvedic Spas, Healing Centers, Practitioners, And Spas Offering Ayurvedic Services

USA

East Coast:
Center for Health and Harmony
Sally Galloway
7013 Backlick Court
Springfield, VA 22151
(703) 912-2901
www.centerforhealthandharmony.com

BodiScience
80 Prospect Street
Peabody, MA 01960
Phone: 978-977-9966
www.BodiScience.com

Sivam Yoga & 9 Stone Body Therapy
400 Columbia Blvd
Cherry Hill, NJ 08002
Phone: 856-482-5183
www.Sivamyoga.com
kathleen@sivamyoga.com

SPAyurveda Medical Spa
213 Loudoun ST, SW
Leesburg, VA 20175
703-779-7789
spayurveda.com
info@ayurvedicmd.com

The Spa Center, Inc.
PO Box 1305
Hillsborough, NC 27278
919-732-1164
info@thespacenter.com

Midwest:

Dayst, ar Center for Well-Being
204 Woodlawn Avenue or 44 Summit Ridge Drive
Tahlequah, OK 74464
918-456-6388
shivanichase@yahoo.com

Jon Alan Atelier
7172 N. Keystone Ave. Suite C
Indianapolis, IN 46240
Phone: 317-202-0063
www.jonalanatelier.com

The Raj
1734 Jasmine Ave.
Vedic City, Iowa 52556
Phone: 800-248-9050 or 641-472-9580
www.theraj.com

Tranquility Spa LLC
300 South Broadway
Green Bay, WI 54303
(920) 438-8399
www.tranquilityspasanctuary.com

Northwest:

Ayurveda Plus Rejuvenation Center
3607 SW Corbett Ave.
Portland, OR 97239
800-588-4108
www.ayurvedaplus.com

Healing Waters Skincare
13320 Goodnough Dr. NW
Gig Harbor, WA 98332
Phone: 253-857-6113
www.Jurlique.com
dawnshealingwaters@hotmail.com

South:

Ayurvedic Center for Well Being
3023 Proctor Road
Sarasota Florida 34231
941-929-0999
www.AyurvedicHealers.com
info@AyurvedicHealers.com

Phyl's Garden Retreat: Massage and Spa Services
RR1 Box 2775 Wireglass Road
Folkston, GA 31537
Phone/FAX: 912-496-4168

The Spa at Mandarin Oriental
500 Brickell Key drive
Miami, FL 33131
Phone: 305-913-3841
FAX: 305-913-8326
www.mandarinoriental.com

momia-spa@mohg.com

Southwest:

Ayurvedic Institute
11311 Menaul Blvd. N.E.
Albuquerque, NM 87192
505-291-9698
www.ayurveda.com

FACE, etc
6400 Brisa del Mar
El Paso, TX
915-845-2829
866-322-3382
www.faceetc.com
sales@faceetc.com or
faceetc@sbcglobal.net

Skin Goddess Spacare
1728 N. Alma School Road
Chandler, AZ 85224
480-212-2431
Shanti@SkinGoddessSpa.com

West:

Dr. John Douillard's LifeSpa
6662 Gunpark Drive
Suite 102
Boulder CO 80301
Phone: 303-516-4848 / 866-227-9843
www.LifeSpa.com
Info@LifeSpa.com

Elemental Wisdom
1362½ Alpine Ave
Boulder, CO 80304
(303) 579-0764

The Shirodhara Day Spa
2122 Fort Union Blvd.
Salt Lake City, UT 84121
801-943-3840
www.shirodharadayspa.com
shirodhara2002@yahoo.com

Sweet200
Melanie Orris
2550 Elm Street Dallas Texas
214-823-2485 Or 214-742-2500
Sweet200.com
e-mail Maggiestarfish@aol.com

West Coast:

Akash Healing Center
Sharon Forsyth
Kailua-Kona, Hi 96740 (Big Island)
(808) 331-2276
livinglight@hawaii.rr.com
www.livinglightministry.com

Aqua Day Spa
1422 2nd Street
Santa Monica, CA 90401
Phone: 310-899-6222
www.aquadayspa.com

Ayurveda Healing Center
29621 Mission Blvd.
Hayward, CA 94544
510-727-9891
www.AyurvedaHealingCenter.com
ushakhosla@hotmail.com

Ayurveda Living
Oakland, CA
510-301-5163
www.ayurvedaliving.com
barbora@ayurvedaliving.com

Ayurvedic Spa: Pancha Karma Center
1117A East Main Street
Grass Valley, CA 95945
Phone: 530-274-9100, ext. 217

Blue Sage Sanctuary
P.O. Box 2135
Nevada City, CA 95959
Phone: 888-878-5222
www.bluesage-sanctuary.com

Buddha's Eye Ayurveda
David Wells, C.A.S.
Phone: 323-687-4478
dwellsohm@yahoo.com

The Chopra Center at La Costa Resort and Spa
2013 Costa del Mar Road
Carlsbad, CA 92009
Phone: 888-424-6772 or 760-931-7566
www.Chopra.com

Maharani Ayurveda
1605 Bath St., #4
Santa Barbara, CA 93101
Phone: 805-452-2526
www.maharani.us
ayurveda@maharani.us

Mirabella Mansori
161 S. Highway 101
Solano Beach, CA 92075
Phone: 858-720-1832
www.mirabellamansori.com

Northridge Prana Center
Dr. R.K. Mishra
18527 Devonshire St.
Northridge, CA 91324
Phone: 818-368-3484

Santa Barbara Prana Center
Dr. R. K. Mishra
1605 Bath Street
Santa Barbara, CA 93101
Phone: 805-452-2526

Spa Gaucin
The St. Regis
Monarch Beach Resort & Spa
1 Monarch Beach Resort
Dana Point, Ca. 92629
949-234-3367
www.stregismb.com

Surya Spa
310-459-7715 or 310-459-0677
www.suryaspa.com
martha@suryaspa.com
john@suryaspa.com

Canada

Perfect Health Ayurveda
Steven & Pat Harvey
Box 61171 Kensington PO
Calgary, Alberta T2N 4S6
CANADA
Phone: 403-220-1667
ambienthealth@hotmail.com

Salt Springs Spa and Resort
1460 North Beach Rd.
Salt Spring Island, B.C. V8K 1J4
CANADA
Phone: 250-537-4111
Fax: 250-537-2939
www.saltspringspa.com

Continental Europe

Buddha Bar Spa
Hilton Evian-les-Bains
Quai Paul Leger
74500 Evian-les-Bains
FRANCE
Phone: +33 45 84 60 40
Email: buddhabarspa-evian@buddhabar.com

Energeticum
Dr. Mahindra De Souza
Rosengarten 8
D-22800 Hamburg-Wedel
GERMANY
Phone: +49 (0) 4103/989195

Feng Shui and Health Center Ludwigsburg
Sabine and Christoph Deutscher
Lindenstr. 40
D 71634 Ludwigsburg
Phone: 07141 921266
Fax 07141 901957
Email SabineDeutscher@gmx.de
www.fengshui-und-gesundheitszentrum.de

Yoake
Gullegemsestraat 66
B8501 Kortrijk
Belgium
+ 32 495/23 14 14
www.yoake.be
www.wellnessboat.com
info@yoake.com

Yoga Naturheilzentrum
Dr. Mahindra De Souza
Burgerstr. 16
D-76133 Karlsruhe
GERMANY
Phone: +49 (0)721/26924

Great Britain

London Centre of Indian Champissage International
136 Holloway Road
London N7 8DD
ENGLAND
Phone: +44 (0) 20-7609-3590
          20-7607-3331
FAX: +44 (0) 20-7607-4228
www.indianchampissage.com
www.faceliftmassage.com
kundan@faceliftmassage.com
indianchampissage@yahoo.com

Shymala Ayurveda
152 Holland Park Avenue, London W11 4UH
ENGLAND
Phone: 0207 348 0018
www.shymalaayurveda.com
enquiries@shymalaayurveda.com

The Spa at Mandarin Oriental
66 Knightsbridge
London SW1X 7LA
Direct Tel. +44 (0) 20 7838 9888
Direct Fax. +44 (0) 20 7838 9883
Email. molonspa@mohg.com
www.mandarinoriental.com/london

India

Arth: An Ayurvedic Health Center
1074-E, 11th Main, HAL II-Stage
Indiranagar, Bangalore 560 038
INDIA
+91 80 2528-8630 or 2525-4654
(USA contact) 888-522-6860
www.arthworld.com
arthindia@vsnl.com

Ayushakti Clinic (Mumbai)
Drs. Pankaj and Smita Naram
Bhadran Nagar Cross Road #2
Ofl. S. V. Road, Opp. Milap Theatre
Mlad (W), Mumbai-400 064
INDIA
Tel: 091-22-806-5757/49
FAX: 091-22-806-5748
www.ayushakti.com
ayushakti@ayushakti.com

Dr. J. P. RANADE
Director, VEDikA AYURVEDIC HEALTH CENTRE
B/6, Madhu-Manisha, Anand Nagar, Santacruz (East), Mumbai-400055.
INDIA
Tel: +91-022-26686798 / Mob. 09820232459
E-mail: ayurlife2000@yahoo.com

Mexico

Villa Ananda
Punta Mita Nayarit
Mexico
US Phone: 503-922-1712
Mexico Phone: + 55-53-51-45-59
www.villaananda.com

West Indies

The Spa at Elbow Beach, Bermuda
60 South Shore Road
Paget PG 04
Bermuda
Phone: 441-239-6831
Fax: 441-239-8043

Ayurvedic Educational Materials, Products and Spa Equipment

Educational Materials

Aesthetic VideoSource
P.O. Box 188
West Jordan, UT 84088
801-282-2490
Toll Free 800-414-2434
www.videoshelf.com
info@videoshelf.com
(Ayurvedic and other treatment videos and DVDs)

Ayurvedic Institute
11311 Menaul Blvd. N.E.
Albuquerque, NM 87192
505-291-9698
www.ayurveda.com

Bazaar of India
1810 University Ave.
Berkeley, CA 94703
1-800-261-7662
www.bazaarofindia.com
(herbs, oils, books, videos, Indian handicrafts)

Diamond Way Ayurveda
P.O. Box 13753
San Luis Obispo. CA 93405
www.DiamondWayAyurveda.com
ayurveda8@earthlink.net or ayurveda8@sbcglobal.net
(Ayurvedic face and body oils, lotions, spa equipment, books,
    videos, music)

Natalie Gougeon
519 Redbud
Mt Shasta, CA, 96067
530-926-5985
natalie@ayurvedicare.com
www.Ayurvedicare.com
(Ayurvedic Principles Chart and Video /DVDs
Abhyanga/Massage & Ayurvedic Treatments Presentations)

Internatural
Dept. AS
PO Box 489
Twin Lakes, WI 53181 USA
800-643-4221 (toll free order line)

262-889-8581 (office phone)
262-889-8591 (fax)
Email: internatural@lotuspress.com
Website: www.internatural.com
(Retail mail order and Internet re-seller of Ayurvedic products, essential oils, herbs, spices, supplements, herbal remedies, incense, books, yoga mats, supplies and videos)

Lotus Light Enterprises
Dept. AS
PO Box 1008
Silver Lake, WI 53170 USA
800-548-3824 (toll free order line)
262-889-8501 (office phone)
262-889-8591 (fax)
Email: lotuslight@lotuspress.com
Website: www.lotuslight.com
Wholesale distributor of Ayurvedic products, essential oils, herbs, spices, supplements, herbal remedies, incense, books and other supplies. Must supply resale certificate number or practitioner license to obtain catalog of more than 10,000 items.

Lotus Press
Dept. AS
PO Box 325
Twin Lakes, WI 53181 USA
Ph: 262-889-8561
Fax: 262-889-2461
Email: lotuspress@lotuspress.com
Website: www.lotuspress.com
Publisher of books on Ayurveda, Reiki, aromatherapy, energetic healing, herbalism, alternative health and U.S. editions of Sri Aurobindo's writings.

SWA MA CHI—Sacred Window Ayurveda for Mothers & Children
Postpartum Kayakalpa and Basic AyurDoula Care, Correspondence/ Intensive Training, Herbs & Essential Oils. *The Keys to Postpartum Rejuvenation—42 Days for 42 Years*—Parent's Handbook
PO Box 2276
Alachua, Florida 32616
352-378-3660
www.sacredwindow.com
(Discussion site) www.groups.yahoo.com/mygroups
    "Perinatalayurveda"
EMAIL ADDRESS AyurDoulas@sacredwindow.com

Herbs, Supplements, Tinctures, Oils

Auroma International
Dept. AS
PO Box 1008
Silver Lake, WI 53170 USA
Ph: 262-889-8569
Fax: 262-889-2461
Email: auroma@lotuspress.com
Website: www.auromaintl.com
Importer and master distributor of Auroshikha Incense, Chandrika Ayurvedic Soap
    and Herbal Vedic Ayurvedic products.

Ayur Herbal Corporation
Dept. AS
PO Box 6390
Santa Fe, NM 87502
Ph: 262-889-8569
Website: www.herbalvedic.com
Manufacturer of Herbal Vedic Ayurvedic products.

Ayushakti USA
333 Millwood Rd.
Chappaqua, NY 10514
914-244-8580
www.ayushakti-usa.com
info@ayushakti-usa.com
(Ayurvedic formulas developed by Drs. Pankaj and Smita Naram)

Ayurvedic Institute
11311 Menaul Blvd. N.E.
Albuquerque, NM 87192
505-291-9698
www.ayurveda.com

Ayurveda Living Products
Oakland, CA
510-301-5163
www.ayurvedaliving.com
barbora@ayurvedaliving.com

Banyan Trading Company
6705 Eagle Rock Ave. N.E.
Albuquerque, NM 87113
800-953-6424
www.banyantrading.com
Bulk Ayurvedic herbs, oils, supplements.

Bazaar of India
1810 University Ave.
Berkeley, CA 94703
1-800-261-7662
www.bazaarofindia.com
Herbs, oils, books, videos, Indian handicrafts.

Diamond Way Ayurveda
P.O. Box 13753
San Luis Obispo. CA 93405
www.DiamondWayAyurveda.com
ayurveda8@earthlink.net
Ayurvedic face and body oils, lotions, spa equipment, books, videos, music.

Heal Thyself
213 Loudoun ST, SW
Leesburg, VA 20175
703-777-4203
www.thehealthyselfstore.com
info@ayurvedicmd.com

Floracopeia Inc.
206 Sacramento Street, Suite 304
Nevada City, CA 95959
Phone: 530-470-9269
http://www.floracopeia.com
info@floracopeia.com
Ayurvedic and Tibetan herbal products.

Internatural
Dept. AS
PO Box 489
Twin Lakes, WI 53181 USA
800-643-4221 (toll free order line)
262-889-8581 (office phone)
262-889-8591 (fax)
Email: internatural@lotuspress.com
Website: www.internatural.com
Retail mail order and Internet re-seller of Ayurvedic products, essential oils, herbs, spices, supplements, herbal remedies, incense, books, yoga mats, supplies and videos.

Laughing Coyote Spirit Medicine
John Holmstrom III
shivalchemy@yahoo.com
Quality Ayurvedic tinctures.

LifeSpa Products
6662 Gunpark Drive
Suite 102
Boulder CO 80301
Phone: 303-516-4848 / 866-227-9843
www.LifeSpa.com
Products@LifeSpa.com

Lotus Brands, Inc.
Dept. AS
PO Box 325
Twin Lakes, WI 53181 USA
Ph: 262-889-8561
Fax: 262-889-2461
Email: lotusbrands@lotuspress.com
Website: www.lotusbrands.com
Manufacturer and distributor of natural personal care and herbal products, massage
    oils, essential oils, incense and aromatherapy items.

Lotus Light Enterprises
Dept. AS
PO Box 1008
Silver Lake, WI 53170 USA
800-548-3824 (toll free order line)
262-889-8501 (office phone)
262-889-8591 (fax)
Email: lotuslight@lotuspress.com
Website: www.lotuslight.com
Wholesale distributor of Ayurvedic products, essential oils, herbs, spices, supple-
    ments, herbal remedies, incense, books and other supplies. Must supply resale
    certificate number or practitioner license to obtain catalog of more than 10,000
    items.

OM Organics
3245 Prairie Ave., SuiteA
Boulder, CO 80301
Toll Free: 888-550-8332
www.omorganics.com
Organic teas and bulk herbs.

Planetary Formulas
PO Box 533
Soquel, CA 95073
(800) 606-6226
www.planetherbs.com

Sarada Ayurvedic Remedies
P.O. Box 2425
Toluca Lake, CA 91610

Phone: 877-541-5836 Toll Free Phone
Website: www.tarikausa.com
E-Mail: info@tarikausa.com
Products: Sarada Ayurvedic Remedies Ayurvedic Herbal Body & Massage Oils,
   Tarika Ayurvedic Skin Care, Sarada's Remedies (Herbal Tinctures).

ShopViewNutrition
Dept. AS
3425 Patzke Lane
Racine, WI 53405 USA
email: viewnutrition@yahoo.com
www.shopviewnutrition.com
Retail internet website specializing in natural products including an extensive selection of ayurvedic books, supplements and personal care products.

SLO Chai
1160 17th street UnitB
Los Osos, CA 93402
slochai@sbcglobal.net
Organic, bottled chai tea.

Tara Spa Therapy, Inc.
26384 Carmel Rancho Lane
Suite 203
Carmel, CA 93923
831-624-9570 or 800-552-0779
www.taraspa.com
customerservice@taraspa.com

Veda Enterprises
2351 Sunset Blvd. Suite 170
PMB 236
Rocklin, CA 95765
Toll Free: 800-745-7077
Phone: 916-624-0798
www.vedaenterprises.com
Lakshmi Spa and Beauty products.

Spa Equipment

DarleyUSA Massage tables
612-866-7175
www.DarleyUSA.com
darleyusa@msn.com
(in UK)
01 208 873200
www.darleycouches.net

Diamond Way Ayurveda
P.O. Box 13753
San Luis Obispo. CA 93405
www.DiamondWayAyurveda.com
ayurveda8@earthlink.net
Ayurvedic face and body oils, lotions, spa equipment, books, videos, music.

Gilden Tree
www.gildentree.com
7409 Main Street #10
Omaha, Nebraska 68127
Toll Free: 1-888-445-3368
FAX: 402-339-8826
Quality cotton robes and spa clothing.

Richard Haynes
3607 SW Corbett Ave.
Portland, OR 97239
800-588-4108
Ayurveda Plus Rejuvenation Center
www.ayurvedaplus.com
Shirodhara equipment.

Natural Health Technologies, Inc.
50 N. Third Street
Fairfield, Iowa 52556
Phone: 641-472-0945, ext. 225
www.steamywonder.com
rick@steamywonder.com
Steamy Wonder steam canopies.

New Life Systems
2853 Hedberg Drive
Minnetonka, MN 55305
800-852-3082
www.newlifesystems.com
info@newlifesystems.com
Shirodhara equipment, massage tables, etc.

Tara Spa Therapy, Inc.
26384 Carmel Rancho Lane
Suite 203
Carmel, CA 93923
831-624-9570 or 800-552-0779
www.taraspa.com
customerservice@taraspa.com

TouchAmerica
PO Box 1304
Hillsborough, NC 27278
800-678-6824
info@touchamerica.com
Supplier of massage and spa equipment.

Architects and Building Consultants

VASTUVED INTERNATIONAL 614-472-2157
Michael Borden
P.O. Box 2197
Fairfield
Iowa
52556
vastuved@yahoo.com
www.vastu-design.com
Building and furniture design using Vastu Shastra.

VASTU LIVING
"Creating A Home For Your Soul"
Kathleen Cox
www.vastuliving.com
info@vastuliving.com
Phone: 212-245-4655

THE HOUSE DOCTORS
Marilee Nelson 1-830-238-4589
Consultant for Environmental Sensitivity

SWANSON ASSOCIATES 512-288-9097
George Swanson
Cell 512-653-8624
FAX 512-288-9096
PMB 126, 6705 Hwy 290 W. Suite 502
Austin
TX 78735
website: www.geoswan.com
e-mail: gps@flash.net
Offering specialized consulting services for
"Eco Resorts" and "Eco Spas".

Environmental Home Center 1-800-281-9785
Supplies and information.

Natural Home Magazine 1-800-272-2193
www.naturalhomemag.com

Decorating Products for the Chemically and Environmentally Sensitive

O.S hard Wax 1-800-281-9785
Resists stains used for all cabinets and trim.

East Street Basic Coating 1-800-247-5471
Wood floor finish.

Hydra coat 1-800-229-0934
Kitchen cabinets and treatment room furnishings.

Zip guard environmental water based eurathane 1-800-321-9785
Anything that needs a lacquered finish.

Best 1 1-800-281-9785
Interior paint all Benjamin Moore colors.

Anchor paint 1-800-999-4626
Exterior paint.

Bioshield www.bioshieldpaint.com 1-800-621-2591
All finishes, pigments, plaster, cork flooring and cleaners.

Hydrotile mate thinset 1-800-726-7845 by Bostik
Tiles with no latex.

Ultra Touch 1-480-812-9114
Mold proof insulation.

John Mansfield 1-800-644-4013
Formaldehyde free fiberglass insulation.

Wirsbo 1-800-321-4739
www.wirsbo.com
Radiant heat systems.

Natural Plus Company 1-727-447-2344
Pool supplies.

Solutions 4 You 1-800-301-9911
Laundry powder, fabric softener, bleaches, dish soap, hand soap, window cleaners, carpet and upholstery cleaners, tile and tub cleanser, furniture polish, toilet bowl cleanser, mold inhibitor and disinfectant.

OxiClean 303-740-1909
Great on tough dirt and stains on anything.

The Big Orange Cleaner 880-527-5722
www.carrollco.com
Oil-cutting for surfaces and linens.

Marketing and Ethical Business

Enlightened Business Institute
Gary Hirsch
2523 Huber Lane NE
Olympia, WA 98506
360-357-4823
360-357-6182 (fax)
gary@enlightenedbusiness.com
www.enlightenedbusiness.com

Marta Martine
3905 State Street Suite 7254
Santa Barbara, CA 93105
Phone: 805-967-8279
martcnslt@aol.com

Xsense
Uta Birkmayer
805-549-9005
Email uta@x-sense.biz

Bibliography

Atreya, *Secrets of Ayurvedic Massage*. Twin Lakes, Wisconsin: Lotus Press. 2000

Douillard, Dr John. *The Encyclopedia of Ayurvedic Massage*. Berkley, California: North Atlantic Books 2004

Clifford, Terry. *Tibetan Buddhist Medicine and Psychiatry*. York Beach, ME: Samuel Weiser Inc. 1984

Dash, Vaidya Bhagwan. *Massage Therapy,* New Delhi, India: Concept Publishing 1992

Frawley, Dr David. *Yoga and Ayurveda*. Twin Lakes, Wisconsin: Lotus Press 1999

Frawley, Dr David, Ranade, Dr Subhash and Lele, Dr Avinash. *Ayurveda and Marma Therapy*. Twin Lakes, Wisconsin: Lotus Press 2003

Johari, Harish. *Dhanwantari*. Rochester, Vermont: Healing Arts Press 1998

Johari, Harish. *Ayurvedic Massage*. Rochester, Vermont: Healing Arts Press 1996

Joshi, Dr. Sunil. *Ayurveda and Panchakarma*. Twin Lakes, Wisconsin: Lotus Press 1996

Lad, Dr. Vasant. *Ayurveda: Science of Self-Healing*. Twin Lakes, Wisconsin: Lotus Press 1984

Mehta, Narendra. *Indian Head Massage*. Hammersmith, London: Thorsons 1999

Miller, Dr. Light and Dr. Brian. *Ayurveda and Aromatherapy*. Twin Lakes, Wisconsin: Lotus Press 1995

Morningstar, Amadea. *Ayurvedic Cooking for Westerners*. Twin Lakes, Wisconsin: Lotus Press 1995

Sachs, Melanie. *Ayurvedic Beauty Care*. Twin Lakes, Wisconsin: Lotus Press 1994

Sachs, Robert. *Tibetan Ayurveda*. Rochester, Vermont: Healing Arts Press 1995

Svoboda, Dr. Robert. *Prakriti: Your Ayurvedic Constitution*. Twin Lakes, Wisconsin: Lotus Press, 2003

Rapgay, Dr Lopsang. *The Tibetan Book of Healing*. Twin Lakes, Wisconsin: Lotus Press, 2005

Raichur, Dr. Pratima. *Absolute Beauty*. New York, New York: Harper Collins 1997

Roach, Geshe Michael. *The Diamond Cutter*. New York, New York: Doubleday 2000

Vyas, Kiran. *Le Massage Indian*. Paris, France: Adi Shakti 2001

Warrior, Gopi and Gunawant, Deepika. *The Complete Illustrated Guide to Ayurveda*. Shaftesbury, England: Element Books Ltd 1997

Last thought—

"Give in anyway you can, of whatever you possess,
To give is to love,
To withhold is to whither,
Careless for your harvest than how it is shared
And your life will have meaning
And your heart will have peace"

KENT NERBURN, *LETTERS TO MY SON*

Index